Women and
Culture Series

The Women and Culture Series is dedicated to books that illuminate the lives, roles, achievements, and status of women, past or present.

Fran Leeper Buss
  Dignity: Lower Income Women Tell of Their Lives and Struggles
  La Partera: Story of a Midwife
Valerie Kossew Pichanick
  Harriet Martineau: The Woman and Her Work, 1802–76
Sandra Baxter and Marjorie Lansing
  Women and Politics: The Visible Majority
Estelle B. Freedman
  Their Sisters' Keepers: Women's Prison Reform in America, 1830–1930
Susan C. Bourque and Kay Barbara Warren
  Women of the Andes: Patriarchy and Social Change in Two Peruvian Towns
Marion S. Goldman
  Gold Diggers and Silver Miners: Prostitution and Social Life on the Comstock Lode
Page duBois
  Centaurs and Amazons: Women and the Pre-History of the Great Chain of Being
Mary Kinnear
  Daughters of Time: Women in the Western Tradition
Lynda K. Bundtzen
  Plath's Incarnations: Woman and the Creative Process
Violet B. Haas and Carolyn C. Perrucci, editors
  Women in Scientific and Engineering Professions
Sally Price
  Co-wives and Calabashes
Patricia R. Hill
  The World Their Household: The American Woman's Foreign Mission Movement and Cultural Transformation 1870–1920
Diane Wood Middlebrook and Marilyn Yalom, editors
  Coming to Light: American Women Poets in the Twentieth Century
Leslie W. Rabine
  Reading the Romantic Heroine: Text, History, Ideology
Joanne S. Frye
  Living Stories, Telling Lives: Women and the Novel in Contemporary Experience
E. Frances White
  Sierra Leone's Settler Women Traders: Women on the Afro-European Frontier
Catherine Parsons Smith and Cynthia S. Richardson
  Mary Carr Moore, American Composer
Barbara Drygulski Wright, editor
  Women, Work, and Technology: Transformations
Lynda Hart, editor
  Making a Spectacle: Feminist Essays on Contemporary Women's Theatre
Verena Martinez-Alier
  Marriage, Class and Colour in Nineteenth-Century Cuba: A Study of Racial Attitudes and Sexual Values in a Slave Society
Kathryn Strother Ratcliff et al., editors
  Healing Technology: Feminist Perspectives

Healing Technology

Healing Technology

FEMINIST PERSPECTIVES

Edited by
Kathryn Strother Ratcliff and
Myra Marx Ferree
Gail O. Mellow
Barbara Drygulski Wright
Glenda D. Price
Kim Yanoshik
Margie S. Freston

Ann Arbor
The University of Michigan Press

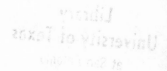

Published in the United States of America by
The University of Michigan Press
Manufactured in the United States of America
1992   1991   1990   1989 4 3 2 1

Library of Congress Cataloging-in-Publication Data

Healing technology : feminist perspectives / edited by Kathryn
Strother Ratcliff . . . [et al.].
    p.   cm.—(Women and culture series)
    Includes bibliographies and index.
    ISBN 0-472-09395-9 (alk. paper).—ISBN 0-472-06395-2 (pbk. :
alk. paper)
    1. Women—Health and hygiene. 2. Medical technology—Social
aspects. 3. Human reproductive technology—Social aspects.
I. Ratcliff, Kathryn Strother, 1944–   . II. Series.
RA564.85.H38   1989
613'.04244—dc20   89-4900
                                                        CIP

Contents

Introduction

Kathryn Strother Ratcliff

The subject of women and health has become a focal concern for academics, activists, and practitioners. Since the 1969 meetings that resulted in the Boston Women's Health Book Collective and the 1971 Women and Health Conference in New York City, a distinct women's health movement has emerged and continued to grow. Participants have criticized the health care provided to women, voiced frustration with the traditional paternalistic doctor-patient relationship, challenged professional authority and expertise, objected to the medicalization of childbirth and the loss of understanding and control of their bodies, called for more humanistic and affordable care, educated each other, and demanded changes in the health and health care of women (Ruzek 1978).

While decidedly activist in orientation, the women's health movement has been unique in its extensive grounding in research and education. In important ways the movement's growth has been propelled by the discoveries of threats to the health of women, of inadequacies in available health care, and of power imbalances in society that affect women's health. As such, the women's health movement has been a particularly fertile ground for the combined energies of academics, activists, and practitioners. This book further develops this important link between research on women and health and the efforts of activists and practitioners to address the health needs of women and to mobilize around issues relevant to the women's health movement.

The special focus of this book is on ways in which changing technologies affect the relationship between women and health. Technology is broadly defined to include devices, drugs, and procedures. Many of the technologies considered here are part of the health care system, but we also look at occupational and environmental technologies that affect women's health. As the contributors to this volume make clear, rapid changes in a range of technologies in recent times have had profound implications for women's health. Our concern with technology stems from a growing recognition of the importance of technology in our everyday life—that it is, on the one hand, ubiquitous and obvious, but, on the other hand, often so accepted as to be rendered invisible. The importance of research on technology and women's health is particularly great, not just because the problems are complex but because values and biases in the larger society tend to obscure our view of how technological changes affect our lives.

Among the key values that shape popular perceptions of technology are a kind of technological determinism and the notion that whatever new technologies emerge are the only options available. Together these two values support the view that new innovations are developed "according to their own inner necessity, from laws that govern the physical and biological world," (Wright 1987, 9) and that it is not relevant to examine political and economic contexts in order to ask why some technologies are produced while others are not. According to this viewpoint, one either accepts all emerging technological innovations or one is antitechnology.

The research approach represented by the authors in this book rejects the validity of this choice. Instead, we see technological change as a process involving constant choices among a wide range of technological possibilities. We see the asymmetries of power, especially in regard to class, gender, and race, as well as the incentives of the economic system as key determinants of the particular technological innovations that are produced. Certainly abundant evidence shows that technology is also shaped by political factors (Bodenheimer 1984; Corea 1977; Scully 1980; Brown 1979; Kaufert and McKinley 1985; Dreifus 1977; Rothschild 1983; Banta and Gelijns 1987; Winner 1985).

In some areas relevant to women, health, and technology, the political struggles have been quite open. The long history of severe restrictions on access to safe contraception and abortion represents an area in which women's health has been directly regulated through the political process. Less overt but certainly still important have been areas in which the political system has been selective in gender-biased ways in regulating experimentation and general utilization of new technologies.

Concern with the political and economic determinants and effects of technology focuses our attention on asymmetries of power—between the middle and upper classes and the lower class, doctors and patients, the scientific community and citizens, men and women, whites and blacks. These asymmetries have both shaped the development of technology and often been increased by technological developments. Health care provides clear examples: technologies such as surgical procedures and monitoring machines reduce the power of the patient as they enhance the power of the professional. In the workplace, asymmetries of power allow technologies to include or exclude workers, as for instance when fetal protection laws exclude women from the workplace or require them to be sterilized, or when research examines the effects of technology on men but not on women. Power asymmetries along gender lines are often operative in both settings.

A concern with the political economy also focuses attention on the incentives built into the economic system. The for-profit intrusions into health care are of particular concern, as they encourage the use of technology and diminish the importance of improved health as the overriding concern in decision making in a setting allegedly trying specifically to improve health. Various chapters in this book document the growth and effects of for-profit forces in health care. Furthermore we examine the profit considerations in the workplace that have diminished the societal surveillance of technology and the concern for possible occupational and environmental health hazards.

In examining technology we certainly take a critical stance. Such a stance is amply justified by the evidence of the negative health effects of many technologies such as Thalidomide, DES, and the Dalkon Shield. The crises produced by these technologies should help us learn about the forces of production and distribution, the social and ethical implications, and strategies for changing the available technologies. It would be incorrect to see this critical stance as antitechnological. Rather, our overall message is not one of halting technological development, but redirecting it and, as the title suggests, "healing" technology in the sense of removing its diseases and defects. Women have, indeed, asked for technological responses to problems and in many instances benefit from new technologies. Women want good contraceptive technology and many want more prenatal information about the fetus. Instead of arguing for an end to technological development, we need to show early, sustained, and organized concern with technological innovations so that women's interests have a greater role in shaping the process. The staying power of particular innovations, even when they are found to represent threats to women's health, must be addressed. At the design and assessment stage critical, wide-ranging, and different questions must be asked. The questions need to be more women-centered and more infused with a concern for ethical and social issues.

It is important that we question technological developments and the directions in which they are moving at their inception because a technological trajectory is difficult to redirect once it is established. "By far the greatest latitude of choice exists the very first time a particular instrument, system, or technique is introduced. Because choices tend to become strongly fixed in material equipment, economic investment, and social habit, the original flexibility vanishes for all practical purposes once the initial commitments are made" (Winner 1985,

30). A major difficulty is that the development of technology often proceeds by incremental steps, thereby discouraging debate on the ethical or social implications, because each change is so small. When debate does occur, the principles used set the stage for approval of later developments that may be more troubling. Once society has ventured forth, it is hard to retreat. We argue for increased and continued vigilance over technology. The biotechnology field offers numerous examples of the need for early vigilance. We are moving in the direction of ever earlier detection of an increasing number of physical problems. Prenatal detection encourages prenatal surgery and potentially raises standards for "acceptable" newborns. Early detection done on children and adults poses the possibility of advance warning of pain and our likely cause of death. We must spend as much time discussing the social and psychological ramifications of that knowledge as we do in producing the technology to obtain it. Our stance is hopeful, in that we see organized activism as influential in altering the contours of public debate and decision making.

Our book contains a range of feminist perspectives. Although the contributors have sought not to align themselves with any particular viewpoint within feminism, there are still certain commonalities of approach. First of these is a more wholistic view of health. Our concern with the health of women is not limited to physical health, and our criterion for physical health is not just being officially certified as disease-free. Health includes mental and emotional well-being and as such particularly includes being active and empowered. Such an inclusive view of health remains a controversial idea, including as it does elements of process and outcome. Central concerns of health become lay involvement in decision making, access to information, humanistic care, and a concern with the overall quality of life.

Second, our analysis is woman-centered. We object to the devaluing of both women and stereotypically female characteristics. Evidence of such devaluing in the history of science (Keller 1985), in corporate decisions concerning health products for women (Mintz 1985), in health care (Ehrenreich and English 1973; Corea 1977), in policy (Parker 1983), in ethics (Tronto 1987), and in other arenas is disturbing. We want to encourage women to be active participants in all aspects of technology and we want their voices heard. We are concerned with the tendency to minimize or exclude a consideration of the impact of technological developments on women of all races and classes, in the United States and abroad.

Third, and closely associated, we are critical of male domination in corporate, government, health care, and educational settings. Although there are signs of change—for instance almost two-fifths of current medical students are women and it is projected that by the year 2000, 20 percent of practicing physicians will be women (Altekruse and McDermott 1988, 66–67)—women remain underrepresented at the top of the field while they are overrepresented at the bottom, comprising 70 to 90 percent of the health workers in lower positions. Authentic involvement of more women in decision making about technology is needed, and this involvement must come from all races and classes.

Fourth, we continue to see choice and informed consent as critical and empowering elements in the use of technology. The full ramifications of such processes challenge professional dominance, and developing them has been central to the women's health movement. Choices need to be real and the information about each alternative must be available and as accurate as possible. Part of making the choices real for any individual is to restructure the discussion of options so they occur in supportive settings, where women are not cast in subservient roles and economic constraints do not preclude choice. Even if we are well informed, we become powerless in the face of the traditional structures (Fisher 1986).

Fifth, we reject the assumption that research or decision making can be value-free. When researchers study the causes of premature delivery and neglect to ask about the nature of the women's employment (Messing 1983, 81) or the government ignores the ethical and social implications of a technology in favor of a quantitatively based cost-benefit analysis, values have entered into the research and changed the direction of technology. Discussions about technology must expose and question the underlying values. We find a devaluing of risks to women evident in the choices of which technologies are to be developed.

And finally, we are committed to change, with the goal of a more healthful and just society for all. Grounding change in grass roots politics and involving the active participation of those who are affected by technology is a practical strategy for change. In addition, such grounding and such participation are valued ends in themselves. Greater participation by women in decision making about the development and distribution of technology, together with better and more informed choices for workers, consumers, and patients, will not automatically produce an optimal set of technologies which have only beneficial results. Such involvement, however, should drastically reduce the number of horror stories of technologies prematurely implemented, poorly reviewed, and ultimately more harmful than helpful to women. In addition, such a process of technological development will be more in line with democratic ideals. The chapters challenge us to raise questions about the development and utilization of technologies, and they argue for collective discussion and action to shape future decisions about technology.

Unlike most writing on women and health, this book is organized around issues raised by technology, rather than around a single health issue (e.g., reproductive technology), or around problems of health care delivery (e.g., the education of obstetricians), or the women's health movement. It is organized around various technologies, only some of which are in the health care setting, but all of which are relevant to women's health. It explores common themes in the development, utilization, and impact of technology on women's health. First, we are concerned with understanding the political and economic contexts within which technologies are designed, produced, and distributed, and in particular the devaluing of health, women, poor people, and minorities in those processes.

Second, we are concerned with the political, social, and ethical implications in the use of these technologies because we are often slow to recognize any unintended impact of technology, and in particular the social and ethical ones. Third, we are concerned with empowering individuals to work for change in the development, assessment, and implementation of appropriate technologies; since technology will remain with us, the issue is reshaping the technology. Our focus on technology examines technology throughout women's life cycles—from conceiving, birthing, and nurturing young children to working and maturing in the middle years to dying. Our intent is to support an activist and feminist agenda throughout the life course.

The book is divided into three parts: reproductive technologies, health care technologies, and occupational and environmental technologies. Each part's introduction discusses the primary themes in the chapters and places each in a broader context. The first part, Reproductive Technologies: Economic and Social Implications, highlights the nearly universal importance of such technologies to women. Historically, the examination of reproductive technologies has been a critical rallying point for feminists (Ruzek 1986, 186). The availability of safe abortion services, the medicalization of childbirth, and new high technology reproductive methods have served to coalesce concerns for women's health. We have deliberately chosen not to feature the new reproductive technologies as such. In vitro fertilization, gamete intrafallopian transfer, surrogate motherhood, and sex predetermination not only affect few women but also have been the focus of several recent books and a new journal. Thus the current data and perspectives on various new reproductive technologies (Lasker and Borg 1987; Corea

1985; Arditti et al. 1984; Spallone and Steinberg 1987; Stanworth 1987; *Reproductive and Genetic Engineering: Journal of International Feminist Analysis,* various issues) are widely available. Several chapters in this volume do discuss these new technologies, but unlike books and articles on them alone, these contributions put the high technology innovations in the context of more widely used reproductive technologies. This highlights the similar forces that determine them and the similar social implications. Further, we examine the new technologies not just in terms of who uses them, but also who does not. We consider, for instance, the implications of in vitro fertilization for women who do not use it and the implications on the moral community of sustaining pregnancy in brain-dead women.

The second part of the book, Health Care Technologies: Political and Ethical Considerations, continues to develop ideas from the first part. Unlike reproductive technologies, these technologies are applied to both men and women and the implications of their use are not so obviously gendered. However, the chapters in this part draw out the gendered meaning of the implementation of technology in health care settings. Gender is especially evident in the power asymmetries of technology use. The political embeddedness of technologies has at its core male control of the production and distribution of technologies and the selling of preventative services to women. Chapters in this part examine the implications of male domination in health care settings for the use of technologies as diverse as mammograms and heart monitors. The inclusion of women as health care providers (e.g., genetic counselors) may bring different perspectives to bear, but even the conscious effort to redirect health care to meet women's needs can be co-opted, as one chapter demonstrates in the case of osteoporosis and breast cancer screening. The process of women becoming political and challenging male domination can take several forms, as the chapters also show: being able to hear critical information, seeking better data, but also reconsidering questions of ethics and values that have been male defined. The ethical questions discussed in this section include patient autonomy, informed consent, and nonmalfeasance, but they are placed in a feminist context in which empowerment is central. These ethical themes are tied to the power theme because it is through authentic participation in decision making that patients in fact become powerful. Power, in our conception, is not necessarily a zero-sum game among people. For instance, in a hospice setting both provider and patient become more powerful. Jointly they shape the use of technology and thereby reject the power of the hospital setting to define use.

Some technologies seem to evoke less gender-specific concerns than even health care systems. Nonetheless, we argue that a feminist perspective on health needs to include a gendered understanding of all sorts of technologies that have consequences for the well being of women and men. In turning to part three, Occupational and Environmental Technologies: Research and Resources for Change, our concern focuses on gender as it structures a variety of social experiences and at times highlights the need to consider gender similarities. Yet, our social system is structured along gender lines. Gender defines power differences, the amount and type of participation in the workplace, at home, and in the community. Because of this gendered reality, the relationship of women to technology is often different than it is for men. Women and men contribute differently to the development of technology and are exposed to it in different ways. On the other hand, this gendered reality is socially constructed and is not a "natural" extension of biological dissimilarities. Laws in the workplace "protecting" the reproductive capabilities of women ignore the fact that men, too, have reproductive systems.

In considering the health effects of the workplace and health care technologies we recognize that both women and men are often subject to the same poorly regulated technology, but highlight the way in which social arrangements distribute these effects. Technology's impact is transmitted via a gendered social reality and gender is relevant in creating the resources for activism in response to technological change. This third part thus ends with two chapters that directly discuss women as worker-, patient-, and citizen-activists reshaping the development and use of technology. The final message is thus not one of doom and gloom but hopeful optimism that a feminist perspective will empower women and men to shape tomorrow's technology in more intelligent and life-affirming ways, to develop technologies that will indeed help to heal not only individuals but society, and to contribute to the preservation of our planet.

NOTE

Healing Technology: Feminist Perspectives is based on the 1986 Conference on Women, Health, and Technology, sponsored by the Project on Women and Technology, a joint endeavor of the Women's Center and the Women's Studies Program at the University of Connecticut. The chapters in this volume include revisions of papers presented at the conference as well as solicited papers. The editors are indebted to the conference keynote speakers, Judy Norisigian and Evelyn Fox Keller, and to the many panelists, participants, and conference organizers for the success of that conference and the exchange of ideas that made this book possible.

The Research Foundation of the University of Connecticut provided a grant helpful in the final stages of book preparation.

BIBLIOGRAPHY

Altekruse, Joan M., and Suzanne McDermott. 1988. Contemporary concerns of women in medicine. In *Feminism within the science and health care professions: Overcoming resistance,* ed. Sue V. Rosser, 65–90. New York: Pergamon.

Arditti, Rita, Renate Duelli Klein, and Shelley Minden, eds. 1984. *Test-tube women.* London: Pandora Press.

Banta, H. David, and Annetine Gelijns. 1987. Health care costs: technology and policy. In *Health care and its costs,* ed. Carl J. Schramm, 252–74. New York: W. W. Norton and Co.

Bodenheimer, Thomas S. 1984. The transnational pharmaceutical industry and the health of the world's people. In *Issues in the political economy,* ed. John B. McKinlay, 143–86. New York: Tavistock.

Brown, E. Richard. 1979. *Rockefeller medicine men.* Berkeley: University of California Press.

Corea, Gena. 1977. *The hidden malpractice.* New York: Harper and Row.

———. 1985. *The mother machine: Reproductive technology from artificial insemination to artificial wombs.* New York: Harper and Row.

Dreifus, Claudia, ed. 1977. *Seizing our bodies: The politics of women's health.* New York: Random House.

Ehrenreich, Barbara, and Deirdre English. 1973. *Complaints and disorders: The sexual politics of sickness.* Old Westbury, New York: Feminist Press.

Fisher, Sue. 1986. *In the patient's best interest.* New Brunswick, N.J.: Rutgers University Press.

Kaufert, Patricia A., and Sonja M. McKinley. 1985. Estrogen replacement therapy: The production of medical knowledge and the emergence of policy. In *Women, health and healing,* ed. Ellen Lewin and V. Olsen, 113–38. New York: Tavistock.

Keller, Evelyn Fox. 1985. *Reflections on gender and science.* New Haven: Yale University Press.

Lasker, Judith, and Susan Borg. 1987. *Coping with infertility and high-tech conception.* Boston: Beacon Press.

Messing, Karen. 1983. The scientific mystique: Can a white lab coat guarantee purity in the search for knowledge about the nature of women? In *Woman's nature: Rationalizations of inequality,* ed. Marian Lowe and Ruth Hubbard, 75–88. New York: Pergamon.

Mintz, Morton. 1985. *At any cost: Corporate greed, women and the Dalkon Shield.* New York: Pantheon Books.

Parker, Alberta. 1986. Juggling health care technology and women's needs. In *The technological woman: Interfacing with tomorrow,* ed. Jan Zimmerman, 239–44. New York: Praeger.

Rothschild, Joan. 1983. Technology, housework and women's liberation: A theoretical analysis. In *Machina ex Dea,* ed. Joan Rothschild, 79–93. New York: Pergamon.

Ruzek, Sheryl Burt. 1986. Feminist visions of health: An international perspective. In *What is feminism: A reexamination,* ed. Juliet Mitchell and Ann Oakley, 184–207. New York: Pantheon.

———. 1978. *The women's health movement.* New York: Praeger.

Scully, Diana. 1980. *Men who control women's health.* Boston: Houghton Mifflin.

Spallone, Patricia, and Deborah Lynn Steinberg, eds. 1987. *Made to order: The myth of reproductive and genetic progress.* New York: Pergamon.

Stanworth, Michelle, ed. 1987. *Reproductive technologies: Gender, motherhood and medicine.* Minneapolis: University of Minnesota Press.

Tronto, Joan C. 1987. Beyond gender difference to a theory of care. *Signs* 12, no. 4: 644–55.

Winner, Langsdon. 1985. Do artifacts have politics? In *The social shaping of technology: How the refrigerator got its hum,* ed. Donald MacKenzie and Judy Wajcman, 26–38. Philadelphia: Open University Press, Milton Keynes.

Wright, Barbara D. 1987. Introduction. In *Women, work, and technology: Transformations,* ed. Barbara Wright, 1–22. Ann Arbor: University of Michigan Press.

Part 1
Reproductive Technologies:
Economic and Social Implications

Introduction

Barbara Drygulski Wright

A *Time* magazine advertisement features a sober-faced, boyishly dressed infant and the caption reads "Are you my mother?" The text that follows announces that "for a growing number of childless couples, making babies is no longer strictly a 'family affair.' It's a business collaboration whose partners could be any combination of expectant parents, doctors, donors, surrogates and lawyers." With apparently unconscious irony, the magazine then cites its own "enterprising" reporting on this "business collaboration" as a reason to buy *Time* magazine (October 26, 1987, 60). As growing numbers of couples have turned to "startling techniques" to achieve their "desperate dreams," growing numbers of feminists have been startled, as well—by the connections they have found between reproductive high tech and high profits. At the same time, feminists have begun to examine the social and political ideologies that sanction the virtually unrestrained development of reproductive technologies, and they have begun to analyze the way these ideologies in turn have been changed by the availability of reproductive technologies. For women's reproductive health and autonomy, the results have been mixed.

These complex interactions are the subject of this part on women and reproductive technologies. When we attempt to sort out the tangled threads that come together here, we find, first, a Western faith in the usefulness and benevolence of medical technology that can be fairly described as technophilia—and I use this term in deliberate contrast to the "technophobia" which skeptics of modern technology are constantly accused of. Though modern medical technologies have been questioned by critics ranging from Ivan Illich to Ralph Nader, from Elizabeth Bing to Barbara Ehrenreich and Deirdre English, the technophilia of medical researchers, physicians, the business establishment, government, and the general public has made it possible for reproductive technologies to be developed with little or no control or oversight, and to be implemented with little or no testing of their effectiveness or hazards.

Second, we have a Western-dominated market economy that knows very well that technological innovation can be exploited for an economic return. The market economy has a vested interest in turning technological discoveries into marketable commodities, exaggerating their benefits, minimizing their risks, and expanding the potential clientele for a given product to include as many people as possible. Business turns enormous profits from the marketing of medical technologies, and in a kind of symbiosis, those profits then help to finance further research.

Finally, there are the social values, relationships, and responsibilities, the lines of gender identity, class, and power out of which reproductive technologies emerge, and which they in turn have the power to reaffirm or reconstruct. The *Time* advertisement suggests there *was* a time when "making babies" was "strictly a 'family affair' "; it evokes nostalgia for those supposedly simpler days, and it promises to lead us through the legal and technological labyrinth back to private bliss. Yet since time immemorial, sexual behavior has been structured by social sanctions and taboos while female fertility has been linked, one way or another, with agricultural cultivation, economic prosperity, political power, and military might. *Time* argues that we are living in a period when "concepts of birth and parenthood are conceived faster than dictionaries can define them." But it is not only birth and parenthood that are being redefined; the meanings of childlessness, of safety, risk, and individual choice are also being renegotiated. So, perhaps, is the relationship between genders, generations, and classes. What is old and what is genuinely new in all of this?

What does it mean, in the face of new reproductive technologies, to have a child of "one's own"? Why are couples (usually white and affluent) willing to go so far for this kind of child, and why is society as well as the research community so supportive? How do we rationalize the fulfillment of supposedly natural desires by such highly artificial means? And why are we simultaneously so disinterested in the kinds of prosaic public health measures advocated by Ruth Hubbard (1985) and others—things like nutrition programs, prenatal checkups, immunization, and removal of environmental hazards—that would improve the survival rates and health of millions of mothers and infants? Given the link between infertility and delayed childbearing, why are we fascinated by individualized technological or legal fixes like surrogacy or in vitro fertilization (IVF), instead of calling for structural changes like adequate child care and effective maternal leave policies that would make delayed childbearing unnecessary in the first place? The chapters in this part, which range from theory to case study and from a focus on economic factors to social and ideological ones, help us to raise and begin to answer questions like these.

The first part of the book opens with Elisabeth Beck-Gernsheim's contribution on reproductive technology and reproductive ideology. She dispells some of the seeming uniqueness and mystery of reproductive technology, with its sudden emergence and eager acceptance, by relating it to sociological theories of modernization. Using the example of the birth control pill, Beck-Gernsheim argues that in the twenty years since its introduction, women's individual "freedom" to reliably control their fertility has become a social compulsion to do so. On the personal level, the process of decision making has been reversed: whereas "previously people had to go to great lengths to find a means of preventing pregnancy, today they have to make a conscious decision to discontinue their use of contraceptives when they want to have a child." And on the social level, "planned parenthood, at first a new option, now turns into a kind of duty." It is worth noting that in the United States today, this "duty" weighs most heavily on particular groups of women, i.e., the impoverished and the unmarried. For them, condemnation of their sexual activity as "immoral" has been largely replaced by the social stigma of "irresponsibility," "selfishness," and "greed."

Next, Beck-Gernsheim turns to more recent reproductive technologies, in particular in vitro fertilization, and asks what changes in ideology are likely to flow from them. She suggests, first, that whereas before, infertility was "destiny," with the availability of IVF it becomes a "choice" and the decision to cease IVF treatment becomes not a failure of reproductive physiology but a failure of personal will. She notes, second, that to justify the extraordinary physical and emotional stresses of IVF as well as the tremendous expense, medical researchers are wont to emphasize the central importance of motherhood in a woman's life. So, one imagines, are the couples undergoing treatment; and surely this underlying afffirmation of motherhood is a major reason for the sympathetic and approving coverage which "test-tube babies" enjoy in the media.

But Beck-Gernsheim's concerns do not end here. She foresees the day, once IVF has become routine, when *all* men and women may become potential clients. The techniques will not be limited to the problems they were originally developed to solve, but will be used for other purposes: for "prevention," for selective breeding, or to allow genetic reproduction after a partner has been sterilized. The implications for social ideology are clear: there is the question of who will define "quality" for purposes of human breeding, and there is the risk that in this process of "rationalizing" reproduction, the reproductive capability of all women may become subject to technological interventions and legislative control.

But our imaginations can race even beyond that point, to more far-reaching connections between economics, social ideology, and reproductive technology. Ecofeminists have suggested that the "peaceful" use of atomic energy has been consciously promoted by governments and economic interests as a convenient pretext to raise the money and build the facilities that could support atomic energy for military purposes on a massive scale (Gambaroff et al. 1986, 106). Similarly, as research on genetic engineering and reproductive technology proceed, grim possibilities present themselves: for example, the creation of human beings with strategically useful characteristics, such as heightened immunity to atomic or chemical warfare; the reproduction of human beings using uncontaminated eggs and sperm from before a nuclear war; or the ability to correct—or at least detect and destroy—genetic mutations after a nuclear holocaust (SIPRI 1985). Do such speculations sound hopelessly paranoid? In fact, it was precisely the possibility for tactical advantages such as these that inspired Gordon Rattray Taylor to argue two decades ago in his widely acclaimed book, *The Biological Time Bomb,* that the West could not afford *not* to pursue reproductive research (Taylor 1968).

With her detailed case study of the development and marketing of the electronic fetal monitor (EFM), Judith Kunisch brings us back to the here and now. Corroborating the four-step model presented in the preceeding chapter, Kunisch shows how EFM technology has changed both the social and economic context of childbirth in the United States. For the vast majority of doctors, nurses, and insurance companies, the EFM within a few short years became an essential part of the "standard of care" for birthing women—not merely for the 10 percent to 15 percent diagnosed as at high risk, for whom the technology was originally designed, but for all pregnant women. In other words, Kunisch provides us with a textbook example of Beck-Gernsheim's principle of "universal implementation" or "everybody . . . defined as client." When every pregnant woman becomes a client for the technology, the market for the technology becomes vastly inflated and far more lucrative. Apart from financial interests, however, the virtually universal adoption of EFM over a period of less than five years was made possible by a willingness to *believe* that EFM technology could improve infant survival rates; no adequately large-scale, controlled tests by impartial investigators were ever conducted before aggressive marketing began. Again Kunisch corroborates Beck-Gernsheim, who describes this bias toward "uncontrolled implementation" as the "inner politics of medicine."

EFM did succeed in reducing the incidence of death or injury to high-risk infants, and that is all to the good; but the impact of the technology has far exceeded the good it is able to accomplish. Since the development of EFM, social and economic changes have occurred that support its continued use, and that make the removal of EFM from the labor and delivery room far more difficult than its introduction ever was. Machine-generated data has acquired greater status and validity than the information that a nurse or doctor could obtain from a physical examination of the birthing woman, to the point where all participants in the birth are now afraid to forego this technology. And whereas the large-scale introduction of the technology was motivated largely by the developers' desire for financial gain, it is now insurance companies' fear of financial loss that keeps it there. "Compulsory implementation," to quote Beck-Gernsheim again, has occurred informally rather than formally, but it is highly effective nevertheless.

While Kunisch demonstrates the intersection of medical technology and economic interests using a single, local example, Kim Yanoshik and Judy Norsigian present a similar argument from an international perspective. Surveying a vast range of new contraceptive technologies aimed at women, they find the medical imperative of "uncontrolled implementation" and the economic imperative of "universal implementation" at work on a global scale. Yanoshik and Norsigian trace the typical path of many contraceptive drugs and devices, from testing in the Third World, to marketing in the United States and western Europe, to dumping in the Third World when serious health hazards emerge. The authors discuss the population control policies which, at least in part, allow such testing and dumping to occur, and they describe the disregard, indeed contempt, for women's reproductive health and personal autonomy which often accompanies such policies. Clearly, in the face of international population policy and multinational pharmaceutical companies, the women's health movement, too, must become international.

In their chapter on low-income women, particularly women of color, and their access to new reproductive technologies, Laurie Jefferson and Elaine Hall consider not only economic issues but also the social definition of reproductive problems that are perceived as requiring medical intervention. First they demonstrate, not surprisingly, that women who must rely on Medicaid, the Maternal and Child Health Program, or Community and Migrant Health Centers for health care have significantly limited access to reproductive technologies in comparison with middle-class women who enjoy other kinds of medical coverage, and they argue the illogic as well as the inhumaneness of these restrictions. For example, at publicly funded clinics in Vermont the waiting period simply to enter prenatal care is fourteen weeks—a circumstance that makes early detection and treatment of some conditions impossible. And in some states or regions, ironically enough, women may have access to prenatal screening tests but no access to a state-funded abortion, should the test results indicate a problem.

However, in Jefferson's and Hall's view the social definition of what constitutes a reproductive "problem" and what constitutes appropriate "treatment" of that problem is an even more fundamental issue than inadequate funding. They argue that there are profound cultural and philosophical differences between the perceptions and values of the educated, upper middle-class providers of reproductive services and those of their poor or minority clients, and these differences raise further barriers to appropriate reproductive care. For example, physicians or counsellors may be oblivious to clients' concerns, they may withhold or skew information, and they may counsel directively.

Even more challenging, however, is Jefferson's and Hall's assertion that poor women, including women of color, may actually suffer *higher* rates of infertility than middle-class women—yet infertility has been *defined* as a white middle-class problem, and the high-tech solutions to infertility that have been developed have been pitched to an affluent, educated audience of private individuals. In other words, the problem and its solution are seriously out of joint, for reasons that have to do with economics, but even more with ideological judgments about who may or should reproduce. The flip side of "universal implementation" for economic gain turns out to be "selective implementation" based on ideological criteria. Jefferson's and Hall's perspective on infertility is acutely relevant, not merely to poor women who need infertility services, but to all women who may find themselves allowed or denied access to reproductive technologies they do not control.

The whole question of access, in fact, suggests a link from Yanoshik's and Norsigian's chapter on contraceptives in the Third World to Jefferson's and Hall's contribution on poor women and infertility in the United States to Francoise Laborie's (1989) critical examination of IVF in France—and at the same time the relationship between reproductive technologies and eugenics becomes a little clearer. Noting the serious physical risks involved for the women, as well as the very low rates of success, Laborie interprets the activities at IVF centers in France not as "treatment" but as research, with women serving as the unwitting experimental subjects. It seems unlikely that the medical research community would be able either to raise the money it needed, or to obtain the permission for experimentation with human subjects that would be required, if IVF were not being sought out and paid for by couples willing to volunteer themselves for the procedures.

At what point, we are forced to ask, does the "privilege" of access to a new reproductive technology turn into the exploitation of a client as a human guinea pig? And who gets access to what? Poor women in both the United States and Third World, vulnerable to coercion and politically powerless, have had little trouble gaining access to devices that would *prevent* them from reproducing; on the contrary, in testing programs they have often been the unlucky first to use new contraceptives. To advance research on technologies that *promote* reproduction such as IVF, however, a different kind of female guinea pig seems to be required, one that Laborie describes as cooperative, motivated, and wealthy enough to pay for the treatments: "As opposed to mice or monkeys, women are intelligent and can talk. They are conscious of how and when their ovulation occurs; they can observe and describe to the doctors the effects of different medications; they don't have to be purchased, fed, or kept in a clean cage; they come to the hospital all by themselves, on the right day, at the right time, and . . . they pay for that privilege (sometimes exorbitantly)!" (Laborie 1988). Not only that, but they produce offspring who most likely will belong to the physicians' and scientists' own race and class.

A different aspect of the social construction of women's reproductive experience comes to the fore with Lynne Garner's and Richard Tessler's contribution on the use of technology in childbirth and its effects on postpartum moods. Garner and Tessler discovered that the more medical technology was used during the birth, the "bluer" women tended to feel one week postpartum. Even more fascinating, however, is the authors' suggestion that "postpartum blues" as such may be a figment of our social imagination. Contrary to all expectation, Garner's and Tessler's respondents reported feeling approximately the *same* shortly before and after the birth. Both immediately before and after a birth, the authors point out, women frequently experience both anxiety and physical discomfort. While crying did peak at one week postpartum, women *also* reported a peak in positive feelings about the birth at that time, including pride, excitement, and joy. Whereas scientific literature has often cited "hormones" as the cause of postpartum moods, the authors' respondents tended to view hormones as the cause of their crying *before* the birth; afterward, reasonably enough, they cited feeling overwhelmed by caring for the new baby and by other responsibilities.

What is curious here, of course, is the extent to which women's own descriptions of their affective state just before and after childbirth differ both from popular wisdom and the scientific literature. We need to probe gently at this discrepancy to see what it can offer—about the projection of emotional states onto women, about our expectations for mothers, about social understandings of the mother-child bond, or perhaps about our tendency to blame the maternal victim of medical technology or social indifference.

The final chapter in this part deals with the difficult question of whether pregnancies in brain-dead women should be sustained. In it, Julien Murphy continues the focus on social meanings and values: how they influence the implementation of technology; and even more, how the use of technology affects values and changes the social definition of what pregnancy is. Murphy examines some of the medical questions as well as the moral and legal contradictions surrounding postmortem maternal ventilation (PMV), a procedure that can sustain a pregnant cadaver for weeks or even months until the fetus reaches maturity. She argues with other authors in this part that PMV, like other new reproductive technologies, is a procedure "that threatens to separate pregnancy from women's control while altering the social meaning of 'pregnancy.' " Like other authors, Murphy foresees ways in which this procedure, applicable to only an infinitesimal number of pregnancies, could affect the reproductive experience of all women as all pregnant women come to be viewed as potential candidates for the procedure. And as with other reproductive technologies, this one, too, suggests futuristic scenarios: if the procedure became widely accepted, cadavers might be used for egg farming or might receive embryo transplants in lieu of the artificial womb which thus far has eluded scientists.

As a philosopher, however, Murphy is most interested in analyzing how PMV might affect the discourse about pregnancy, including assumptions about pregnancy, the legal and moral status of the pregnant woman, and the influence of these on social policy. The centerpiece of Murphy's thesis is a feminist definition of pregnancy as an activity requiring consciousness and resulting from the exercise of free choice. It follows that a mandatory policy of PMV will violate women's reproductive freedom; however, a voluntary PMV policy is also objectionable in Murphy's view because it will be based on arguments such as the analogy to organ donation, which she considers specious. Her ultimate concern is that the practice of PMV reduces women from ends to means, thus diminishing women's personhood and undermining the moral community; her ultimate position is that the practice of PMV should not continue, even with the voluntary consent of the mother.

In current media discussions of genetic engineering, reproductive technologies, and high-tech birth, as well as in medical and scientific publications, the emphasis lies on bringing private happiness to the infertile couple with the "desperate dream" of having a child of "their own," or help to the woman whose pregnancy is at risk. At the same time, contraceptive technologies offer the fertile the chance to control reproduction in accordance with their desires and means. As legitimate as the desires or preferences of these individuals may be, it is apparent that the medical technologies discussed in this part have more complex origins and more far-reaching consequences than private happiness.

If private happiness is the text, the subtext is economic gain. Clearly, economics has played a prominent role in determining the course of development that reproductive technology has followed. But economic motives have not operated in a vacuum, and the search for profit has not been the only source of problems. We also need to be aware of the social meanings that are embodied in reproductive technologies when they are developed, and the social meanings that are constructed as a result of our use of reproductive technologies.

Nowhere, it can be fairly argued, is the seemingly personal more political than in the realm of new reproductive technologies. On the one hand, we tend to think of sexuality, reproduction, and family life as the most intimate and private parts of our lives; yet at the same time, these same areas are subject to economic pressures and social regulation, and they are precisely the areas that, in the twentieth century at least, have sparked the most bitter and emotional responses in the political arena, from the first wave of the women's movement and the eugenic policies of the 1930s and 1940s to the ongoing struggles over abortion today. The wish of all the authors in this part is that women—their health, their dignity, and their needs—become at least as prominent in the discussion of reproductive technology as scientists, physicians, politicians, judges, or fetuses have been until now. It seems little enough to ask.

REFERENCES

"Are you my mother?" (Advertisement). 1987. *Time* 130, no. 60 (October 26): 60.
Gambaroff, Marina, Maria Mies, Annegret Stopczyk, Claudia von Werlhof et al. 1986. *Tschernobyl hat unser Leben verändert. Vom Ausstieg der Frauen,* (Chernobyl changed our lives: Why women have had enough). Reinbek bei Hamburg: Rowohlt Taschenbuch Verlag.
Hubbard, Ruth. 1985. Lecture at University of Connecticut Medical Center, Farmington, Connecticut, October.
Laborie, Francoise. 1988. New reproductive technologies: News from France and elsewhere. *Reproductive and Genetic Engineering* 1, no. 1: 77–85.
Stockholm International Peace Research Institute (SIPRI), eds. 1985. *Gentechnik als Waffe. Rüstungsjahrbuch 5* (Genetic technology as weapon.

Armament yearbook 5). Reinbek bei Hamburg: Rowohlt Taschenbuch Verlag.

Taylor, Gordon Rattray. 1968. *The biological time bomb*. New York, Cleveland: World Publishing Company.

From the Pill to Test-Tube Babies: New Options, New Pressures in Reproductive Behavior

Elisabeth Beck-Gernsheim

Since the early 1960s, an astonishing array of new reproductive technologies has appeared. The new techniques include biomedical interventions for women and men who want to have a child as well as measures for those who decide against having a child. The spectrum ranges from new forms of birth control that are nearly 100 percent effective to spectacular ways of treating infertility such as in vitro fertilization (IVF). These new technologies have not only affected human reproductive physiology; within a relatively short time, they have also profoundly altered prevailing patterns of reproductive behavior.

In this chapter I examine the new reproductive technologies with a view to determining their social and psychological impact on women and men—their life-styles and motivations, their hopes and fears. The discussion falls into two parts. In the first, I will describe the new reproductive technologies and contrast the medical perspective with a sociological one. Instead of examining only the biological implications of these new techniques, I argue that there are predictable social processes involved in their propagation and use. The impact lies not only in the medical pressures that are created to use these new reproductive technologies, but also and more significantly in the *social* transformations that accompany their use. In the second part, I go on to a more detailed discussion of two particular examples of techniques for controlling reproduction, one relatively "old" and one new, namely the birth control pill and interventions designed to treat infertility. In both these instances, the central questions will be: What new options and what new pressures are produced by these new technologies? And how do they reshape the lives of women and men and the relationship between them?

In order to find a key to the consideration of these questions, I would like to begin with the debate in the social sciences over "modernization." The framework for this debate is the transformation of premodern society into modern industrial society. A number of modernization theories describe and analyze the developments that characterize this historical upheaval—for example, changes in the forms of

23

production, increases in mechanization, the disintegration of the family as an economic unit, the decline of religious values and faith, and the rise of geographical and social mobility (e.g, Beck 1986; Berger 1986; Berger et al. 1975; Durkheim 1977; Weber 1984). In all of this a question appears over and over again like a kind of leitmotiv: What exactly is the meaning of this change in the forms of working and living that occurs in the transition to modern times? Does the change bring liberation for human beings—or does it simply create new forms of oppression? Let us look more closely at the two sides of this controversy.

The common assumption on both sides is that in the transition to modern society, the traditional ties between people are loosened. At this point, however, views diverge sharply. Some authors argue that the dissolving of traditional bonds represents an increase in freedom for the individual. They understand modernization primarily as broadening the scope of life, as a net gain in opportunities for action and choice. "Modernity has indeed had a liberating effect. It has freed human beings from the narrow control of the family, the clan, the tribe, or the small community. It has opened to the individual possibilities for choice and paths of mobility which were hitherto unknown" (Berger et al. 1975, 168).

But having said that, the other side will argue, we have only described a part of this development. Along with the new freedoms, there arise new forms of dependency, control, and oppression. When the family ceases to function as an economic unit, individuals are cast upon the labor market with its demands, they become dependent upon cycles of business activity, and they are threatened by economic crises. As birth and social standing become less important, social mobility increases, but so do the pressures to compete and the danger of downward mobility. As ties to neighbors and relations grow weaker, one's horizon becomes wider, but then one may lack a social network and suffer isolation and uprootedness. In short, the new "freedoms . . . carried a high price" (Berger et al. 1975, 168).

A closer look at individual issues suggests a characteristic chronology in this discussion of modernization and its consequences. At the beginning, the focus is primarily on the positive outcomes of change; during later phases, in contrast, the focus shifts to drawbacks. This shift of focus can be found in many contemporary areas of debate, from computer technology to ecology or genetics. Today, many people have lost their faith in seemingly unlimited "progress," a faith which originally lay at the heart of the development of modern industrialized society.

Now, what does this discussion of modernization tell us about reproductive technologies? What can we learn from the one about the other? I suggest the following answer. First, reproductive technologies can be viewed as *one of the most recent products in the long history of modernization*. For they, too, represent a release from traditional bonds. Here, too, human beings are disregarding the limits supposedly set by nature, intervening ever more deeply in the process of reproduction, and seeking to plan, direct, and control the process according to their own aims. Second, keeping in mind the preceeding discussion of modernization, we can assume that the coin of these new reproductive technologies will always have *two sides*. Undeniably, they bring certain freedoms—for example, protection from unwanted pregnancy, or help with unwanted infertility. But on the other hand, they also create new forms of dependency and oppression—for example, control by doctors, the impersonality of medical technology, and coercion to become a "career patient." Third, we can assume that the development and application of reproductive technologies will follow the established historical pattern. At the beginning the positive side, the promise of liberation, stands in the foreground, just as it did with the automobile and nuclear energy as well as IVF. Only later does it become apparent that liberation also has its price, and that with each of these achievements we also take on a burden of new risks and dangers.

The purpose of this contribution, then, is to help us gain a perspective on the "two faces" of reproductive technology.

The New Reproductive Technologies: Jekyll and Hyde?

The common characteristic of the new reproductive technologies is that they remove barriers to sexuality and reproduction imposed by nature. Thus this central area of human life becomes more and more open to planning and decision making. The pioneers of biomedical research see nothing but progress in this. In recent years, however, a new coalition has emerged with a critical viewpoint (e.g., Hubbard 1982; Arditti et al. 1984; Corea 1985; Corea et al. 1985; Spallone and Steinberg 1987; Stanworth 1988). These critics emphasize the unplanned and unintended side effects of technological change. They argue that the changes not only open up new options but simultaneously close down older ones.

According to them, the new reproductive technologies do more than simply increase our freedom of choice. Implied in the new freedom are new controls, new constraints, and new compulsions. Thus they argue that it is naive to assume technology is neutral in its impact on socially accepted ways of behaving. On the contrary, technology reshapes the very process of decision making, which involves available options and expectations as well as social norms and legal regulations. To paraphrase Max Weber, "modernization is not just a taxicab from which you can hop out whenever you please."

Advocates of the new reproductive technologies do not deny the possibility of risk or abuse. But they begin by assuming that users, researchers, and practitioners are free, ethical, and responsible human beings. No one, they assert, is forced either to take risks or engage in abuse. Only individual misuse can be blamed for resulting problems (e.g., Bräutigam and Mettler 1985). Opponents of the new techniques respond that this point of view is simplistic and narrow. Technology is embedded in social institutions, and individual choices are made within a social system that rewards some choices and punishes others.

In short, the controversy over the course of technological development centers on the relative weight of individual decision versus socially prescribed choices and pressures. In the following discussion, I will use the arguments involved in this general debate related specifically to the implementation of new reproductive technology in order to derive a four-step model of change. This framework applies to the social processes of technological change in all areas, but it is illustrated here by the specific effects of reproductive technologies.

Step One: Secret Implementation; or, Revolution Like the Fog Comes on Little Cat Feet

Most often, the development of new technology is a gradual process. Each step, taken by itself, seems trivial. No single point marks a historic transformation, a qualitative leap forward (Kuhn 1962). Yet when seen as a whole, these steps form a continuous process, pushing ever onward and leading to deep transformations. What goes on before our very eyes, without our realizing it, is a subtle, silent, and long-lasting revolution (e.g., Jonas 1985; Baele 1985, 1986). For example, in the 1960s and early 1970s, artificial insemination—a relatively "low-tech" technique—began to be used with increasing frequency; this helped to break down many emotional barriers to the manipulation of reproduction and created precedents for dealing legally with offspring born of "alien" genes. Thus in a very concrete sense, artificial insemination prepared the way for subsequent substitutions of egg or womb or both. Other "low-tech" factors developed separately included fertility drugs and laparoscopic surgery, which legitimized non-disease-related handling of women's reproductive systems. None of these effects implies a conspiracy, but rather an ongoing process of gradual and partial change that by its nature tends to be invisible. Each change in medical practice had effects upon social relations and expectations, but no single change was dramatic enough to excite controversy at first.

Step Two: Uncontrolled Implementation; or, the Inner Politics of Medicine

Democracy is the institutionalization of the idea that the important issues of society and its future should not be decided clandestinely by small numbers of people with a monopoly on power, but should be negotiated openly through the channels of public discourse. Of course, this principle has frequently been violated during the course of history, from the earliest beginnings of democracy. Today, however, we have reached a new stage.

With the growth of modern technology, central questions of human life are decided without the direct intervention of the institutions of democracy. They are introduced long before parliaments, officials, or judges can exert their power, often before they even realize what is going on. This is precisely what has happened with the new reproductive technologies, which have become the center of a process of "subpolitics" that transforms the very foundations of human life, yet bypasses elections, parliamentary votes, or political controls (Beck 1986). "Because of its built-in structure of action, medicine has a free ticket to test and apply its innovations. It can override public criticism and debate about what a scientist or professional may or may not do by a simple policy of 'fait accompli' " (Beck 1986, 335).

Designation of a technology as "experimental" is a social device used by science and medicine to protect innovations from public scrutiny in their early (and most vulnerable) stages. Judges and lawmakers only enter in to regulate use once the technology has ceased to be experimental and has come into common use—or, as in the case of Baby M, when they are faced with trying to get the lid back on Pandora's box. At that point, the technology is already diffused and cannot be undeveloped. New entities literally never before seen in nature are produced and entered into social and political relations, where they must be dealt with in some fashion. One potential social response is to define these new creations as *products* that can be profitably bought and sold. Laws of supply and demand, rather than of collective social choice in democratic political systems, are then the only regulations seen as appropriate. The restrictions that can now be imposed are only efforts to channel the social effects, not to undo medical or scientific discoveries.

Step Three: Universal Implementation;
or, Everybody Defined as Client

With the arrival of new options and opportunities, standards of behavior gradually begin to change. The same act that once seemed totally impossible, and later possible but taboo, may appear today as an interesting novelty and tomorrow perhaps as routine. Eventually, it may even become *the* legally sanctioned course of action. In many ways, technology has a self-fulfilling prophecy built into it. The pattern has been described as one in which "wants are awakened by possibilities" (Jonas 1985, 22). It is characteristic that new technologies, once available, produce new standards of what we "ought to have." Wishes become reality that in the past were hardly even dreams. In medicine, orthodontic care, preventive checkups, or good prenatal care are only a handful of examples. With the advance of medical knowledge and the development of social institutions such as health insurance, these things have become part of the standard package of middle-class life. Routine amniocentesis is but the next step in prenatal care. Routine artificial insemination and test-tube babies lie not too far ahead. Medical technology, like other technologies, creates its own market. It offers and sells an ever-growing range of products, and it needs to continually awaken and stimulate demand for what it sells (Jonas 1985, 22).

Thus over time, measures initially designed to cure infertility are likely to become transformed into universal procedures in reproductive medicine. This development follows a script with several distinct acts. At first, new biomedical interventions are introduced into a limited market confronting immediate problems of health. Then a period of transition and normalization sets in and the potential applications become considerably wider. At some point, the probability arises that all women and men will be defined as potential clients for their use, because by then the procedures will no longer be restricted to the treatment of particular physical problems. Rather, the new techniques will seem superior to the old ways: more effective, and the next logical step in correcting the accidental and unpredictable ways of nature (e.g., Amendt 1986; Corea 1985; Corea et al. 1985; Testart 1988). Many forms of surgery on women's reproductive systems have already been marketed as routine and virtually essential: hysterectomy, caesarean section, and episiotomy are well-known examples.

This same marketing approach has already begun to be applied to the newest reproductive technologies. In the last few years, the indications for in vitro fertilization have multiplied. Initially, IVF was intended specifically for women whose fallopian tubes were blocked or no longer present. In the meantime, however, IVF has also come to be used in the case of couples where the reproductive system of the woman was fully normal, but where the sperm quality of the *male* partner was not optimal (e.g., Lorber 1987; Testart 1988). Likewise IVF is resorted to as the "last chance" for couples where the cause of infertility remains undiagnosed (Amendt 1986; Testart 1988). In vitro fertilization has already been depicted by some authorities as the ideal method of reproduction for the future, desirable because of its potential for decreasing the incidence of birth defects—or to put it more bluntly, the incidence of *children* born with defects (see Corea 1986, 24). In addition, some pioneers working in the field of in vitro fertilization find it paradoxical, if not downright anachronistic, that humans "use" sperm of "inferior" quality, while with cattle we select for the highest quality (see Corea 1984). It has been proposed that it would be a great aid to women and men working in industries with high risk to genetic material if their eggs and sperm were to be deep frozen before their exposure (see Corea 1986, 23; Amendt 1986, 27).

Furthermore, before sterilization, men increasingly ask whether they may deposit sperm in a sperm bank to make it possible for them to have children, should they change their minds (or maybe move on to a new wife) (Friederich 1985). Some couples have asked whether they could use donated sperm or eggs to have a child because they are not wholly satisfied with the appearance or personality of the husband or wife (Corea 1986, 24). Individuals can be "blamed" for these choices, but the medical marketing of reproductive technologies as a solution to a wide variety of medical *and social* problems creates the social context in which these desires and choices are produced and legitimated.

**Step Four: Forced Implementation;
or, from Promise to Threat**

"As 'choices' become available, they all too rapidly become compulsions to 'choose' the socially endorsed alternative" (Hubbard 1982, 210). In the beginning, new technologies come as options. Whether we take them or leave them is up to us. But gradually they become part and parcel of the socially accepted and expected pattern of behavior. In many ways, subtle or not so subtle, choice turns into pressure (Daele 1985, 1986; Jonas 1985).

The questions and problems raised by the new reproductive technologies "are important for *all* women. Because female biology is exploited in *all* spheres of *all* women's lives. Whether we want children or decide to remain childfree, or are beyond our childbearing years, and whatever is our sexual preference, we are *all* at risk of becoming Test-Tube Women—at risk of being subjugated to a variety of controls: from technological interference when we are pregnant, to legal regulations that declare the fetus and the woman bearing it to be two separate 'patients,' to workplace policies that pressure women employees to become sterilized" (Arditti et al. 1984, 6–7).

Does this seem too pessimistic a picture? Then consider the following example. Today, some scientists praise reproductive technologies as the high road to family planning: "Parents could soon be in a position to plan their family totally, from control over the size of the family to determining the sex of their offspring and the sequence of male and female children" (Rosenzweig and Adelman 1976). Similarly, some popular books see reproductive technologies as a new form of self-determination for women: "Now science promises to put the very definition of mother, father, family lineage, and even human life in our hands. We'll decide not only if and when, but whose eggs and sperm will be used, where fertilization will take place, whose womb the fetus will grow to birth in, what sex it will be, what defects call for abortion or correction, and eventually, what genetic improvements in intelligence, character, or appearance we want to make" (Keeton 1986, 213). But contemplation of such prophecies leaves an unpleasant aftertaste. In this way, family planning could quite possibly turn into social surveillance and regulation of the family. To this end a whole spectrum of interventions stands ready, some of them mild, others less so, from "the myth of free will" (Corea 1985), that is, slanted information and directive "educational" efforts or counseling, all the way to monitoring, sanctions, and punishments. At the end of this line of development we may find what the well-known geneticist Bentley Glass has predicted: "Unlimited access to state-regulated abortion, together with perfected techniques for detecting chromosomal abnormalities . . . will relieve us of a certain percentage of those births which today reveal irremediable birth defects. . . . In this future, no couple will have the right to burden society with a misshapen or intellectually unfit child" (quoted in Löw 1985, 179).

In summary, the advocates of the new reproductive technologies see their use or nonuse as a matter of individual choice, relating to a person's preferences and responsibility, and emphasize their liberating potential. The critics, in contrast, stress the personal costs and the many new social pressures involved in all forms of modernization. Social processes of technological change, in the reproductive field as in other areas, move inexorably from secret development to uncontrolled implementation to universal use and finally coerced deployment. Humanity, once it develops a new technology, mounts an escalator that brings it into new worlds in a manner beyond control. What this process means in concrete terms for the users will be shown in the following section using two examples of reproductive technology: the birth control pill, and new methods of treating infertility.

Here again we will be confronted with the experience that we are already acquainted with from the history of modernization. Here it will become apparent that the loosening of traditional bonds has two faces. Obviously, that process can mean liberation for the individual and greater autonomy vis-à-vis the limits of nature. In a word, now biology is no longer destiny. But the loosening of traditional bonds can also lead to new hierarchies of power and create new controls, new dependencies. The less willing we are to accept the limits of nature, the more fully we are placed under the domination of medicine and technology.

The Pill: From Optional to Compulsory Contraception?

From the earliest times people have tried a variety of means, from herbs to witchcraft, to prevent unwanted pregnancies. However, in the past these measures all too often proved unreliable. One big change came during the early twentieth century with the arrival of new and more effective means of protection, like the diaphragm; and the development of the contraceptive pill during the second half of the twentieth century brought even greater changes. Since the 1960s we have had a method of contraception that is readily available, relatively simple to use, and which offers close to 100 percent protection.

We can now prevent many forms of suffering characteristic of earlier days, including the constant fear of unwanted pregnancy which haunted so many marriages and love affairs of the past, or the constant exhaustion of women who had to live through, and sometimes succumb to, an endless series of pregnancies and births. The choices that followed accidental pregnancy were always bad and sometimes terrifying: single motherhood, "shotgun marriage," abortion. In light of these problems, it is no wonder that on its arrival, the pill was welcomed by many, liberals and feminists in particular. To them it marked a new era of liberation and reproductive freedom.

Today, roughly two and a half decades later, some of these earlier advocates have begun to have second thoughts. Not that they wish to return to the old days with their fears and burdens. Rather, they have begun to realize that with the new freedoms, new problems have arisen. This shift is especially marked within the women's movement. In the beginning, the pill seemed to free women from the chains of biology. But later, the side effects and drawbacks emerged. First, there are serious health risks, especially to those women who use the pill continuously over long periods of time. Although the new freedom in sexuality is shared by both sexes, it is only women who experience the risks. In addition, the liberalization of sexuality has brought new psychological problems, and again, it is mostly women who pay the price. Now it is women, for example, who become both more readily available and disposable, because the sexual relationship is "without consequences." Men, on the other hand, are relieved of even more responsibility than before. Not infrequently, the pressure of sexual expectations has increased, in some cases culminating in a "throw-away relationship" with a woman as sex object. "The liberating pill has become the compulsory pill. The positive possibility of engaging in intercourse without fear of pregnancy has become the obligation to engage in intercourse" (Helferich 1983, 94).

Furthermore, we know from history that a new invention or technology is by no means a neutral instrument; it has a program of social change built into it. And so it is with the pill: it brings new pressures and new forms of behavior follow. While previously people had to go to great lengths to find a means of preventing pregnancy, today they have to make a deliberate decision to discontinue their use of contraceptives when they want to have a child. Thus the decision-making process has been turned around. And along with the new possibilities of contraception, corresponding attitudes, norms, and expectations begin to change. I suggest the following pattern.

Because of the speed with which news of the pill made headlines and the intensity of the public discussion that followed, a new consciousness arose. From big city to remote village, people came to realize that biology was no longer destiny, and that they could *decide* whether to have a child or not. Suddenly, as questions and viewpoints were raised in public debate, having a child became a matter of evaluating the pros and cons. Gradually a change in prevailing mores set in. Planned parenthood, at first a new option, now turned into a kind of duty (Häussler 1983). More precisely, contraceptive technology became contraceptive ideology. "The new morality calls for conscious, rational, technically reliable contraception. It is oriented to the enlightened, modern individual who deals responsibly with the act of procreation. . . . In an age of unlimited contraceptive possibilities, the individual who does not make use of them becomes suspect. Contraception is transformed from necessary evil into the duty of every responsible and enlightened citizen" (Häussler 1983, 65).

"Then what about the decision *not* to control fertility?" (Rothman 1984, 27). The medical pioneers of reproductive technology speak only of the choices they open up but do not seem to see that at the same time they have closed down other options. In an age of planned parenthood and unlimited contraception, those who do not want to use contraception or who want a large family gradually become "different," then "suspect" (naive, backward, irrational). Now the *nonuse* of contraception becomes stigmatized. Medical sociologist Barbara Katz Rothman was one of the first to notice and analyze this development. She provides a vivid example, describing first her own experience:

> I have been troubled in recent years by reactions, including my own, to unlimited fertility. A woman I see each summer was pregnant this year. Again. It was her fourth baby in five years. I know that she is having problems with money (and who wouldn't be, with four kids?). I know she is overworked and tired. . . . Four babies, I thought. My god. And then we talked. She's the classic case: the woman who has gotten pregnant with every birth control method, in place, used correctly. This last pregnancy, the doctor said, "C'mon, I'll abort it right now; you can go home not pregnant and forget it." She was tempted, sorely tempted. But no, she chose not to abort. . . . It was a choice she made, an unpopular reproductive choice, one which is not, in her community of friends, socially endorsed. . . . While on the one hand we worry, with very good reason, about losing the option of legal abortions, on the other hand we are losing the option not to abort. (Rothman 1984, 27)

We become caught in a kind of vicious circle. As more people make use of contraception and families become smaller, our social institutions become geared to couples with fewer children, or no children at all. This in turn makes life more difficult for those who want a large family. On many levels, from housing to economic capability, they run into obstacles and experience discrimination. Because of this, some will resign: they refrain from having another child. They use contraception. And so they further strengthen the trend. As Rothman explains, "the choice of contraception simultaneously closed down some of the choices for large families. North American society is geared to small families, if indeed to any children at all. Everything from car and apartment sizes to the picture book ideal of families encourages limiting fertility. Without the provision of good medical care, day care, decent housing, children are a luxury item, fine if you can afford them. . . . Does the choice not to be burdened with continual childbearing have to be paid for with the choice to have larger families?" (Rothman 1984, 28).

Such examples make it apparent that if we look at contraception in isolation, we are taking much too narrow and limited a view. Because if we do that, the foremost, the central question never gets considered at all: namely, *why* do women practice contraception, *why* do they decide against having children? Is this really a free decision, or is it not all too often dictated by political, economic, or social considerations—say, the conditions of the workplace, or housing, or transportation—which are entirely removed from our control? Put even more bluntly, "Do you have a choice if there are no viable options?" (Hanmer 1984, 441). Or to quote Rothman again, "it is a choice all right that contraception gave us . . . but it may be a somewhat forced choice. In its extreme, legislation has been repeatedly introduced to punish 'welfare mothers' by cutting off payments if they have more children. Sterilization abuse is the flip side of the abortion battle: the same sorry record" (Rothman 1984, 28).

What enters our field of vision here is the framework of social conditions—and the structures of power and dependency that stand behind that framework—that influences the decision for or against children. This insight is of central importance, because in the political arena it is otherwise easy to get caught in a kind of boomerang effect. It could happen, for example, that women are allowed to decide against children—but that at the same time, the decision for children becomes increasingly difficult. It could happen that the individual woman is saddled with all the burdens associated with having a child, because she has "freedom of choice." From this perspective, society is then released from all responsibility and from the pressure to take any action. Why bother with day care and parental leave and all the rest, why even consider ways to make scientific-technological society less hostile to children? None of that is necessary; after all, it's the woman's own choice to have a child or not.

New Ways of Treating Infertility: From Hope to Burden?

Many new ways of treating infertility have been introduced in the recent past. They range from hormonal stimulation, a routine part of gynecological practice now, to methods like in vitro fertilization, which seems spectacular today but may become routine tomorrow. But whether routine or spectacular (these labels change so quickly), such measures serve a common aim. They bring new hope to couples who are eager to become parents but who have tried in vain to achieve that goal, often for years on end. Now, through advances in reproductive medicine, involuntary childlessness may come to an end, along with the suffering and despair that accompany it. Now such couples may see their heart's wish come true—a child of their own.

Or so the pioneers of reproductive technology say. How much of this picture is true? And does it give the whole truth? To determine this, we must know more about the procedures involved than we can derive from sensational success stories in the mass media. We need detailed information about the whole process of medical intervention. Only then can we see how it affects the lives of women and men caught up in striving for parenthood.

To begin with, let us examine more closely the routine measures of fertility treatment today, the daily charting of the woman's temperature and hormonal stimulation. Under such a regime, sexuality becomes, in large part, subject to medical control. It becomes a combination of dutiful exercise and competitive sport, to be performed according to strict technical rules (when, when not, how often, in what position). It is regulated and disciplined, reduced to a biological act. Lost are its other technically "irrelevant" aspects: sensuality, spontaneity, love. With the constant pressure of following the rules, joy turns into frustration. Both self-esteem and the relationship between partners may be considerably damaged (Pfeffer and Woollett 1983, 144). For example, one interviewee explains, "The major problem of going through infertility is making love to order. It takes all the spontaneity out of it. I went through a stage of only wanting him in the fertile time; it seemed pointless on other days." And another says, "It got to the stage where sex was up a gum tree; it really didn't count for much. It was a bit squeaky and not very exciting; a bit frenetic. I had it all organized" (Pfeffer and Woollett 1983, 38).

With the more spectacular measures, more problems arise. The treatments may go on for months or even years. They will be time-consuming and expensive and may involve considerable risk to health and emotional stability. Take, for example, in vitro fertilization. Two physicians, Hans Bräutigam and Liselotte Mettler, provide the following description.

The procedure begins with hormone stimulation, continuously supervised by laboratory controls. When an increase in levels of hormones is established, the eggs are removed. This requires "the abdomen to be cut open." Then four hours later, according to schedule again, the sperm is obtained by means of masturbation, "which many men find embarrassing." Then comes test-tube fertilization, followed by "quality control of embryos," "in order to make sure that only those embryos will be reimplanted that appear to be regular." Under the microscope the embryo is "evaluated on a scale ranging from 1 to 5."

If the embryo passes this "check list of embryo quality," it is implanted into the uterus. Then the woman "has to remain lying in a sloping position for fourteen hours, womb upward, head downward." Additional hormones may be given at short intervals. But in many cases the implantation is not successful and no pregnancy results. Or the implantation may work but be followed by a spontaneous abortion. Clearly, we must consider "the hope and disappointment, the physical and emotional pain for thousands of women and men who, when admitted to the reproduction program had thought that they were close to the fulfillment of their wishes." And what about those women who do actually become pregnant and whose pregnancies develop normally? Even for them, the ordeal is not over since half will have to undergo a caesarean section. "This is to prevent the possibility that after such a demanding and difficult process the success of the treatment will be placed in jeopardy by problems during delivery." The price to be paid is risk to the women, since "the mortality rate of a caesarean section is three to four times higher than that of a normal delivery."

Is this a horror story handed out by obstinate foes of progress? Not at all. This is a matter-of-fact description of the actual treatment, given by those who know it best: two pioneers of in vitro fertilization (Bräutigam and Mettler 1985, 54–68).

And after undergoing such trials, how many women and men see their wishes come true? The truth contained in the statistics is sobering. The majority of couples seeking medical help will not achieve the hoped-for result, that is, a child. And this is particularly true with in vitro fertilization, the object of so many desperate hopes today. Here the rate of success is very low: not more than 15 percent to 20 percent at best (Daele 1985; Bräutigam and Mettler 1985), and much lower according to some sources (Corea 1985; Laborie 1988; Testart 1988). To quote again from the pioneers of reproductive technology, given the current rates of success (or rather, of failure), the rapid increase in the number of laboratories offering IVF "may prove disastrous for the couples experiencing infertility" (Bräutigam and Mettler 1985, 65).

Beyond this, even when the treatments do not bring the hoped-for result, they often have other consequences. For those women and men who remain infertile—and remember, this is the majority—the medical intervention does not relieve the suffering but will, instead, increase it (Testart 1988). Iatrogenic suffering, i.e., suffering caused by the medical treatments themselves, will have been added; and the couple will suffer from the identification as "patients" and as "physically deficient." As a result, self-esteem and self-confidence may be injured; the couple's relationship will be subject to considerable strain. Often social life will diminish. All is the consequence of the medical treatments, which demand such effort and energy that they leave but little room for other interests and activities. And then the dream of having a child of one's own becomes the center of all thought, emotion, and action, only to be disappointed time and time again.

Of course it might be argued that after all, anyone is free to hop off the carousel, to stop trying to have a child. This may prove far more difficult than it appears at first glance. Some part of this difficulty is produced by the very process of medical progress. As a by-product of advances in technology, infertility is redefined as a "curable" condition. When there are so many ways of treating it, how can one in good conscience stop trying? In Rothman's words, "all of the new treatments for infertility have also created a new burden for the infertile—the burden of not trying hard enough. Just how many dangerous experimental drugs, just how many surgical procedures, just how many months—or is it years?—of compulsive temperature-taking and obsessive sex does it take before one can now give in gracefully? When has a couple 'tried everything' and can finally stop?" (Rothman 1984, 31).

In former times, infertility was destiny. Today, it becomes, at least in part, a kind of choice. If you give up before trying the latest procedure, an endless rat race, it is your own fault. You *could* have continued to try. Rothman struggles with this issue of guilt and blame: "At what point is it simply not their fault, out of their control, inevitable, inexorable fate? At what point can they get on with their lives? If there is always one more doctor to try, one more treatment around, then the social role of infertility will always be seen in some sense as chosen: they chose to give up. Did taking away the sense of inevitability of their infertility and substituting the 'choice' of giving up truly increase their choice and their control?" (Rothman 1984, 32).

Last but not least, it is the pioneers of medical research themselves who contribute to the redefinition of fertility. In order to legitimize the enormous costs of their efforts, they stress motherhood as central, even predominant, in women's lives. For example, Kurt Semm, director of the leading embryo transfer team in West Germany, says, "It is the very task of women to have children. This is women's reason for being, to preserve the race, the species. . . . Anything else that is added, be it work or whatever, is secondary to this goal. If a woman is unable to achieve the goal of having a child, her main task in life remains unfulfilled" (quoted in Idel 1986, 63).

Then what about those women who do not succeed in fulfilling their "main task"? Faced with such definitions, they are bound to feel useless and inferior, in short, failures. As the motto of the Sheba Hospital IVF clinic in Israel puts it so nicely, combining promise and threat, "You're not a failure till you stop trying" (quoted in Solomon 1988, 43). Most probably, some women will prefer to shop around for yet another treatment rather than live with such labels. And so the very measures that were designed to help infertile women are now being turned against them. Eventually they produce new social definitions, new forms of social stigmatization, which make women more and more dependent on the medical system. Thus women are trapped in the endless circles of the infertility career. As with the pill, reproductive technology becomes reproductive ideology.

N O T E

This is a revised version of a paper presented at the symposium initiated by Kurt Lüscher, "Familiale Lebensformen und Familienpolitik im Übergang zur Postmoderne" (Forms of family life and family politics in the transition to the post-modern era), in Constance in 1986; and of a later version presented at the Third International Interdisciplinary Congress on Women, Dublin, 1987.

I wish to thank Bernard Mausner, who helped with the translation; and the women on the editorial committee, especially Myra Marx Ferree and Barbara D. Wright, who made many useful comments and clarifying suggestions.

R E F E R E N C E S

Amendt, Gerhard. 1986. *Der neue Klapperstorch. Über künstliche Befruchtung—Samenspender—Leihmütter—Retortenzeugung* (The new stork: On artificial fertilization, sperm donors, surrogate mothers, test tube reproduction). Herbstein: März Verlag.

Arditti, Rita, Renate Duelli-Klein, and Shelley Minden, eds. 1984. *Test-tube Women: What future for motherhood?* Boston: Pandora Press.

Beck, Ulrich. 1986. *Risikogesellschaft. Auf dem Weg in eine andere Moderne Zeit* (Society of risk: On the way to a new modern age). Frankfurt: Suhrkamp.

Berger, Johannes, ed. 1986. *Die Moderne—Kontinuitäten und Zäsuren* (The modern age: Continuities and discontinuities). *Soziale Welt,* special issue, vol. 4. Göttingen: Schwartz and Co.

Berger, Peter, Brigitte Berger, and Hansfried Kellner. 1986. *Das Unbehagen in der Modernität* (The modern age and its discontents). Frankfurt: Campus.

Bräutigam, Hans Harald, and Liselotte Mettler. 1985. *Die programmierte Vererbung. Möglichkeiten und Gefahren der Gentechnologie* (Programmed heredity: Possibilities and dangers of gene technology). Hamburg: Hoffmann und Campe.

Corea, Gena. 1984. Egg snatchers. In *Test-tube women,* 37–51. *See* Arditti, Klein, and Minden, eds.

―――――. 1985. *The mother machine.* New York: Harper and Row.

―――――. 1986. *Die Zukunft unserer Welt* (The future of our world). In *Die Grünen im Bundestag* (The Green Party in parliament), ed. AK Frauenpolitik: Frauen gegen Gentechnik und Reproduktionstechnik, 22–26. Cologne: Kölner Volksblatt Verlag.

Corea, Gena, Rita Duelli-Klein, Jalna Hanmer, Helen B. Holmes, B. Hoskins, M. Kishwar, J. Raymond, R. Rowland, and R. Steinbacher. 1985. *Man-made women: How new reproductive technologies affect women.* London: Hutchinson.

Daele, Wolfgang van den. 1985. *Mensch nach Maß? Ethische Probleme der Genmanipulation und Gentherapie* (Custom-made man? Ethical problems of genetic manipulation and genetic therapy). Munich: Beck.

―――――. 1986. Technische Dynamik und gesellschaftliche Moral. Zur soziologischen Bedeutung der Gentechnologie (Technical dynamics and social morality: On the sociological meaning of gene technology). *Soziale Welt,* nos. 2–3: 149–72.

Durkheim, Emile. 1977. *Über die Teilung der sozialen Arbeit* (On the division of social labor). Frankfurt: Suhrkamp.

Friederich, Wolfgang. 1985. Samenbanken. Hintertüren der Sterilisation (Sperm banks: The back door to sterilization). *Pro familia magazin,* no. 3: 22–24.

Häussler, Monika. 1983. Von der Enthaltsamkeit zur verantwortungsbewußten Fortpflanzung. Über den unaufhaltsamen Aufstieg der Empfängnisverhütung und seine Folgen (From abstinence to responsible reproduction: On the irresistible rise of contraception and its consequences). In *Bauchlandungen. Abtreibung, Sexualität, Kinderwunsch* (Belly landings: Abortion, sexuality, the desire for children), ed. Monika Häussler, Cornelia Helfferich, Gabriela Walterspiel, and Angelika Wetterer. Munich: Frauenbuch Verlag.

Hanmer, Jalna. 1984. A Womb of One's Own. In *Test-tube women,* 438–48. *See* Arditti, Klein, and Minden, eds. 1984.

Helfferich, Cornelia. 1983. Mich wird es schon nicht erwischen. Risikoverhalten und magisches Denken bei der Verhütung (It can't happen to me: Risk taking and magical thinking with regard to contraception). In *Bauchlandungen. Abtreibung, Sexualität, Kinderwunsch* (Belly landings: Abortion, sexuality, the desire for children), ed. Monika Häussler, Cornelia Helfferich, Gabriela Walterspiel, and Angelika Wetterer. Munich: Frauenbuch Verlag.

Hubbard, Ruth. 1982. Some legal and policy implications of recent advances in prenatal diagnosis and fetal therapy. *Women's Rights Law Reporter,* 7, no. 3 (Spring): 201–18.

Idel, Anita. Gentechnologie und einige Folgen (Gene technology and some of its consequences). In *Die Grünen im Bundestag* (The Green Party in parliament), ed. AK Frauenpolitik: Frauen gegen Gentechnik und Reproduktionstechnik, 64f. Cologne: Kölner Volksblatt Verlag.

Jonas, Hans. 1985. *Technik, Medizin und Ethik. Zur Praxis des Prinzips Verantwortung* (Technology, medicine and ethics: On the application of the principle of responsibility). Frankfurt: Insel Verlag.

Keeton, Kathy. 1986. *Women of Tomorrow.* New York: St. Martin's Press.

Kuhn, Thomas S. 1962. *The Structure of Scientific Revolutions.* Chicago: University of Chicago Press.

Laborie, Francoise. 1988. New reproductive technologies: News from France and elsewhere. *Reproductive and Genetic Engineering* 1, no. 1: 77–85.

Lorber, Judith. 1987. In vitro fertilization and gender politics. *Women and Health* 13, nos. 1–2: 117–33.

Löw, Reinhard. 1985. *Leben aus dem Labor* (Life from the laboratory). Munich: Bertelsmann.

Pfeffer, Naomi, and Ann Woollett. 1983. *The experience of infertility.* London: Virago Press.

Rosenzweig, Saul, and Adelman Stuart. 1976. Parental determination of the sex of offspring: The attitudes of young married couples with university education. *Journal of Biosocial Sciences* 8:335–46.

Rothman, Barbara Katz. 1984. The meanings of choice in reproductive technology. In *Test-tube women,* 23–34. See Arditti, Klein, and Minden, eds. 1984.

Solomon, Alice. 1988. Integrating infertility crisis counselling into feminist practice. *Reproductive and Genetic Engineering* 1, no. 1: 41–49.

Spallone, Patricia, and Deborah Lynn Steinberg, eds. 1987. *Made to order: The myth of reproductive and genetic progress.* Oxford: Pergamon Press.

Stanworth, Michelle, ed. 1987. *Reproductive technologies: Gender, motherhood and medicine.* Minneapolis: University of Minnesota Press.

Testart, Jacques. 1988. *Das transparente Ei* (The transparent egg). Frankfurt and Munich: Schweitzer.

Weber, Max. 1984. *Die protestantische Ethik I. Eine Aufsatzsammlung* (The protestant ethic: A collection of essays). Ed. Johannes Winckelmann. Gütersloh: Gütersloher Verlagshaus Gerd Mohn.

Electronic Fetal Monitors: Marketing Forces and the Resulting Controversy

Judith R. Kunisch

Contemporary childbirth is defined as an acute event requiring aggressive medical management with frequent pharmacological and surgical interventions. For most women, childbirth has lost its personal and familial character. The childbearing mother has become a passive patient directed through the birth experience by an assortment of medical professionals. These health care professionals take control of the pregnancy away from the birthing woman, asserting that medical management is superior to the natural biology of the event.

This transformation in the character of childbirth has occurred over the past one hundred years. It is a result of moving birth from home into hospital, eliminating midwives as primary caregivers to parturient women, creating obstetrics and perinatology as medical specialties, and designing a multitude of scientific machines with medical applications. It is the masculinization of American medicine which is above all responsible for these changes.

The changed definition of childbirth has been dictated by obstetrical practices developed by men who operate in a society that believes more technology makes better medicine. From a psychological point of view, male obstetricians may find it easier to identify with the fetus than with the mother, and this may explain their tendency to focus on the fetus rather than on the birthing woman. The current model for obstetrical care incorporates traits of aggressiveness and a need for control that are common to males in this society, together with a symbiotic relationship between male obstetricians and machines which may be congenial to men who view the machine as enhancing their power and control. The result of this dominance of males and male values is a move away from a biological focus to a technological one. The contemporary merger of business and health care systems represents another male alliance that further defines childbirth for women and controls the experiences of childbearing families. Both these male-dominated systems regard women as passive objects for whom the birthing experience must be controlled, regulated, and manipulated according to scientifically "credible" practices of organized medicine. Women have been denied the freedom to define their own birthing experiences.

Using the example of the electronic fetal monitor, this chapter describes the impact of the technology explosion on the definition of childbirth in the United States, and it looks at the alliance between business and health care systems that has emerged during the past two decades. This paper examines the role of business and health care in manipulating marketplace forces, and how the two together created the perception that electronic equipment is essential in providing safety to mothers and babies, the perception that technology is better able to monitor the birthing process than human attendants, and the perception that without such technology, safety and well being are jeopardized. In essence, health care practitioners, patients, and their insurors, all came to believe that without the assistance of electronic fetal monitors, the birth experience is dangerous.

The story of the electronic fetal monitor (EFM) provides us with an excellent case study of how business joined with health care practitioners in creating a standard of care. The rapid acceptance of EFM into labor and delivery rooms throughout the nation was assured through a well-organized and well-executed marketing effort conducted primarily by one small company, Corometrics Medical Systems, Inc. of Wallingford, Connecticut. The obstetrical community eagerly embraced the machine at a time when other medical specialties were also becoming increasingly technological. In addition to marketing strategies, product promotion, and capitalization from investment sources, this chapter surveys the controversies that resulted from rapid introduction of EFM, as well as issues related to inadequate regulation of medical devices.

This is a story of male dominance in defining the birthing of infants. Men dominated in the creation of EFM technology, in the sales and marketing of the machine, and in the excited investment community which financed product development and sales growth, as well as in the medical setting where it was employed. The story of the EFM is the story of a machine that is now a part of the labor and delivery experience of virtually every woman in the United States who gives birth in a hospital. It is the story of the failure of a regulatory agency designed to protect health care consumers. And finally, it is the tragic story of women subjected to needless interventions and surgeries, a story of the violation of one of the most profound of female experiences.

Electronic Fetal Monitors

"Electronic fetal monitoring has emerged as the most effective screening technique available for detecting the fetus which is already asphyxiated or at risk for intrapartum hypoxia" (Banta and Thacker 1978).

This statement from the early 1970s best describes the perception of medical providers who decided to use the electronic fetal monitor in the management of women's labor. An electronic fetal monitor is a machine that evaluates the status of the fetus during labor. It is used to identify cases of fetal distress. Proponents of this technology see labor as a time of stress to the fetus due primarily to the rigors of uterine contractions. The stress of labor may produce adverse consequences to the infant from a lack of oxygen to the fetal brain, including brain damage, tissue damage, and even death. Others agree stress is present but see it as a normal part of birth. Monitoring is conducted either externally, through the mother's abdomen, or from inside the uterus itself. Two measurements are usually obtained: the fetal heart rate, and the strength of maternal uterine contractions. External monitoring is accomplished by placing two belts across the lower abdomen of the laboring woman. One belt attaches an ultrasonic transducer to the abdomen for measurement of fetal heart rate. The second belt attaches a sensing device to measure the strength of uterine contractions. Internal monitoring is utilized after rupture of the amniotic membrane. In this case, electrodes are passed through the vaginal canal and cervical opening into the uterus. One electrode measures the force of uterine contractions. The other, a small device which is screwed or clipped to the fetal scalp, obtains fetal electrocardiogram readings. Internal monitoring is the more precise of the two methods.

Prior to development of EFM technology, fetal status during labor was monitored by periodic auscultation (i.e., listening to the fetal heartbeat using a fetoscope, similar to a stethoscope). Uterine contractions were measured for duration, frequency, and intensity by a labor attendant using manual palpation. This technique required professional attendance at the bedside of the laboring woman and consistency in recording maternal and fetal response to labor.

The designers of EFM equipment produced a machine that was portable, simple to operate, and as inexpensive and reliable as the producers deemed acceptable. With EFM, the fetal heart rate and strength of contractions are displayed on an oscilloscope for immediate viewing and simultaneously recorded on paper. Health professionals are able to obtain at a glance the current condition of the mother and fetus, as well as review what has previously occurred by reading the paper tracing. Today, an EFM machine used in an urban hospital costs approximately $8,000.

Introduction to the product line of a central display system installed in the nurses' station provided for expanded surveillance of one to four women simultaneously. In this way, one nurse or physician could monitor four women and fetuses without even leaving the desk. Most recently, portable monitors have been developed for use at home. Women deemed at risk for premature labor attach themselves to a home monitor and use specially designed telephone modem equipment to send in a tracing to a central office, where specially trained nurses interpret fetal and uterine activity.

The advantages of EFM are its ability to provide continuous read-out of data, and avoidance of human error in counting fetal heart beats and evaluating uterine contraction strength. It reduces personnel needs for each laboring woman. The EFM paper tracing record also provides reference to ascertain patterns of heart rate and uterine contractions as labor progresses, and creates a "paper trail" for insurors of both doctors and patients.

The disadvantages of EFM include limited movement for the woman attached to a monitor. Most women are monitored throughout their labor, and this requires the woman to remain in bed, unable to move about or change position, for this will disturb the belts across her abdomen. Forced immobility and unnatural position in bed lead to discomfort and lack of control over labor management by women, and may actually cause problems in labor. An additional disadvantage with use of EFM is that professional attention is directed to readout data supplied by the machine and there is less "laying on of hands" by labor attendants. After introduction of EFM, it became common to enter a labor room and find the physician or nurse, back to the patient, focused on the machine. The machine, rather than the woman herself, has become the most significant source of information regarding her labor.

In the case of internal monitoring, an additional disadvantage is that doctors tend to artificially rupture the amniotic membranes in order to attach electrodes. This induced, premature rupture occurs all too frequently, resulting in needless acceleration of the labor and removal of the natural cushioning effect of the amniotic fluid against the fetal head. Documented cases of infection caused by Group B strep virus at the site of insertion of the screw-type electrode have caused concern among medical professionals and consumer groups alike. This commonly occurring pathogen may cause serious illness in the newborn in 1 of 100 cases (Sweet 1985).

The significance of recording and documenting progress through labor became even greater in the early 1980s with an emergent malpractice crisis in obstetrical care. Large monetary awards were made to families of infants injured during birth. Medical practitioners were advised by insurance companies and members of the legal profession to secure documentation of as much of the labor and delivery event as was possible. The paper record of EFM became admissible evidence in court and physicians would not take the risk of managing labor without it. Thus more and more women found themselves in bed, strapped to monitors, because of defensive medicine.

Development of EFM Technology

Development of EFM technology began in the 1960s in the United States, Germany, and Uruguay. The technology makes use of the Doppler effect, a phenomenon described in the science of physics. The Doppler effect provides information to an observer from moving objects. As an object moves toward or away from a receiving source the frequency of sound waves produced by the object changes. This physical event is employed in radar detection in which radio waves are emitted and then measured as they strike an object and bounce back. The Doppler effect was originally employed in military applications for detection of enemy movement under cover of darkness. Early developers of electronic fetal monitoring employed military research in designing the technology.

EFM employs high-frequency sound waves rather than radio waves, as in radar. To measure fetal heart beats, the movements of the fetal heart muscle are bombarded by "ultra" sound waves that bounce back to a receiving source. As the fetal heart contracts and relaxes, a change in frequency occurs. However, the human heart has many different movements in its various chambers that occur simultaneously as the heart carries out its beating function. Therefore, many sound receptions must be differentiated in order to ascertain the fetal beat. EFM measures three separate heart sounds (blood flow, muscle, and valve signal) and then averages the rate to produce a beat-to-beat record of heart activity.

Patent Documents

Examination of patent documents written over a twenty-year period shows a continuous upgrading and improvement in EFM's ability to accurately measure fetal heart rates. By inference, these patents reveal a technology that was originally shockingly primitive and unreliable. The degree of reliability continues to be an issue today. What is most alarming is that while inventors attempted to improve machine accuracy, marketers were selling the EFM to a medical community that relied upon it—despite its significant shortcomings—as the major source of information for decision making.

Patents awarded in the late 1960s and early 1970s refer to the development of filters to block out other sounds in an effort to receive only the three major heart sounds used in beat counting. An early German patent, assigned to Hewlett-Packard in 1971, describes an apparatus that includes error detection and correction circuitry. The major concern of the inventor was that fetal beats could be missed due to movements of the fetus, sounds of maternal heartbeat, intestinal and respiratory activities, and changes in intrauterine pressure (from contractions) during labor. All of these sounds were blocking out or obscuring the heart sounds being measured and, therefore, impeded reliable results. The missed heartbeats resulted in readings of "decreased frequency which may cause confusion and may even induce an attending physician to follow unnecessary emergency procedures" (U.S. Patent no. 3, 581, 735).

While early patents focused on problems of obtaining all fetal heartbeat sounds, the ability to count accurately dominates patent refinements in the later 1970s and 1980s. Selective filters, tachometers, counters, and circuit refinements were added to improve EFM effectiveness. Still, the problem continued. A patent assigned to Gould, Inc. in 1975 refers to spurious counts and multiple counting. "It has been found that beat-by-beat information can be quite misleading" (U.S. Patent no. 4, 143, 650). In March, 1979, a document for a patent assigned to Hoffman–La Roche, Inc. relates that "present Doppler arrangements are at times unable to reliably provide from such complex [heart] signals the accuracy desired in the medical profession. . . ." (U.S. Patent no. 4, 143, 650). Finally, a patent assigned to American Home Products Corporation in March, 1986, alerts us that counting problems continue to nag designers and engineers:

> Fetal motions as well as motions of maternal tissue surfaces introduce large artifacts in the echo signals which greatly complicate the task of deriving useful information of fetal heart activity therefrom. . . . It is thus necessary to select the towards or away echo components for producing a heart beat event signal and the selection of a component representing noise can result in a failure to detect one or more subsequent heart beat events. . . . Consequently, when the fetal heart is in the range of 50–105 beats per minute, prior art techniques often detect the fetal heart rate at twice the real rate . . . and double counting occurs. (U.S. Patent no. 4, 573, 479)

The significance of this quotation as late as 1986 is profound. Often during a uterine contraction, the fetal heart rate may normally drop to between 50 and 105 beats per minute. Double counting of such a heart rate may indicate fetal distress where, in fact, none exists. The physician or nurse does not know that the information being provided by an EFM tracing during a woman's labor is incorrect, and unnecessary emergency procedures in response to this false information may begin. Clearly, even in 1986 an alarming gap between the myth and the reality of EFM reliability existed. Yet medical professionals continued to exhibit a remarkable faith in the use of the machine as a basis for decision making.

How is this possible? At least part of the answer lies in the implications of the patenting process. Legal protection through a patent of a particular device implies the validity of claims made for such a device. As each development of EFM received a right of manufacture through the patent from the United States government, EFM technology became further legitimized as part of the standard of care in obstetrics. In the early 1960s and 1970s, at a time when regulation of medical devices was inadequate, EFM was able to gain acceptance in the industry of health care machinery through the patenting process itself. EFM was welcomed as a sign of progress and improvement in patient care through technology.

Chronology of Events

A brief chronology of events will assist the reader in understanding the rapid acceptance of EFM as a part of the obstetrical standard of care. Roberto Caldeyro-Barcia, M.D., of Uruguay, is a pioneer in electronic fetal monitoring. An early report he wrote in 1966 for *Medical World News* was entitled "Monitoring Fetal Hearts for the Beat of Distress." At a 1986 convention of the International Childbirth Education Association, I discussed electronic fetal monitors with him. Dr. Caldeyro-Barcia noted that while he was among the first users of the technology, it was never his intention that such a device be applied to all laboring women. Rather, EFM was originally designed for and considered suitable for use in the 10 to 15 percent cases of high-risk labor that do occur.

Publication of early work related to fetal heart monitoring in the international medical press brought attention to the device in the United States and Germany. In this country, research and development was conducted both within the nonprofit and profit-making sectors. Major developers of EFM worked at the University of Southern California and Yale University. Private companies, notably Hewlett-Packard on the west coast and Corometrics Medical Systems on the east coast, joined in the development.

Caldeyro-Barcia's early experiment with electronic monitoring of fetal heart rates in high-risk situations gave way in the early 1970s to rapid application of the technology to low-risk laboring women, as well. By the late 1970s, virtually all United States hospitals had purchased electronic fetal monitors, and they were routinely used in all cases, regardless of the risk status of the mother and infant (Dolin 1973). The bias in obstetrics to assume that any birth was high risk until proven otherwise was reinforced. EFM provided protection, should anything indeed go wrong.

Two factors led to this rapid inclusion of EFM in standard birthing procedures. First, production of EFM moved out of the research laboratory and into the health industrial complex. Commercialization of EFM was largely accomplished by Corometrics Medical Systems, Inc., which began manufacturing monitors in the late 1960s. The first five years of the seventies represented not only increased use of the product, but also tremendous sales growth for the company (*Wall Street Journal* 1974). As each hospital purchased more machines and as physicians came to rely on machine-generated data, additional machines were bought and each labor room became so equipped, until EFM was an accepted part of the standard of care. The presence of the machine in the labor room in turn increased the likelihood that it would be used.

Second, physicians were able, for the first time, to obtain continuous information about the fetus during labor. The physician was able to enter a labor room and read the complete record of everything that had happened while he/she was gone. Since labor may take many hours, observation by machine was viewed as quite practical and helpful. Indeed, the machine came to be perceived as providing more reliable information than nursing attendants in monitoring maternal and fetal status. This preference may in part be due to a physician bias concerning nurses and their professional abilities. Or it may represent a false confidence that machines protect us against human error. But in this way, of course, technology was placed ahead of biology, and obstetrics came to rely even more on a male definition of machine-oriented manipulation of biological events.

At the same time, other influences on birthing practice emerged. During World War II, there had been tremendous progress in pharmacology. Drugs were invented that could sedate a laboring woman and effectively remove her from the labor and delivery experience. Largely male obstetricians assumed that a woman would not want to experience the pain of childbirth. It became common for women to be heavily medicated with drugs such as scopolamine, which produced a twilight sleep, but in this way women were prevented from participating in what was going on. In addition, babies were born drowsy from the heavy medication. Both mother and infant took two to three days to recover from the residual effects of the medication (Haire 1972). Then with publication in the fifties of such popular books as *Thank-you, Dr. Lamaze* by Marjorie Karmel and Grantly Dick-Reid's *Childbirth Without Fear,* women began to demand the kind of birth experience in which they could be active participants. In the 1960s women actually began to take control of birth.

The introduction of awake and aware childbirth in this country by such pioneers as Marjorie Karmel and Elizabeth Bing brought to labor rooms a new definition of practice. Women began to learn about the physiology of birth, to participate actively, and to control events surrounding the birth itself. Consumer groups sprang up around the country and couples began taking classes to prepare themselves mentally and physically for the rigors of birthing. Women became active consumers of health care and were no longer content to settle for passivity in receiving care. Birth was redefined as a natural function for a female body, and women demanded a role as equal member of the health care team (Young 1982).

For many physicians, this change in attitude, together with renewed popularity of home birth and midwives, was highly threatening. Obstetricians resented having alert patients who asked questions and requested information. Many were highly indignant that women no longer were intimidated by the medical training required for obstetrical specialties. These women viewed birthing as a natural event requiring little or no intervention. To make matters worse, husbands and boyfriends were accompanying women into labor and delivery. The physician was no longer the central figure. Everyone's attention was directed to the birthing couple. What better way to regain control than by bringing in a machine that only a sophisticated physician could read and interpret. Once again, the obstetrician was indispensable, his/her word was authority, and woman was reduced to passive object.

Corometrics Medical Systems, Inc.

This clarifies the demand factors behind the rapid adoption of EFM, but there were significant supply-side factors as well, orchestrated primarily by Corometrics Medical Systems, Inc. Between 1968 and 1975, this small company was able to create tremendous demand for its sole product—the electronic fetal monitor. How did one company, which eventually acquired 75 percent of market share for EFM, do it?

Corometrics Medical Systems, Inc. was formed as a Delaware corporation in June, 1968. Its sole business was manufacturing and marketing of electronic fetal monitors and the paper and electrode disposable products used with the machines. Throughout the early and mid-1970s, Corometrics held 75 percent of the market. Hewlett-Packard held another 20 percent, and the rest was divided among smaller companies.

Corometrics' early growth was remarkable. Revenue statements for 1969 show sales of $467,000. Four years later, in 1973, sales had reached $5 million, almost a 1,000 percent increase.

In order to finance product research and development, Corometrics issued common stock to the public market. The stock was traded on the OTC market and the company was regarded as an excellent investment. Companies listed on the OTC market generally tend to be innovative, and investors look here for opportunities to get in on the ground floor during a company's early growth period. For investors, a tremendous opportunity exists at this point to make large profits.

Investment literature written in the early 1970s describes the company accordingly: "Corometrics offers investors the extremely rare and highly profitable opportunity of investing in an emerging growth company in an emerging growth industry" (Dolin 1973). Or: "We can see the time when the fetus will be monitored from several months after conception until birth by a series of electronic devices able to monitor a variety of fetal functions. When this happens, the market for equipment and disposables will be in the billion dollar range" (Dolin 1973).

Such interest and enthusiasm from the investment community led to capital inflow as investors purchased Corometrics stock. Capital inflow meant expanded operations, enlarged research and development capability to improve technology, and aggressive product marketing. Research and development allocations in 1973 account for 6 percent of revenue, a high percentage. It was management's goal to upgrade and improve their product.

In moving EFM out of the research laboratory, with strict scientific application, and into the arena of the health-industrial complex, the strategies for successful profit making become incorporated into product promotion. Marketing is essential in promoting sales and use of any product, and Corometrics' marketers played a crucial role in setting the obstetrical standard of care. The Corometrics marketing plan was a highly effective one.

Corometrics management made several crucial assumptions concerning industry potential and marketability of their product. First, they assumed there existed in society a tendency to equate "better medicine" with "more technology." Second, they assumed no parents will take the risk of not using technology and jeopardizing their infant's well being. Third, they knew insurance companies would tolerate the expenses for care to become more "scientific" and "safe." Finally, they knew that charges for use of EFM equipment, after covering the cost of purchase, would become a source of profits for hospitals and physicians.

Based on these assumptions, Corometrics made yearly sales projections for the United States and world markets. Sales of equipment and disposable products for a total worldwide market were estimated at $194.8 million per year. With these projections, Corometrics had every intention of seeing that their product was used by everyone. This view was in marked contrast to the view of Dr. Caldeyro-Barcia, who developed EFM. Yet that is exactly what happened.

Corometrics' marketing plan aimed for attainment of a leadership position in the monitor market. The company employed their own sales force rather than depend on salespersons from larger medical-supply distributors. These salespersons were supposed to be well informed, able to respond immediately to customer requests, and capable of assisting with technical and service problems (Blyden 1973). This strategy probably contributed to Corometrics' success in penetrating the market.

Sales efforts were directed to large metropolitan and university hospitals. Here, larger numbers of births occur and the product was immediately put to use. Additionally, the more complicated, high-risk births are brought to these locations. At the universities, medical professors were quick to try the new machines as an addition to the "science of childbirth." A secondary gain of this sales focus is that many large hospitals act as purchasing agents, or at least recommend purchases, for smaller hospitals in their areas. This is especially true if smaller hospitals refer patients to the larger ones and need compatible equipment.

In the early and mid-1970s regionalization of obstetrical care was occuring. Hospitals were designated according to their ability to handle complicated obstetrical cases. The highest level high-tech hospitals were often associated with universities and always located in larger metropolitan areas. Regionalization called for patient referral to the next higher level of care should complications develop. The smaller, lower-level hospitals needed compatible equipment in order to communicate with the larger medical centers. And it is likely that physicians in smaller, lower-level hospitals desired higher technology as they attempted to emulate the larger ones.

In order to gain physician acceptance of its product, Corometrics employed a number of strategies already acceptable to the medical community. First, three well-credentialed physicians were on Corometrics' board of directors: Dr. Edward Hon of Yale, called the "Father of EFM" in Corometrics promotional literature; Dr. Orvan Hess, also of Yale, and Dr. Barry Schifrin of Harvard.

Management capitalized on the prestige of Yale and Harvard in connection with their directors. Dr. Hon conducted extensive studies on fetal heart rates and published results in medical journals. Other articles by Hess and Schifrin provoked the interest of medical professors as well as other obstetric practitioners. These articles were published in journals frequently read by practicing physicians. Corometrics was able to associate its product with this published research. As company spokesmen said, this educational effort, plus "having its product in major urban and university hospitals was seen by the company as Corometrics' best assurance that the next generation of obstetricians will learn to depend on fetal monitors" (Dolin 1973).

Another tactic employed by Corometrics was to conduct training on the use of its product in seminars in various parts of the country (Dolin 1973). This IRS-approved, tax-deductible educational technique, if held in a desirable location such as Florida or Las Vegas, guarantees physician participation in the seminar and exposure to the product. Often physicians will attend such seminars, then return to the hospital where they practice and request purchase of the product. Needless to say, Corometrics salespersons were also in attendance at medical conventions and meetings catering to obstetrical practitioners.

The final component of the marketing plan was Corometrics' guarantee of its product only if Corometrics disposable products (electrodes and paper) were used. This limited guarantee not only captured the disposables market but also assured a continuing relationship with the purchaser. Corometrics estimated a five-year obsolescence period for its monitors, and this continued exposure to the client allowed for promotion of new products as they were developed. As indicated, the company's investment in research and development was substantial and new products were continually forthcoming.

By the end of 1973, the tangible net worth of the company was over $1.9 million. There was no long-term debt, a sign of financial health, and Corometrics became an attractive candidate for acquisition by a larger company (*Wall Street Journal* 1974a, b, c). In 1974 Corometrics was purchased in a common stock exchange by American Home Products, Inc. (*Wall Street Journal* 1974). This large conglomerate company is highly respected for its marketing capability. It is interesting to note that over 50 percent of Corometrics stock was held by company insiders, the very men who worked so hard to promote the product as a standard of obstetrical care. Once purchased by American Home and now a subsidiary company, Corometrics disappeared from the business literature. However, in American Home annual reports, Corometrics is identified as a leader in the field of fetal and neonatal monitoring and continuously active in new product development.

1976—Controversy Begins

A chronological time line of events surrounding introduction and use of EFM shows 1976 as a key year. By this time EFM was firmly established as a standard of care in obstetrics. Corometrics had created a market and defined its product in terms of its necessity for labor management. In 1976, however, a major controversy emerged regarding use of the machine. It was reported that caesarean birthrates in the United States had tripled between 1968 and 1976. The 1976 annual report of the American College of Surgeons, which reports the ten most frequently performed surgeries, for the first time showed caesarean delivery as the tenth most common surgical procedure (American College of Surgeons Annual Report 1976). Caesarean delivery accounted for 20 percent of all births and the number and proportion continued to increase. Reports from some of the most technologically sophisticated hospitals showed caesarean rates of up to 50 percent of all births (Caesarean Childbirth Consensus Conference 1981).

Caesarean birth is major abdominal surgery causing increased risk to both mother and infant. Iatrogenic conditions, i.e., problems resulting from the medical treatment itself, can occur. Such problems include blood loss, pain, infection, increased immobility, and difficulty in recovering from anesthesia. Caesarean births are costly to society. They cost more in health care dollars, they necessitate increased physician service, they increase the amount of time women require to recover, and they decrease women's ability to work or to care for children. Obstetrics-gynecology is a surgical subspecialty, and caesarean delivery is a common solution to problems in labor—one that further tilts the balance of power in the delivery room in the physician's favor.

The large increase in caesarean births caused health care professionals and consumers to examine what had changed in childbirth experience to cause such a drastic rise in surgical delivery. What stood out was the rapid introduction and diffusion of EFM into the labor experience (Caesarean Childbirth Consensus Conference 1981). Health care professionals and consumers asked the same question: "Was there a sudden rise in infant distress in labor, or might the monitor be pointing out signs of fetal reaction to labor that, although they look abnormal, in fact occur routinely during the course of the labor experience?" The debate that followed was a lively one; the participants fell into two distinct groups.

The first group was composed of advocates of EFM, primarily male physicians and health care professionals. The legal profession did not enter the debate until the 1980s. This group claimed that it was necessary to monitor all infants during labor in order to protect against potential damage from hypoxia or oxygen deficiency (International Childbirth Education Association 1981). The group's inclination was to view birth as a medical situation requiring aggressive management. All fetuses were seen as potentially at high risk; therefore, all women require EFM.

The second group opposed fetal monitoring for all but the 10 to 15 percent of women who were high risk. The proponents of this position were some health care professionals and consumers, many of them women, who had had caesarean deliveries and were questioning the necessity for the surgery. This group defined childbirth as a low-risk event until proven otherwise. They considered EFM itself to be dangerous, for it contributed to major surgery and through use of the scalp electrode was also a source of infection for the fetus.

Both sides agreed that the rapid introduction and widespread use of EFM was responsible for an initial increase in caesareans. Some physicians, unfamiliar with interpretation of the heart rates being recorded, misread the information and often rushed into surgery. What both groups did not know, however, was the extent to which machine error had been responsible for variations in fetal heart-rate readings as seen in the section on EFM patents. These machine errors, even more than human error, were likely responsible for unknown numbers of unnecessary surgery.

Additionally, physicians received their training in the use of the machines from Corometrics staff, a group clearly biased toward a finding of fetal distress. Finally, and most significantly, there was a startling lack of large-scale clinical trials from which to gather information concerning the efficacy of EFM. In 1978, in a report prepared for the National Center for Health Services Research, David Banta, M.D., and Stephen Thacker, M.D., of the Centers for Disease Control, wrote on the costs and benefits of EFM. They concluded that EFM provided little benefit in low-risk labors and that it was a costly and dangerous procedure. Their estimate of annual expenditures related to EFM, including caesarean surgery, was $411 million (Banta and Thacker 1978).

For women, these reports added to their anger and frustration at increased caesareans and use of EFM. Unnecessary surgery became the ultimate in lack of control over birth. Consumer activist groups such as C-Sec., Inc. sprang up nationally. Their message to women was to take control of birthing through required informed consent procedures, self-knowledge and participation, and formation of cooperative relationships with physicians of their choice. A rise in home birth and use of lay and certified midwives also were symptomatic of consumer flight from the high-technology environment of hospital birth.

By 1981, caesarean rates had leveled off as physicians gained sophistication and experience in using EFM technology. Studies conducted to assess the relationship between EFM and caesarean birth found a complementary relationship, if not one of cause and effect. Use of the machine was indicated for high-risk women, but its application in low-risk situations remained an area of concern. A 1981 Consensus Development conference on Caesarean Childbirth was sponsored by the National Institutes of Child Health and Human Development. This provider and consumer-representative group presented an assessment of eighteen studies looking at the relationship between EFM and caesarean birth. The assessment concluded that women who are monitored during labor have higher caesarean birth rates with no improvement in outcome over those who are not monitored (Caesarean Childbirth Consensus Conference 1981).

Helen Marieskind conducted a study in 1979 to assess physician motivation in performing caesarean delivery. Her study found that primary motivation for performance of caesarean was threat of malpractice litigation (Marieskind 1979). As noted above, the crisis in obstetrics malpractice was beginning by this time, and physicians were increasingly fearful of lawsuits. Obstetricians felt they must provide patients with the "best" that technology and science could produce. The second most common reason for caesarean delivery turned out to be for repeat surgery; caesarean delivery for the woman whose prior delivery was surgical. This finding supports the standard in obstetrics, "Once a caesarean, always a caesarean." Threat of rupture of the scar was the potential problem. Here, one must ask, "How many of the primary surgeries were performed due to machine error or misinterpretation of fetal heart rates?" Meanwhile, by 1983, caesarean delivery had become the second most common surgical procedure in the United States, a development that is attributed to the high number of repeat caesareans (American College of Surgeons 1983). And finally, just as Corometrics had planned, the third most common reason for performance of caesarean delivery was a "lack of obstetrical training in management of normal obstetrics for residents, with an emphasis in training on use of sophisticated equipment such as EFM (Marieskind 1979). Practitioners simply could not get along without it.

Medical Technology Assessment

The introduction of EFM occurred at a time when *no legislated mandate existed* to test and evaluate medical devices before they were put into use. This hands-off policy allowed the manufacturers of EFM to produce their own studies to "document" use and efficacy of the product. These tests were conducted on small-sized populations, often by biased researchers. Obviously, the Corometrics company would benefit only if such studies showed the usefulness of fetal monitoring in improving outcome of delivery.

It was not until 1976 that the Medical Devices Act required FDA assessment of electronic devices for patient care. By this time, Corometrics had become a leading marketer of EFM, the company had been purchased by American Home Products, EFM was incorporated into the standard of care, and most ominously, caesarean birth had become the nation's tenth most common surgical procedure. But the Medical Devices Act did not have the ability to regulate or assess medical technology after it was put into broad-based use. Corometrics' position seemed secure.

By 1976, however, independent studies were being conducted to test the efficacy of the device. One of the first, a randomized clinical trial conducted by A. D. Haverkamp at Denver General Hospital, compared high-risk laboring women divided into equal-sized groups monitored with or without EFM. The two groups did not differ in neonatal deaths, Apgar scores (assessment of the newborn infant), or blood oxygen levels in umbilical cord samples. However, the monitored group's caesarean section rate was more than double that of the auscultated group, and the monitored group had a three times higher rate of postpartum infections (Haverkamp et al. 1976).

Two government-sponsored studies conducted by David Banta, M.D., and Stephen Thacker, M.D., of the Centers for Disease Control were very enlightening. The first, released in 1978 and written for the U.S. Department of Health, Education and Welfare, was entitled "Costs and Benefits of Electronic Fetal Monitoring." As noted above, it concluded that EFM provided little benefit in low-risk labors and that it was a costly and dangerous procedure. Their estimate of annual expenditures related to EFM, including caesarean delivery, was $411 million. To Banta and Thacker, "The diffusion of EFM into virtually every obstetrical setting represents a failure of public and private policies and officials" (Banta and Thacker 1978).

Banta and Thacker next directed their attention to the failure of government to protect the public in not requiring large-scale testing of devices before use. Their second report, issued in 1979, was entitled, "The Premature Delivery of Medical Technology: A Case Report." This was prepared for the U.S. Congress Office of Technology Assessment. The report not only points out the failure to assess for safety, as well as social and ethical consequences of using the machine, but also cites a lack of indications for use, cost, and cost-effectiveness (Banta and Thacker 1978).

Finally, researchers at the National Center for Health Services Research reviewed over 600 studies on fetal monitoring. They concluded that there was no scientific evidence that continuous EFM prevents brain damage or improves infant health except in the case of very small babies (Institute of Medicine Committee for Evaluating Medical Technologies in Clinical Use 1985). It was not until 1981 that a large-scale study of low-risk women was conducted. This group of 13,000 women in Dublin, Ireland showed no benefit in terms of reduced mortality, no difference in caesarean rates, and only a suggested decrease in neurologic damage to infants (Institute of Medicine Committee for Evaluating Medical Technologies in Clinical Use 1985). *This first large scale trial comes more than fifteen years after introduction of the monitor.*

The interactions of government, the private sector, and health care providers have impeded an orderly assessment of EFM technology. As the story of the EFM clearly demonstrates, the development and testing of medical devices cannot proceed "objectively" when the financial support for such work is provided by those who stand to profit from manufacturing and marketing the products. This bias needs to be recognized and corrected.

In 1983, the House Subcommittee on Oversight and Investigations issued a report regarding the Medical Devices Act of 1976. While the Act calls for regulation through the FDA, the report reveals an astounding lack of action and failure to carry out the law itself (Network News 1983). Certainly, in the case of EFM in which retrospective analysis would be necessary, the new law was meaningless. The embrace of technology, the willingness to accept technology, and the assumption that more technology makes better medicine seem to dominate the assessment as well as research and development.

Summary

Initially, consumers, physicians, and nurses all regarded the EFM as a welcome addition to the management of labor. One does wonder whether the machine brought greater stress to the labor room with its focus on reliable, concise, up-to-the-minute data. My own experiences and perceptions tell me that EFM did in fact create an additional element of acuteness in the labor experience. Emergency surgery increases the drama in the delivery suite, and obstetrical care givers, particularly those who work in labor and delivery room areas, perceive themselves as specialists in dealing with emergency situations. This crisis mentality has replaced the more traditional idea of birth attendants who support a woman through the slow process of normal birth. Two studies that measure the psychological acceptance of monitors by mothers show a largely positive response to EFM use, with laboring women finding the monitor reassuring. When the labor is prolonged, however, discomfort and forced immobility begin to cause increased stress on the part of the mother and infant (Verney 1985).

One cannot deny the important contribution of electronic fetal monitoring to management of high-risk cases. The information gained from the monitor on the high-risk fetus's response to the rigors of labor has contributed significantly to reduction of morbidity and mortality in the labor and delivery experiences of thousands of women. For those women whose pregnancies are complicated by illness and jeopardized fetal well being, the electronic fetal monitor has been but one of many technological advances helping them to secure the safest birth possible. These are the cases referred to by Dr. Caldeyro-Barcia when he talks of the appropriate use of the monitor.

In examining the story of the electronic fetal monitor, however, we see more than this. We learn something about the impact of technology on our society and about the interactions of business and health care systems as well as government regulatory bodies that allow technology to exert that impact virtually unchallenged. The example of the development and marketing of the EFM teaches us to question technology and to think carefully about where its introduction may lead us. In this case we see how a well-designed and executed marketing plan promoted by one small, well-organized company, profoundly changed the practice of obstetrics and the lives of millions of women.

Understanding the methods and motivations involved in promoting use of fetal monitors, can we ever again accept the idea that someone else knows best for us? Can we trust health care practitioners to fully understand the process by which technology is "sold" to them? As women, we must remain vigilant against the control of our birthing experiences by others. We must remain firm in our conviction that birthing is a biological process and not a technological event. The story of electronic fetal monitors mandates us to regain our loss of control and to weigh critically the benefits of technology against both medical and human costs.

BIBLIOGRAPHY

American College of Surgeons. 1976. Annual Report.
————. 1983. Annual Report.
Banta, David, and Stephen Thacker. 1978. *Costs and benefits of electronic fetal monitoring*. U.S. Department of Health, Education and Welfare, National Center for Health Services Research Publication, Unnumbered.
————. 1979. *The premature delivery of medical technology: A case report*. U.S. Congress Office of Technology Assessment.
Blyden, Arthur J. 1973. Corometrics Medical Systems, Inc. *Wall Street Transcript*, 3 December: 35217.
Caesarean Childbirth Consensus Conference. 1981. National Institute of Child Health and Human Development. National Institutes of Health Publication no. 82-2067.
Dolin, Fred. 1973. Corometrics Medical Systems, Inc. *Wall Street Transcript*, 7 May: 32873.
Haire, Doris. 1972. *The cultural warping of childbirth*. A special report for the International Childbirth Education Association, Minneapolis, Minnesota.
Haverkamp, Albert D., Horace E.Thompson, John G. McFee, and Curtis Cetrulo. 1976. The evaluation of continuous fetal heart rate monitoring in high risk pregnancy. *American Journal of Obstetrics and Gynecology* 125, no. 3: 310.
Institute of Medicine, Committee for Evaluating Medical Technologies in Clinical Use. 1985. *Assessing medical technologies*. Washington, D.C.: National Academy Press.
International Childbirth Education Association. 1981. Position statement on electronic fetal monitoring. Minneapolis, Minn.
Marieskind, Helen. 1979. An evaluation of caesarean section in the USA. *ICEA News* 18, no. 4: 1.
National Women's Health Network. 1983. FDA fails to protect public from defective devices. *Network News* 8, no. 4 (September/October): 6.
Sweet, Richard L. 1985. Chlamydia, Group B streptococcus and herpes in pregnancy. *BIRTH* 12, no. 1: 17.
U.S. Department of Commerce, United States Patent Office, Washington, D.C. 1968 June 12. Patent 3,581,735.
————. 1975 October 7. Patent 3,910,259.
————. 1979 March 13. Patent 4,143,650.
————. 1986 March 4. Patent 4,573,479.
Verney, Thomas R. 1985. The psycho-technology of pregnancy and labor. *Neonatal Network* 3, no. 5: 12.

Wall Street Journal. 1974. Corometrics Medical Systems earnings reports. January 23 (a): 18.
_____. June 17 (b): 21.
_____. September 19 (c): 24.
_____. September 30 (d): 7.
Young, Diony. 1982. *Changing childbirth, family birth in the hospital.* Rochester, New York: Childbirth Graphics Limited.

Contraception, Control, and Choice: International Perspectives

Kim Yanoshik and Judy Norsigian

Throughout history, women have devised methods to control their own fertility. Herbal preparations, abortion, and abstinence were among the early techniques women used. In the past women worked among themselves to develop, disseminate, and employ the means to control their fertility. As men increased their presence in and control over the healing professions, the power that women exercised in preventing and giving birth was wrested away from them. However, the dislocation of women from healing and the increased control by men over women's reproductive lives and choices did not occur without resistance. Women have continually sought to regain control over their health and their reproductive lives. The women's health movement of today is the most recent manifestation of this struggle.

This chapter examines the development and marketing of today's contraceptive technologies. In order to do this, we must first try to understand the social forces that shape women's contraceptive choices and experience. The first section of this chapter will discuss these social forces. Western medicine is the first of these forces, an institution that often operates to further the social oppression of women (Fee 1983; Corea 1985; Scully and Bart 1978) through efforts to medicalize as many aspects of human existence as possible (Zola 1972; Illich 1976). A second influence is the population control establishment, which has dominated the development and distribution of contraceptives since the 1950s. Although born in part out of feminist struggles, population control organizations today are more concerned with limiting the size of poor and Third World populations than with assisting women in meeting their individual fertility needs (Bell 1984; Hartmann 1987). A third factor is the multinational pharmaceutical industry that constantly seeks new ways to maximize profits and increase consumption of its products. Together these forces are strong enough to shape most governments' policies on reproductive health, and, so shape women's lives indirectly as well as directly. Although we present medicine, the population control establishment, and the pharmaceutical industry as separate entities, an ideology of population control and the workings of patriarchy (or men's control over women) are so pervasive that the divisions among the three are often blurred.

Over the last thirty years there has been an explosion of new technologies aimed at preventing conception. Theoretically, this should be a boon to women in our search for more ways to control our own fertility. However, because western medicine, the population control establishment, and the pharmaceutical industry are more interested in controlling population and making money than in ensuring users' safety or creating woman-centered options, the effects of many of the contraceptive technologies have proven to be catastrophic. Millions of women's lives have been adversely affected by following advice or orders to use such new "miracle" technologies as the Dalkon Shield, oral contraceptives, Depo-Provera, or hormonal implants. The second section of this chapter will examine several specific contraceptive technologies. Through these case studies we will see how gender, class, and race biases guide the development and implementation of contraceptive technology and lead to actions that are often contrary to women's needs and health.

In the last section of this chapter, we will discuss the significance of the contemporary feminist health movement as it attempts to right the reproductive wrongs that have been committed against women. Despite the diversity of today's feminist health movement, it has grown into an international force of resistance and change on contraceptive issues. Around the world, women's health activists are increasingly questioning the practices and the policies of contraceptive research, development, and service delivery.

The Rise of Western Medicine

The first major force limiting women's own control over reproduction is the medical establishment. In the Western world, the early 1800s brought men increasing power over medicine in general and increasing control over women's reproductive lives in particular. Women's traditional role as healers was usurped by white upper-class men (Ehrenreich and English 1972). The main mechanism by which men monopolized control over the practice of healing was through the professionalization of the physician (Starr 1982). Correspondingly, medicine became increasingly associated with science. This association extended the limits for the social control of women. Women were equated with the natural world that (male) science by right should dominate (Merchant 1980). Kathryn Ratcliff (in this volume) discusses how the glorification of science by medicine, combined with the pursuit of capital, has encouraged the health care system to pursue technological innovation even at the expense of human needs. What has transpired with respect to birth control has occurred within this context of western medicine. The contemporary birth control story is a prime example of what happens when professional dominance and technological sophistication are placed ahead of women's health and safety.

One result of the increased power of the medical profession and the control of health care by male physicians was a patriarchal ideology regarding health and reproduction. This ideology, which still exists today, is characterized by the belief that women do not know what is good for them and therefore must rely on what (male) experts decide. Moreover, the art of healing underwent a change. Natural, noninvasive practices and techniques were replaced by heavy reliance on surgery, drugs, and other new techniques. These changes have created a western medical model that is structurally hierarchical, curative (as opposed to preventive), intrusive, and technologically oriented. The specific case of contraceptives reflects these characteristics of western medicine.

Like healing, birth control was once a decentralized, woman-controlled, woman-centered practice. As male-dominated medicine expanded its influence, women's practice of birth control became subject to moral and legal prohibitions. The prohibitions did not put an end to women's use of birth control. "Rather it forced women underground in their search for reproductive control. It transformed traditional behavior into criminal behavior" (Gordon 1976, 47).

From the mid nineteenth to early twentieth century, birth control activism in the United States was a radical feminist movement based on the belief that women had the right to control whether or not they would have children (see Gordon 1976). At the turn of the century, this activism became more militant, typified by the work of Margaret Sanger and Emma Goldman, both of whom identified the demand for birth control as part of the class struggle (Gordon 1983). Perhaps because birth control was traditionally a woman-centered and woman-controlled practice, physicians were not initially open to the idea of women's right to contraception. In fact, in the early 1920s most doctors in the United States opposed contraception with a "revulsion so hysterical that it prevented them from accepting facts. . . . Many doctors believed that they had a social and moral responsibility to fight the social degeneration that birth control represented" (Gordon 1976, 259–60). However, other doctors believed that if they could control birth control they would be able to further their profession and use their expertise to decide social values. Eventually, the latter physicians won out. The "doctors-only bills" of the 1920s and 1930s served to remove the techniques of birth control from women and legally enshrined medical domination of birth control in the West.

By the beginning of the twentieth century, birth control became associated with medicine and medical science. Prior to this, birth control functioned as part of "the folklore and folk culture of nearly all societies" (Gordon 1976, 26). Birth control techniques and technologies were passed down by women through generations. Interestingly, some of the early techniques adapted to the change from folk culture to medical culture. For instance, vaginal sponges, which had been used for several thousand years, were commonly prescribed by doctors in birth control clinics during the 1930s (Gordon 1976).

Today birth control is almost completely identified with medicine. Furthermore, the contraceptive technologies that are being the most aggressively developed are highly dependent on medicine. Since these technologies often involve potent drugs and invasive techniques, medical personnel are necessary for screening, administration, follow-up and referral should adverse effects occur. This association and dependence on medicine is problematic for women for at least two reasons. First, from development to utilization, women are no longer at the locus of control. Secondly, sophisticated contraceptive technologies may be indiscriminately promoted and applied, thus increasing the likelihood of harmful outcomes. Although all women are subject to these problems, women particularly endangered are those with inadequate access to health care or women who have not been fully informed of possible risks.

The Exportation of Western Medicine

As the institution of medicine has grown, so have its levels of technological sophistication, economic complexity, and political power. Western medicine is often viewed as the ideal throughout the world. However, while western medicine and its technology sometimes improve the quality of life, the hegemonic rise of the institution of western medicine often bodes ill for the peoples of the world, especially the women. One reason for this is the lack of sufficient resources to support the capital and personnel requirements of conventional western medicine. For the vast majority of the world, resource deficiencies are staggering: there are not enough educated people to train as western-model nurses, technicians, and physicians; and there is not enough money to maintain high-tech equipment, to compete with western salaries in retaining the educated elite of providers, or to support a clinic- and hospital-based health care delivery system. In spite of this, many Third World countries and international health groups direct the limited resources they have into urban, capital-intensive medical systems. This money could be better spent on programs aimed at meeting basic human needs such as nutritious food, clean water, adequate housing, simple medicines, and decentralized health care delivery systems.

Clearly, under such circumstances the export of modern western-style contraceptive technologies can be both inappropriate and potentially hazardous, for many of today's contraceptive technologies require access to adequate health care. But in "many countries the modern health services tend not to be where the majority of the people are and they do not serve equally those in greatest need" (Elling 1980, 31). Indigenous birth control methods, regardless of their effectiveness and safety, are regarded as primitive and unscientific. In Africa, western techniques "do not appear to be very popular, arguably because they are expensive and, besides, dramatically reduce sexual enjoyment" (Cutrufelli 1983, 136). Despite the lack of popularity, western birth control techniques, specifically invasive high-tech methods, are the forms of birth control promoted and administered in family planning programs. In Africa, Latin America, and Asia many international development organizations require countries to have population control programs (using western methods) operating before loans are approved. For example, the International Bank of Reconstruction and Development requires that a country that receives one of their loans must invest part of it in a family limitation program. The World Bank has openly threatened to withdraw its credits from countries that are not embarked on a birth control policy (Cutrufelli, 1983). Such external pressure on Third World countries demonstrates the enormous influence of both western medicine and the population control establishment.

From Birth Control to Population Control

The second major force that has shaped women's contraceptive choices and experience is the population control establishment. Like the medical establishment itself, population control organizations are dominated by physicians. This domination began during the first part of the twentieth century.

The feminist and radical orientation of the United States birth control movement of the late nineteenth and early twentieth century was undermined by certain historical forces. World War I brought with it a tremendous political swing to the right. Feminism was one of the fatalities of that swing. Birth control activists lost their political foundation; many of these women turned their energies toward social work (Gordon 1983). As new professionals they often welcomed and sought out the aid of established "experts"; and on matters of birth control, physicians and eugenicists replaced feminists and radicals as the advocates. When professionals entered the birth control movement, the movement shifted from one based on self-determination for all people to a campaign "infused with elitist values and operated in an elitist manner" (Gordon 1983, 151). Even Margaret Sanger, early in her career a socialist and feminist, gave in to the prestige and authority of medicine and the ideology of the eugenics movement (Gordon 1976; Davis 1981). By the 1920s the birth control movement, which once emphasized class struggle, women's control, and equality, had become a physician-dominated movement that believed "more children from the fit, less from the unfit—that is the chief issue of birth control" (Sanger 1919, as quoted in Gordon 1976, 281). Today, this orientation still shapes contraceptive research and development and many family planning programs, but it has taken on an international dimension.

The so-called contraceptive revolution of the 1950s and 1960s was stimulated by a growing acceptance of a population control ideology by governmental officials, and the scientific and business communities (Mass 1980; Hartmann 1987). The guiding image was of a "population bomb."

> The population bomb threatens to create an explosion as disruptive and dangerous as the explosion of the atom, and with as much influence on prospects for progress or disaster, war or peace. (Griessemer 1954, 1)

Such language often encouraged a sense of desperation and urgency in which normal precautions were discarded and a quick solution to the world's rising population "problem" was favored.

During the 1950s, government officials in the United States and western Europe began to relate their country's security to the raw materials they received from the world's less industrialized countries. The 1950s, as we know, was a time of a sometimes fanatical concern about the "spread of communism." The involvement of the United States in Korea reinforced this fear of communism, and theories that associated an "excess population" with political instability gained more and more acceptance. Policy makers began to regard population growth in the less industrialized world as a serious threat to national and global security (Mass 1980).

In this atmosphere, the population control perspective began to flourish. In 1952, under the sponsorship of the National Academy of Science, John D. Rockefeller III convened a conference to establish an international council for population planning. From this conference came the Population Council (PC). The initial board was composed of politically and economically prominent men such as the head of the

United Nations' Office of Population Research and John D. Rockefeller himself. Illustrative of the council's connection to the earlier eugenics movement was Frederick Osborn, a prominent eugenicist, who served as the first vice-president of the council and later succeeded Rockefeller as president. Notable charter members of the Population Council included General Dwight D. Eisenhower, the secretary of commerce, and the head of the U.S. Council on Foreign Relations (Mass 1980, 186).

Along with the Population Council other groups such as the Ford Foundation, the American and International Planned Parenthood Federations, the Hugh Moore Fund, the Pathfinder Fund, and Laurence Rockefeller's Conservation Foundation became increasingly concerned about population growth. Many of these private groups began to finance population studies at U.S. universities. This financial backing facilitated the development of what has been referred to as "a powerful cult of population control" in U.S. academia (Hartmann 1987, 102). According to development economist Charles Wilber,

> The influence of this "cult" is such that most Western development economists have not thoroughly investigated the evidence [on populations] for themselves . . . dubious assumptions were not questioned and contradictory evidence was explained away or ignored. (Hartmann 1987, 102)

The crisis mentality of the population control ideology has encouraged concern for effectiveness and efficiency to overwhelm questions of safety or free choice. The story of the birth control pill reflects the quick-fix bias of the population control advocates. Gregory Pincus, who developed the first commercially successful oral contraceptive, writes that in 1951 he was visited by Margaret Sanger, who urged him to devise a "foolproof method" for stemming the population explosion in the less industrialized areas of the world (Pincus 1965).

Among the groups that were targeted for the pill's initial clinical trials were poor women in Haiti and Puerto Rico. These women received doses and combinations that are now known to be extremely hazardous; however, their health was not foremost in the minds of the researchers. According to Dr. Frederick Robbins, "The dangers of overpopulation are so great that we may have to use certain techniques of contraception that may entail considerable risk to the individual woman" (as quoted in Seaman 1979, 11). Thus the pill was designed as an instrument of population control, not as a means by which to help women find a safe and effective contraceptive method. Funding for research on the pill included "every major international population control institution" (Petchesky 1984, 171).

Today the fear of a burgeoning population, both in the Third World countries and among the poor and people of color in the industrialized world, still guides contraceptive research and development. The doomsayers press for greater urgency. A recent article warns that the next "contraceptive revolution" will be postponed because the U.S. and other developed-country governments are not yet sufficiently convinced of the grave social and health consequences of unintended pregnancies in their own countries, or of the worldwide adverse social and economic effects of high rates of population growth in the Third World" (Atkinson, Lincoln, and Forrest 1986, 19).

The Growing Dominance of the U.S. Government

From the 1940s to the 1960s the primary funders of contraceptive research were private foundations and pharmaceutical companies. During the 1960s, the idea of population growth as a threat to world security became widely accepted. Gradually the United States government assumed a much greater role in funding both contraceptive research and population control activities (LaCheen 1986). In 1964 the U.S. Agency for International Development (AID) established an Office of Population. Although this office started out small it grew rapidly; the allocation to AID for population activities increased nearly four-fold in one year, from $9 million in 1964 to $35 million in 1965 (LaCheen 1986, 95). In 1985 they spent $250 million (LaCheen 1986, 104). Today AID is by far the largest single funder in the world of population research and activity. About half of AID's Office of Population budget goes to private groups such as the International Planned Parenthood Federation (IPPF), the Population Council, and the Pathfinder Fund; a quarter goes directly to the United Nations Fund for Population Activities (Hartmann 1987, 112); and the remaining quarter goes primarily to foreign governments in the form of direct assistance for family planning programs.

In the late 1960s Congress authorized the creation of organizations like the Center for Population Research in the National Institutes of Health to conduct contraceptive research. Contraceptive manufacturers have welcomed this increased role of government and argue that tough U.S. drug-approval regulations, patent policies, and proconsumer product liability laws make it too expensive for the industry to develop new contraceptives (LaCheen 1986, 103).

The Business of Birth Control

The third main factor influencing women's contraceptive choices is the pharmaceutical industry. The contraceptive business took off during the late 1930s with the winning of widespread public support for artificial contraception and U.S. court approval for distributing contraceptive information (Berkman 1980). For the pharmaceutical industry, contraceptives became a promising new venture. Increased concern over the "population explosion," discussed above, greatly assisted in the development of new technologies. Worldwide, contraceptives became "big business."

Although exact figures are not available, it is estimated that in 1982 nearly $3 billion was spent on contraception and abortion in the United States alone; about $2.4 billion of this was spent on preventing pregnancy (Family Planning Perspectives 1986, 37). It is estimated that the worldwide market, excluding China, is about double the U.S. market (LaCheen 1986, 108).

Today's contraceptive market is composed of five major segments: hormonal contraceptives (such as the pill, injectables, and implants), intrauterine devices (IUDs), condoms, diaphragms, and spermicides. Although some contraceptives like injectables, implants, the morning-after pill, and RU-486 (a once-a-month antiprogestin pill) are not approved for contraceptive use in the United States, these methods are being used in other countries. Judging from what one finds in both the scientific literature (e.g., medical and family planning journals) and in the popular press (*Time, Newsweek, Good Housekeeping, Ms., Mademoiselle,* etc.) most of these methods will soon enter the U.S. market.

In the United States and in much of the world, the contraceptive market is dominated by large pharmaceutical corporations. This dominance means that

> production and distribution of contraceptives . . . is driven by the goal of profit maximization and not a concern for reproductive health. Selling contraceptives to the largest number of people, despite health risks, cultural suitability or the users' needs, is the primary goal of the contraceptive industry. (LaCheen 1986, 105)

This goal of profit maximization has paid off for the industry. For many years the drug industry profit rates have been among the highest for all manufacturing industries both in developed and developing countries (Silverman, Lee, and Lydecker 1982, 99). Within the drug industry contraceptives are extremely profitable. In fact, oral and injectable contraceptives are among the most lucrative of all pharmaceuticals (LaCheen 1986, 108). In 1982, about $1.1 billion was spent in the United States on oral contraceptives (including the costs of physicians/clinic visits). This far exceeds the $760 million spent on sterilization, the $270 million on diaphragms, the $100 million each on condoms and IUDs, and the $57 million spent on spermicides (La-Cheen 1986, 108).

Contraceptive Research and Development: Where the Money Goes and Why

> Basically, current research goals in contraception are often set to meet corporate goals and the perceived needs of society rather than the expressed needs of individuals. (Potts 1981, 28)

Each year millions of dollars are spent on research and development (R and D), and promotion of technologically sophisticated contraceptives despite known and suspected health risks. Research on improving or expanding the selection of safer and simpler barrier and natural methods is virtually ignored. In 1983 worldwide expenditures in basic reproductive research, contraceptive research and development, and the evaluation of the long-term safety of existing contraceptive methods totalled $167 million (Atkinson, Lincoln, and Forrest 1985). Of this amount the United States spent almost 85 percent of the total worldwide expenditures with most of this money funneled through AID. United States contributions include almost 60 percent by the U.S. government, 21 percent by U.S. industry, and 4 percent by U.S. foundations. Other industrialized countries contributed 14 percent of the world's total, with the vast majority of that amount coming from governmental sources. Less industrialized countries contributed 1.4 percent, with almost all these funds originating from government sources (Atkinson, Lincoln, and Forrest 1985, 204).

   With respect to the distribution of R and D money according to the type of contraceptive method, almost 60 percent of expenditures went toward female "high-tech" methods (such as oral contraceptives, steroid injectables, steroid implants, vaginal rings, etc.); only slightly over 3 percent of R and D funds went toward female barrier methods, spermicides, and natural fertility control methods. About 7 percent of R and D money went toward developing male methods. The remaining 30 percent went toward research that could not be attributed to a single type of method and was classified as multiple. This included funds for the synthesis of new compounds that could be used in a variety of methods, and general purpose grants made for contraceptive research (Atkinson, Lincoln, and Forrest 1985, 198). Given the history of contraceptive research, however, it is likely that most of these "multiple methods" center on the female reproductive system.

Contraceptive Biases

Both the spending patterns for contraceptive research and development and the composition of the contraceptive market reveal two prominent biases. First, they overwhelmingly concentrate on the female reproductive system. Forrest Greenslade of the Population Council puts it bluntly when he states that women are targeted "because of sexism" (Hartmann 1987, 167). Throughout the contraceptive field men dominate in both numbers and in the positions of power. Like most of society, these individual men also hold the view that reproduction is primarily a woman's concern. As the majority of scientists, researchers, developers, physicians, drug company vendors and executives, and governmental officials, men control the way contraceptive research is developed and implemented. These men "never have to subject themselves to the very pills, devices, implants and injections they are promoting" (Cowan 1980, 38).

The second bias lies in the fact that the contraceptive field is geared toward systemic and surgical methods of birth control. These long-acting methods include such things as injectables, implants, vaccines, and sterilization; they are viewed by medical researchers and population control advocates as the wave of the future. Long-acting techniques are preferred because of the ease by which they can be administered and because they are highly effective in preventing accidental pregnancy. They require little initiative by the user, and involve a minimum of interaction between providers and users.

However, the convenience and control they offer to providers undermines women's own control. The minimal role for users' (women's) choice and autonomy is their chief attraction to medical personnel and population control advocates. This has led to coercive use of these methods. (Examples will be provided later.) Typically, these methods pose the greatest known and suspected health risks to the very groups of women who have the least access to adequate health care. Moreover, these methods cannot be easily discontinued should women experience side effects or wish to have a child.

These two biases, one toward the control of the female reproductive system and the other toward invasive technologies, stem from the confluence of western medicine, the population control establishment, and the pharmaceutical industry. The preference for high-tech approaches to birth control allows these groups to maintain or to increase their control over women. This is done by selecting the specific types of contraceptives to research and develop, and through the type of information that is distributed to women in the promotion and marketing of these methods. Thus these three social forces always attempt and often succeed at orchestrating women's contraceptive options to suit their own needs.

It ought to be noted that not all birth control methods can be accurately classified as medical technologies nor are they controlled by medicine, the population control establishment, or the pharmaceutical industry. Methods such as the condom, some vaginal barrier methods (such as the sponge), abstinence, herbal techniques, withdrawal, and certain forms of natural fertility control (e.g., cervical mucus observation) are not medical technologies, because they require no prescription or physician involvement. These nonmedical methods are vitally important to both women's reproductive choices and overall health. For instance, in the case of condoms, protection is offered against AIDS and sexually transmitted diseases (STDs).

Development and information about woman-centered, woman-controlled methods of birth control is sometimes suppressed, and the amount of research and marketing devoted to these options pales when compared to the amount of work done on invasive other-directed methods. The most popular methods and those that are being most vigorously researched, developed, and promoted rely on a significant level of medical expertise for development and administration. Like all technological innovations, contraceptive technologies are not neutral constructs. Rather, they embody and are shaped by the values of their creators. In the case of contraceptive technology, development is influenced more by the pursuit of strategic population control, medical-scientific prestige, and corporate profit than by women's need for safe birth control.

Interestingly, illegal abortion, often self-administered, is the main form of birth control worldwide. Illegal abortions are also the main cause of death among women of childbearing age in numerous underdeveloped countries. This fact underscores women's need and demand for safe methods of birth control. Unfortunately, the social forces directing contraceptive research and development have not developed such safe methods. This could change if women assume a greater involvement in deciding what types of contraceptives should be researched and developed, what kind of information on contraceptives should be sought, and how this information should be shared.

Case Studies

Abundant examples exist of the harm to women's health caused by the rush for profits by drug companies, combined with an ideology of population control and a patriarchal approach to health and reproduction. This discussion will examine just four cases: intrauterine devices (IUDs), oral contraceptives, injectables, and implants. These technologies have often been presented as the keys to liberation for women. In the West they have been considered responsible for women's large-scale entry in the paid labor force and the so-called sexual revolution. In the Third World these technologies are heralded as the answer to unwanted pregnancies, high birthrates, and high maternal mortality rates. Yet the unbridled enthusiasm that accompanies the introduction of these technologies has often worked to obscure their drawbacks. In terms of health and safety, these technologies expose women to serious risks and unknowns. Furthermore, the normal practices of the health care and population control establishments have prevented many women from learning about these problems. Through an examination of these four specific contraceptive technologies we will see how medicine, the population control establishment, and the pharmaceutical industry's overarching goal of controlling birth control has actually worked to diminish women's own control over their own fertility and the quality of their lives.

Intrauterine Devices (IUDs)

Perhaps the most notorious IUD is the Dalkon Shield. It was marketed between 1971 and 1975 by the A. H. Robins Company. The entire history of the Dalkon Shield is fraught with deception and a nearly total disregard for women's health and safety (see Mintz 1985). First, the Shield was tested on poor women in the United States without proper consent and without proper research protocols (Dowie and Johnston 1977). Second, women who developed Shield-related complications were frequently told that their lifestyle, not the device, was the problem. This explanation, often accepted unquestioningly by physicians, was based on Robins's "scientific" research efforts. Third, the company falsely advertised a pregnancy rate of 1.1 percent when the actual rate was more likely between 5.5 and 7.2 percent (Mintz 1985; Fugh-Berman 1985). In the United States alone the Shield killed at least twenty women, and worldwide tens of thousands of women have been seriously injured. In just five years over 4.5 million devices were distributed in eighty countries (Mintz 1985).

The company was aware that there were dangers to women. Only six weeks after Robins began marketing the Shield, a doctor wrote a letter to the company stating that he had just inserted his tenth Dalkon Shield and "found the procedure to be the most traumatic manipulation ever perpetrated upon womanhood. . . . I have ordered all Shields out of my office and will do the same in all clinics with which I am affili- ated" (Mokhiber 1986, 43). Internal warnings were disregarded, such as reports from a company microbiologist about the possible "wicking qualities" of the Shield's multifilament tail.[1]

Such emergent problems led Robins to anticipate a drop in U.S. sales. Thus in 1972 they decided to market the Shield internationally. The company began by offering AID a 48 percent discount on bulk packages of unsterilized Shields (Hartmann 1987, 203). In the United States the IUDs were sold in individual sterilized packages with a ster- ile disposable inserter. The fact that Robins and AID distributed un- sterilized IUDs in the Third World reveals a blatant devaluation of foreign lives. Moreover, sterilization instructions were attached only to every set of 1,000 Shields, and printed only in English, French, and Spanish despite distribution to forty-two countries (Hartmann 1987, 203).

The rising number of lawsuits concerning the Shield and increasing reports of serious injuries and even deaths eventually forced Robins to stop U.S. sales in June, 1974. Yet Robins continued foreign sales for another year, and evidence indicates that insertions went on in some Third World countries through 1980 (Fugh-Berman 1985). However, the Shield did not stop maiming or killing women. In April, 1983, be- cause of mounting evidence that women were still wearing the Shield and being harmed by it, the National Women's Health Network filed a citizen petition requesting the government to formally call for the removal of Dalkon Shields in women. In August, 1985, A. H. Robins Company filed a Chapter 11 bankruptcy petition, an action that limited the company's liability and set a deadline for women filing claims. By the deadline, 300,000 claims had been made from over fifty countries (National Women's Health Network 1986).

The Dalkon Shield is just one of many kinds of IUDs. All IUDs place women at risk. IUDs may become embedded in or perforate the uterus and cause infections, excessive bleeding, cramping, and/or infertility (Bell 1985, 252). Should an IUD user get pregnant, she runs a 5 percent chance of ectopic pregnancy, a serious problem that can cause hemorrhage and lead to infection, sterility, and sometimes death.

Today IUD use is declining in the West. In the United States only one IUD remains on the market; however, there are plans to introduce a new copper-6 IUD in 1988 or 1989. Domestic production of other IUDs has stopped, primarily because of liability problems and mount- ing consumer dissatisfaction. The IUD is now the least popular con- traceptive in the United States, used by only 7 percent of contraceptive users. The declining use of the IUD in the West has been offset by the increased exportation of the devices to the Third World. Over twenty-five different kinds of IUDs from abroad are being used in India, and modified IUDs based on Indian women's experience "hardly exist at all" (Savara 1983, 223).

However, the poor health conditions prevailing in many Third World countries exacerbate the risks and complications associated with IUDs. Because of the increased risk from infections, septic abortions, and untreated ectopic pregnancies, the mortality rate from IUDs in the Third World is double that in the West (*Population Reports* 1982, A-211). In spite of the risks, IUDs are heavily promoted in many Third World family planning programs. IUDs are attractive to many family planning programs because they are both effective in preventing pregnancy and because women lack control over the device. Removal of an IUD requires a visit to a health clinic, a journey many women find difficult to make. Women's lack of control is aggravated because even if a woman goes to the health clinic, there is no guarantee that the doctor will remove the IUD (Hartmann 1987, 206). According to some researchers, IUD continuation rates "are probably a reflection of involuntary continuation," not satisfaction with the method (Hutchings 1986, 252).

IUDs have been seriously misused in Third World family planning programs. For instance, in India mass campaigns promoting IUDs have been common. Women are lined up in assembly-line fashion and IUDs are then inserted. Many, if not most, women are not given a medical examination before insertion and little effort is made to tell women about side effects or to treat them later. At a clinic near Bombay, women are told that their uterus is being "cleansed" when they suffer from heavy bleeding (Hartmann 1987, 205).

In China IUDs are the most common birth control method, followed closely by female sterilization (Wolf 1985). Women are routinely X-rayed to check that their IUDs are in place. Furthermore, Chinese varieties of IUDs do not have tails, perhaps because the government does not want women removing the device themselves. China and India are just two examples of IUD use and misuse. These cases illustrate both how the IUD is often an inappropriate technology for the Third World and how this approach to contraception removes the locus of control from women to doctors and governments.

Oral Contraceptives

Certainly the birth control pill has been no stranger to controversy. The initial research trials on the pill used primarily poor and Third

World women because risks were expected (Petchesky 1984). In spite of clinical literature that associated estrogen with carcinogenesis, a decision was made to manufacture a high dosage estrogen pill. Additionally, case reports appeared soon after the pill was marketed in 1960 that linked it with sometimes fatal thromboembolisms. Yet this information was ignored, minimized, or suppressed by researchers, drug companies, and physicians (Petchesky 1984). However, during the late 1960s, women and consumer health activists, in concert with well-publicized Congressional hearings, made information about oral contraceptives public. Subsequently reforms occurred, such as a reduced estrogen content. Additionally, there are now progestin-only pills, which were developed to avoid estrogen-associated complications. Although oral contraceptives have been improved, they are still powerful drugs that expose users to serious health risks. Among the remaining risks of today's oral contraceptives are: blood clots, heart attacks, strokes, high blood pressure, liver and gall bladder disease, cervical dysplasia, diabetes, and depression (see Bell 1985 for more discussion on oral contraceptives' risks and advantages).

Despite the "vociferous opposition of organized medical groups" (Silverman et al. 1982, 77) the Food and Drug Administration (FDA) began in 1970 to require that package inserts describing appropriate use and contraindications accompany all oral contraceptives. Although the FDA ruling applies only to the United States, most other developed countries have followed the FDA's lead.

The pill's use has declined or leveled off in the industrialized world. This decline is due to the increased knowledge about, and unacceptability of, its side effects. Manufacturers of oral contraceptives have therefore turned to the Third World as their growth market. Most Third World countries continue to provide little or no information on possible side effects. In the Third World the pill's adverse effects are "shrugged off with references to high rates of maternal mortality, or hardly mentioned at all" (Hartmann 1987, 179). Clearly, the goals of population control supercede the health concerns of Third World women.

The pharmaceutical industry has been quite successful in the Third World. The significant involvement of the United States AID in family planning has helped the United States pharmaceutical industry gain access to Third World markets. In 1967, in order to get established in the market, four of the biggest manufacturers of oral contraceptives, Searle, Syntex, Ortho, and Parke-Davis, began supplying AID with pills free of charge (LaCheen 1985, 110). This tactic paid off. In 1972 AID spent $10 million on birth control pills (compared to $7 million on all other contraceptives). Since the mid-1970s the yearly average for the pill is about $15 million (LaCheen 1985, 110). Currently AID provides family planning programs with about 100 million cycles of pills annually; other donors provide another 20 million cycles (*Population Reports* 1982).

The lack of local regulations, combined with heavy promotion by AID and other population control agencies, has created a situation in which oral contraceptives are distributed or sold without prescription and with little if any screening or follow-up (Hartmann 1987; LaCheen 1985). Under the recommendation of the International Planned Parenthood Federation, at least eight countries have dropped prescription requirements since 1973. These countries include the Philippines, Pakistan, Bangladesh, Antigua, Chile, Fiji, Jamaica, and South Korea (LaCheen 1985, 116). More often, a prescription requirement exists but is disregarded. "In a growing number of countries the requirement is honoured more in the breach, and the *de facto* situation differs considerably from the *de jure*" (Paxman and Cook 1979, 230). Among the countries where this *de facto* practice prevails are Bolivia, Brazil, Colombia, Ecuador, El Salvador, Egypt, Ghana, Indonesia, Ivory Coast, Lebanon, Malaysia, Mexico, Nigeria, Panama, Thailand, Turkey, and Venezuela (Paxman and Cook 1979, 230).

A strategy known as social marketing has developed that takes advantage of this very lack of regulation. Social marketing programs "are a hybrid—public health oriented social action programs grafted onto commercial distribution and marketing systems" (*Population Reports* 1980, J-393). Contraceptive social marketing programs appear to be a growing trend within the family planning field. Contraceptives, donated by AID or some other group, are sold in a Third World country at a subsidized price through already existing local vendors or shops. Social marketing programs benefit the contraceptive industry by allowing their products to reach more and more remote areas at no added cost to them. Programs actually advertise various products, through billboards, radio, and television advertisements, or signs, thus eliminating one sizable expense for the industry. Funding for social marketing programs comes from a wide array of population control interests, such as AID, IPPF, private foundations, and so forth. (For a more thorough discussion of social marketing refer to *Population Reports* 1980.)

Viewed as "cost effective" by population control groups, social marketing programs distribute contraceptives to more people at a lower cost "by cutting out expensive services like health clinics" (LaCheen 1985, 115). Yet because these programs explicitly target individuals who do not have access to health care, their ultimate health costs may be great. Women with high-risk characteristics may be more likely to use the pill, and follow-up care may be more difficult to find in event of dangerous side effects.

Despite these problems, the pill is an important contraceptive option for many women. Over 60 million women take the pill, making it the most widely used reversible female contraceptive. When used correctly, oral contraceptives are very effective in preventing pregnancy, quite easy to use, and do not interfere with sex. Furthermore, since oral contraceptives are under a woman's direct control, she takes responsibility each day for the decision to continue or not. Should she suffer from acute adverse effects, she can stop immediately. However, pushing the pill indiscriminately on women who frequently are undernourished, have restricted access to health care, have not been screened to determine pregnancy, and have a tradition of extensive breast-feeding increases the likelihood of serious health consequences for these users.

Injectable Contraceptives

As with the pill and IUD, injectables have met with controversy. They are likewise heavily promoted by family planning programs. The International Planned Parenthood Federation and the United Nations Fund for Population Activities are the primary suppliers of injectables (Hartmann 1987, 187). AID has been unable to supply them directly to family planning programs, since no injectable has been approved for contraceptive use in the United States.

At this time two injectable contraceptives are widely available: depot-medroxyprogesterone acetate (DMPA, commonly known by its trade name, Depo-Provera), manufactured by Upjohn, a U.S.-owned multinational; and norethindrone enanthate (NET-EN, trade name, Noristerat or Norigest), manufactured by the West German multinational Schering (*Population Reports* 1983). Although several other injectables are in various stages of development and testing, our focus will be on Depo-Provera and Norigest, since they are the best known.

Although injectables have not been registered or approved for contraceptive use in the United States, Depo-Provera is licensed as a contraceptive in eighty-four countries and Norigest is marketed in forty countries (Hall and Holck 1982). One or both injectables are in use in about one hundred countries. Use is most widespread in Jamaica, Thailand, Sri Lanka, and New Zealand (*Population Reports* 1983). Estimates of women who currently receive injectables range from 1.5 million to 5 million (War on Want 1984; *Population Reports* 1983; Corea 1980, 108). Injectables have become an essential component of family planning programs in Africa and Latin America (CED 1983). According to the World Health Organization (WHO), 98 percent of the women who used injectables in 1982 used Depo-Provera (Hall and Holck 1982, 2). However because of the controversy surrounding Depo-Provera, researchers and family planning organizations have since shifted their attention to Norigest (War on Want 1984).

Both Depo-Provera and Norigest are progestins but belong to different groups of steroids. They both appear to work by inhibiting gonadotropin production in the pituitary gland, which prevents ovulation. Studies indicate that the drugs also have an effect on the production of cervical mucus, on the fallopian tubes, and on the lining of the uterus, all of which reduce fertility (WHO 1982). The major difference between the two injectables appears to lie in the level of steroid found in the blood. Norigest both increases and decreases in concentration rapidly and is usually undetectable by about 10 weeks after injection. Depo-Provera, on the other hand, gradually reaches peak concentration and declines more slowly. It is often detectable more than thirteen weeks after injection. Therefore, Depo-Provera tends to inhibit ovulation for a longer period of time (WHO 1982). Depo-Provera is usually given in a three-month dose of 150 mg, and less often in a six-month dose. Recommended dosage for Norigest is 200 mg at either eight-week intervals or every eight weeks for the first six months and then every 12 weeks (*Population Reports* 1983, K-36). Both injectables are highly effective. Annual pregnancy rates are less than one per one hundred users (*Population Reports* 1983).

Schering began testing its injectable, Norigest, in 1957. Major field trials were conducted in Peru, and smaller studies were conducted elsewhere. Norigest went on the market in Peru in 1967 but was withdrawn in 1971 after pituitary and breast nodules were found in rats that had been given Norigest (War on Want 1984). But when many researchers maintained that the rat data were not applicable to humans, Norigest came back on the market.

While Schering was experimenting with Norigest, Upjohn began developing Depo-Provera. Upjohn began clinical trials of Depo-Provera in 1963 and by the late 1960s had begun marketing it in several countries. Although Upjohn started later than Schering, it quickly came to dominate the injectable contraceptive market. Depo-Provera's main advantage is that a single shot prevents pregnancy for three to six months, while Norigest needs to be administered more often.

To many, injectables are a desirable method because they are highly effective in preventing pregnancy, easy and quick to administer, and minimize the woman's involvement and responsibility. Women whose male partners object to birth control can be given an injection surreptitiously during a quick visit with a family planning worker. Further-more, in many areas of the Third World there exists an "injection mystique." Injections are associated with safe, effective, modern medicine.

However, the very qualities that make injectables attractive can also be viewed as being potentially detrimental to women. Freedom from responsibility can also mean loss of control. From a feminist perspective this lack of control is disempowering. Should a woman suffer from adverse effects, she cannot withdraw the drug from her bloodstream nor can she change her mind and simply elect to change methods—she must wait the two, three, six, or even eight months it takes for the drug to leave her system. The injection mystique can also lead to abuse. If a group unquestioningly trusts injections, it is easier to administer the drug without explaining its effects.

The most common side effects of Depo-Provera and Norigest are disturbances in the menstrual cycle. According to a WHO study, "fewer than one-third of women receiving DMPA [Depo-Provera] report hav-ing a normal menstrual cycle during the first year of use," and with Norigest approximately one-half of the users did not have a normal menstrual cycle (WHO 1982b, 17). Irregularities can take two forms: either frequent bleeding and/or spotting or an absence of bleeding. For undernourished women, heavy bleeding can be particularly serious because of iron and blood loss. Furthermore, in many Third World countries menstrual blood is considered "unclean" or "polluting." Therefore, women who experience frequent bleeding suffer physical inconvenience, potential danger, and various "taboos and practices that separate [them] from the family" (CED 1983, 5).

Other effects reported include headaches, backaches, abdominal discomfort, weight gain, skin disorders, tiredness, nausea, depression, hair loss, loss of libido, diarrhea, and delayed return to fertility (CED 1983; War on Want 1984; Hartmann 1987). Too often these effects are dismissed as "minor," but to the women suffering such reactions their problems may be far from minor. Gena Corea poignantly points out, "Depression is a minor side effect that merely destroys the entire qual-ity of a woman's life." She also notes that as many women lose weight on Depo-Provera as gain it. For thin, undernourished women, this weight loss can be an extremely serious health threat (Corea 1980, 109). Depo-Provera has proven to be an effective male contraceptive, but male complaints of loss of libido have kept it from being promoted as a male contraceptive. Yet the same side effect is casually dismissed when it occurs in women (Corea 1980). This underscores the bias to-wards female-based methods and the devaluing of women's experience.

The possible long-term adverse effects of Depo-Provera are similar to those of the pill: the risk of birth defects should the drug be administered while a woman is pregnant; a potentially negative impact on infant development from ingesting the hormone in breast milk; and a possible link to breast, endometrial, and cervical cancers (Hartmann 1987, 189).

Another disturbing aspect of injectables is their history of abuse. This abuse generally involves problems with informed consent and deliberate misuse. Women around the world have been given shots without their true informed consent; for instance, most often women are not informed of potential risks. Sometimes women are not even made aware of their shot's contraceptive properties, having been led to believe it was simply a remedy for some ailment. In the countries where Depo-Provera is not approved for contraceptive use, such as the United States, England, and Scotland, its availability for other medical treatments has allowed it to be misused as a method of birth control by some individual doctors (Rakusen 1981). Low-income women, blacks and other ethnic minorities, mentally retarded women, incarcerated women, and drug addicts have been special targets (Rakusen 1981; Hartmann 1987). Though the FDA board of inquiry has repeatedly denied requests by industry and population establishment for approval, a member of the FDA board has recommended that Depo-Provera be approved for limited use on retarded women and drug addicts, even though he admitted it was not sufficiently tested for use on "human subjects" (Hartmann 1987, 192).

In the Third World, similar reasoning underlies the drug's promotion and the repeated pattern of abuse among the poor and ethnically distinct populations. According to a Chilean doctor, "A long-acting contraceptive would have nearly ideal advantages . . . in populations with low socioeconomic status and low educational attainment" (quoted in Corea 1980, 108). South African black women, who are denied access to decent health care, have been the victims of mass Depo-Provera campaigns. In fact, family planning is the only free health service available to blacks, and Depo-Provera is the most widely used contraceptive (Hartmann 1987, 193).

In an article detailing the current campaign to stop the widespread introduction of Norigest into India, an Indian health activist notes that the Indian

literate middle class has been brainwashed into believing that population growth is the country's most serious problem. It is quite common to see letters to editors advocating compulsion and coercion to "save" the country from disaster. . . . Birth control as a human right has been submerged under an ideology of family planning as a "patriotic duty" essential to the

"national interest." The feeling . . . is that the illiterate and the ignorant
need contraception desperately and that the "benefits" do indeed outweigh the risks. The question they fail to ask is: whose benefit, whose
risk? (Balasubrahmanyan 1986, 154).

Thailand has one of the longest experiences and the highest percentage of injectable use in the world. However, it is unclear how many
women using it are aware of its potential risks. A Thai health activist
states that injectables are popular among rural Thai women "not only
because the people don't know the adverse effect of the drug, but also
because they are told the drug is good, safe and effective" (quoted in
Hartmann 1987, 192).

In many parts of the Third World injectables are administered
without adequate supervision. Mexico's relaxed regulations allow the
drugs to be sold over the counter in pharmacies and to be given by
"injectionists" who have little or no formal training. Medical personnel
in the Third World report that they themselves were never informed of
possible side effects and never saw any physician package insert accompanying the drug (Hartmann 1987, 193).

The patterns of abuse, the known adverse side effects, and the
large number of possible risks have led many health activists and members of medical communities around the world to action. For instance,
in India there is a legal challenge to the government's proposed program
for mass distribution of Norigest. Due to the vigilance of women's
health advocates in the United States, the FDA has repeatedly turned
down requests by pharmaceutical companies and population groups to
approve injectable contraceptives. In Canada, a coalition of groups is
strategizing on how to respond to the recent approval of Depo-Provera.
Great Britain is the headquarters for an international campaign against
Depo-Provera. Some groups call for a complete worldwide ban on the
drug. Others, acknowledging that injectables do provide another contraceptive option, are demanding a thorough reevaluation of the way
injectables and other high-tech methods are tested, evaluated, marketed, and administered.

Implants

The newest high-tech contraceptive on the market is Norplant, and
now, Norplant II, a subdermal time-released hormonal implant which
lasts five years. Although it is not yet approved by the FDA, clinical
trials in the United States are underway. So far, Norplant is approved
in Finland, Sweden, Thailand, Indonesia, and Ecuador. In 1986 the

International Planned Parenthood Federation added it to its list of available contraceptives (Population Council 1986).

The first contraceptive implants were developed in the 1960s and were made of flexible, nonbiodegradable tubes filled with hormones and placed under the skin. Most often implantation occurs in the inside of the upper arm or forearm. Implants are expected to cause fewer side effects than injectables or oral contraceptives as the drug is released continuously and relatively constantly over a five- to ten-year period; injectables, on the other hand, create very high plasma levels of hormones when injected and oral contraceptives produce daily fluctuations of hormone levels (*Population Reports* 1983).

Implants go much further than injectables by extending the period of pregnancy protection for several years. Correspondingly, they also go further than injectables in taking away users' direct control over reproduction. As with injectables, we have another double-edged sword: the longer effectiveness could free a woman from worry over unwanted pregnancy, but women relinquish direct control over their reproductive lives to medical personnel.

Much of the research on implants has been supported by the Population Council (*Population Reports* 1983). In fact, Norplant is their creation. George Zeidenstein, president of the Population Council, believes, "Norplant contraceptive subdermal implants is the most important new contraceptive system since the pill" (Population Council 1983, 4).

Norplant consists of six capsules, each containing 36 mg of levonorgestrel with an effective life of five years. Insertion and removal of the implants requires local anesthesia, sterile conditions, and skilled medical personnel; these are far from simple procedures. Special care must be exercised during insertion, as implants can migrate in muscles and cause difficulties when it is time for removal. Removal is the more difficult procedure, as once capsules are in the body a layer of fibrous tissue forms around them that must be cut away.

Because of the way Norplant is administered, it may be an inappropriate contraceptive technology in many parts of the Third World, where health systems are lacking or poorly developed. Even in well-controlled clinical trials, infections and problems with removal have occurred. It is likely these problems would be more widespread and potentially more dangerous in areas with inadequate health delivery centers.

Norplant's promoters realize the potential problems and are advising that it ought to be introduced only under certain conditions. The Population Council states that Norplant is essentially a clinic-based method, requiring "careful training, supervision, information dissemination, logistics and follow-up" (quoted in Hartmann 1987, 199). That said, the council has also suggested that Norplant could possibly be used in mobile clinics or contraceptive camps, where follow-up is far more problematic. In spite of the precautions of the council, some Third World officials are enthusiastic about Norplant precisely because it could be introduced in regions that lack access to good health care.

The Population Council has also stated that every woman who wishes her capsules removed should be able to schedule this procedure without delay. This sounds admirable, but in actual practice it may be quite unrealistic. Many Third World family planning programs are in "remote areas" where education, communication, transportation, and health systems are poorly developed. There are already reports from Bangladesh of women having difficulty getting implanted capsules removed.

Although in theory Norplant is a reversible method, in practice this is not always so. In addition to the problem of women's requests going unheeded, women may be fearful of having the implants removed. One study reports that 30 percent of women having the implants removed found the procedure painful (*Population Reports* 1983, K-40). In clinical trials in Ecuador researchers note that the high continuation rates they found may be a result of women fearing removal more than being satisfied with the method (Hartmann 1987, 197).

Another feature of the implant may foster its use as an instrument of population control. Particularly in thin women, the capsules are visible under the skin. Therefore, the government could easily identify nonusers, which might facilitate a coercive population control program with the drug. As with the other high-tech methods, the danger lurks here that yet another contraceptive will be administered inappropriately.

Summary

Our discussion of IUDs, oral contraceptives, injectables, and implants reveals persistent patterns. First of all, women often are not fully informed of health risks. In the Third World, health concerns are often shrugged off with references to high rates of maternal mortality, a shorter life expectancy, and the population crisis. Often in family planning programs, women are not adequately screened or given follow-up care, thus compounding the inherent danger of these contraceptives. As the high-tech methods are pushed by most family planning groups, there is a pervasive attitude that women are too "ignorant" or "irresponsible" to use other forms of contraception (Duggan 1986; Balasubrahmanyan 1986).

Secondly, oral contraceptive and IUD marketing shows that corporations are eager to take advantage of the Third World's weak drug regulations and thereby boost lagging domestic sales. Additionally, many family planning programs employ a variety of techniques in order to induce women to participate. These range from so-called social marketing to offering incentives (payment, food, transistor radios, cloth, etc.) to outright coercion through the use of the military.

The largest and best-known campaign of forced family planning took place in India during 1975–77. In this case, millions of men were rounded up by the military and forced to undergo sterilization (LaCheen 1986, 121). However, women have also been targeted. In Indonesia, for example, the military was directly involved in a mass IUD campaign. One study of the campaign reported that almost half of the acceptors stated that they were coerced; many more said they were fearful (as reported in Hartmann 1987, 80).

Regardless of the type, all inducements have a built-in disregard for free choice and women's health and rights. Betsy Hartmann accurately describes the reality of incentives (a supposedly benign inducement) when she writes that for "people who are desperately poor, there is no such thing as free choice. A starving person is unlikely to turn down a loaf of bread, even if it means being sterilized" (1987, 66). Incentives encourage poor women to seek immediate material gain. Vimal Balasubrahmanyan reports on a physician who encountered a woman who had in place three different IUDs, each inserted on a separate occasion, and as a result was suffering from heavy bleeding (1986, 145). In Thailand, at a camp for Cambodian refugees, women have been given a chicken for their families if they agreed to take a shot of Depo-Provera (Goodman 1985). Incentives act to bias contraceptive choices toward a specific technology and all too often prey on the desperation of the poor. Furthermore, some family planning workers are paid according to how many acceptors they sign up. This practice can lead to additional abuses (see LaCheen 1986; Hartmann 1987; Silverman et al. 1982; Goodman 1985 for more information on incentives, coercion, and corruption).

In sum, profits, efficiency, population control, and control over women appear to be guiding principles. However they do not have to remain so. As Betsy Hartmann puts it, "The time is long overdue to challenge the prevailing mentality that the womb of the individual woman is expendable in the general population control scheme of things" (1987,

207). Today the international women's health community is working to change this picture.

Women Working for Change

Around the world, feminist health groups are working to end the reproductive abuses to which women have been subjected; to this end, women are taking bold steps to expand their contraceptive choices. Health activists recognize that societal practices that keep women ignorant about their bodies further the social control of women as they become dependent on the medical establishment or some other social institution for their health and reproductive concerns. Today in countries as diverse as Brazil, India, the United States, Kenya, the Philippines, Canada, Morocco, Bangladesh, and the United Kingdom, women are working to learn more about their own bodies and to take back control of their own health and reproduction. Thousands of groups offer alternatives to the way contraceptive information and techniques have traditionally been disseminated. Alternatives are offered directly in women-controlled health centers, as well as indirectly by organizing women in local communities, networking with other groups, and trying to activate change within the family planning field and the conventional health service system. (For more on how women around the world are taking back control of their reproductive lives, and more generally working to change the dominant health care system, see Tudiver 1986; Diskin 1984; Mellow in this volume.)

In the past few years many feminist health activists have been working to establish dialogues with the very forces that have acted against the reproductive and health well-being of the world's women—the medical establishment, population control groups, and governmental organizations. The premise for this tactic of increased cooperation is that health activists recognize that these other groups have access to important scientific information and service delivery resources that need to be shared with women's health groups. Of equal importance, women's health groups, because of their knowledge and contact with women throughout the world, need to be able to inform and direct the work of health providers and the population establishment (IWHC 1986).

In 1986 the International Women's Health Coalition (IWHC) and the Population Council sponsored a meeting between representatives from the women's health movement (from the United States and developing countries) and the international family planning field (developers of contraceptives, managers of contraceptive introduction, and family planning service providers). The organizers envisioned that by bringing together these two groups, a useful dialogue might begin. It was hoped that solutions to existing problems would be explored. Four problems emerged as needing immediate attention. First, women are denied the right to reproductive choice (with respect to both abortion and kind of contraceptive). Second, women often receive incomplete information (or misinformation) on risks, benefits, and short- and long-term consequences of various contraceptive methods. Third, the Far Right has mounted a concerted effort to curtail reproductive choice throughout the world. Finally, there has been an increase in the violation of human rights in order to achieve reductions in population growth for specific groups.

The results of this meeting were encouraging. The group developed an extensive list of points of consensus with respect to contraceptive development and the quality of care for family planning clients. Such consensus is vital should women's health activists and the population establishment embark on working together. One participant writes that "International family planning is not really getting better. But, for the first time, it shows promise of being able to. Feminist principles are already part of the discourse. The question now is whether the women's health movement itself will engage in that discourse" (IWHC 1986, 100).[2]

Women's health activism takes many shapes. Indian feminist health activists have filed a petition in the Supreme Court of India arguing that it is unsafe to allow new injectables in India, and that unethical experimentation is being done on Indian women without their informed consent (Balasubrahmanyan 1986). In Brazil, a reproductive rights organization has a call-in radio program that candidly answers questions about contraception in a country where the subject of birth control has long been taboo (Hartmann 1987, 286). In Third World countries many women are working to get the safer, simpler barrier methods of birth control incorporated into family planning programs. Feminist activists in these countries are confronting the prejudice against barrier methods on the part of family planning programs. They have identified several roots of this prejudice, among which are: the belief that poor people are too embarrassed and ignorant about their bodies to attempt to use barrier methods; the conviction that these methods are inconvenient and awkward; and the notion that it takes too much time and too many resources to educate people about how to use barrier methods. Whatever problems do surround barrier methods could be overcome, health activists assert, if methods were introduced with sensitive instruction and follow-up and with stress on the fact that both men and women are responsible for contraception. In the United States, in response to U.S. drug companies' reluctance to pursue the relatively unprofitable cervical cap (a popular European barrier method), feminist health groups pressured for government funding for a cervical cap study. In May 1988 the cervical cap was approved for general use by the FDA based on the research conducted at many feminist health centers across the country. We have seen some successes as a result of women-initiated struggles. Among these have been: curtailing sterilization abuse throughout the world; successfully campaigning against the approval of Depo-Provera in the United States; expanding women's right to abortion in a number of countries (sometimes seemingly against all odds); and, creating a worldwide reaction against the Dalkon Shield.

Conclusion

> It is clear that political administrative elites, and not the masses of acceptors, are deciding on the technology to be used. (Hartmann 1987, 179)

As the quote above reflects, individual women's contraceptive choices are not simply a matter of personal choice. Rather, as we hope this chapter has demonstrated, their choices are affected by complex interactions of their personal situations with the operations of medicine, the population control establishment, and the drug industry. To a great extent, these larger social forces shape the properties of today's contraceptive technologies and provide the social context for contraceptive policy.

The last thirty years provide not merely examples of abuses in the area of reproductive choice; they also provide an indictment of the normal workings of the technological orientation of health care, the population control establishment, and the multinational pharmaceutical industry. Although the developments of contraceptive research may provide more options for women, there has been inadequate testing and gross misapplication of some of these technologies. In most cases, control is actually taken away from women and given over to health care or population control professionals. Furthermore, instead of expanding women's choices, the promotion of a certain technology at times supplants other techniques and curtails women's contraceptive choices.

While we need to recognize that there will probably never be a "perfect" contraceptive, we need to expand the range of "good" and safe methods. "Good" is a subjective concept, as a contraceptive will be assessed differently by different users who make varying trade-offs among contraceptive efficacy, safety, and convenience. The trade-offs may be seen differently by others—the funders, researchers, population control advocates, the pharmaceutical industry. But, in the long and short run it is women who need to be able to have the first and final choice; it is women, with all the options before them, who must be able to define what is best for them.

Obviously changes must be made in the direction of contraceptive research, the implementation of family planning programs, how drug companies conduct business, and the conventional approach to health care. High-tech methods, which rely on potent drugs, hormones, and surgery, need to be de-emphasized. Safety and health concerns should not be neglected in favor of effectiveness, convenience, long-term use, and profitability. Emphasis on highly invasive technologies must yield to methods and education that can enhance women's control over their own reproduction and instill a personal sense of responsibility.

NOTES

We thank Kay Ratcliff, Myra Ferree, Barbara Wright, and other members of the editorial collective along with Irving Zola for their helpful suggestions and advice, which greatly improved this chapter.

1. IUD tails are one or more strings that are attached to the IUD. When the IUD is in place the tail extends into the upper vagina. Tails are both an important safety feature and an aid for removal. Women are advised to check the tail at least once a month. A missing tail or one shorter than it should be is an indication of a possible problem (such as embedding, perforation, or expulsion).
2. A copy of the proceedings of the October 8–9, 1986, meeting may be obtained by contacting the International Women's Health Coalition, P.O. Box 8500, New York, New York 10150.

BIBLIOGRAPHY

Atkinson, Linda, Richard Lincoln, and Jacqueline Darroch Forrest. 1985. Worldwide trends in funding for contraceptive research and evaluation. *Family Planning Perspectives* 17, no. 5: 196–207.
———. 1986. The next contraceptive revolution. *Family Planning Perspectives* 18, no. 1: 19–26.
Balasubrahmanyan, Vimal. 1986. Finger in the dike: The fight to keep injectables out of India. In *Adverse effects,* ed. Kathleen McDonnell, 137–58. Toronto: Women's Press.
Bell, Susan. 1984. Birth control. In *The new our bodies, ourselves,* ed. The

Boston Women's Health Book Collective, 220–62. New York: Simon and Schuster.

Berkman, Joyce. 1980. Historical styles of contraceptive advocacy. In *Birth control and controlling birth*, ed. Helen Holmes et. al., 27–36. Clifton, N.J.: Humana Press.

CED (Center for Education and Documentation). 1983. *Injectables: Immaculate contraception.* Counterfact no. 3 (March). Bombay, India.

Conrad, Peter, and Joseph Schneider. 1980. Looking at levels of medicalization. *Social Science and Medicine* 14A, no. 1: 75–79.

Corea, Gena. 1980. The Depo weapon. In *Birth control and controlling birth*, ed. Helen Holmes, Betty Hoskins, and Michael Gross, 107–16. Clifton, N.J.: Humana Press.

—————. 1985 *The hidden malpractice*. New York: Harper and Row.

Cowan, Belita. 1980. Ethical problems in government-funded contraceptive research. In *Birth control and controlling birth*, ed. Helen Holmes, Betty Hoskins, and Michael Gross, 37–46. Clifton, N.J.: Humana Press.

Cutrufelli, Maria Rosa. 1983. *Women of Africa: Roots of oppression*. London: Zed Press.

Davis, Angela. 1980. *Women, race and class*. New York: Random House.

Diskin, Vilunya. 1984. Developing an international awareness. In *The new our bodies, ourselves*, ed. The Boston Women's Health Book Collective, 611–25. New York: Simon and Schuster.

Dowie, Mark, and Tracy Johnston. 1977. A case of corporate malpractice. In *Seizing our bodies*, ed. Claudia Dreifus, 86–104. New York: Vintage Books.

Duggan, Lynn. 1986. From birth control to population control: Depo-Provera in Southeast Asia. In *Adverse effects*, ed. Kathleen McDonnell, 159–65. Toronto: Women's Press.

Ehrenreich, Barbara, and Deirdre English. 1972. *Witches, midwives and nurses*. Old Westbury, N.Y.: Feminist Press.

Elling, Ray. 1980. *Cross-national study of health systems*. New Brunswick, N.J.: Transaction Books.

Family Planning Perspectives. 1986. Contraception and abortion costs are tiny portion of U.S. health spending. *Family Planning Perspectives* 18, no. 1: 37–38.

Fee, Elizabeth, ed. 1983. *Women and health: The politics of sex in medicine*. Farmingdale, N.Y.: Baywood.

Fugh-Berman, Adriane. 1985. Day of our Dalkon. *Off Our Backs*, 15 (May): 6.

Goodman, Amy. 1985. The case against Depo-Provera. *Multinational Monitor* 6, nos. 2–3: 3–22.

Gordon, Linda. 1983. The politics of birth control, 1920–1940: The impact of the professional. In *Women and health: The politics of sex in medicine*, ed. Elizabeth Fee, 151–75. Farmingdale, N.Y.: Baywood.

—————. 1976. *Woman's body, woman's right*. New York: Grossman Publishers.

Griessemer, Tom O. 1954. *The population bomb*. New York: Hugh More Fund.

Hall, Peter, and Susan Holck. 1982. Injectable contraception. *World Health (WHO)*, May, 2–4.

Hartmann, Betsy. 1987. *Reproductive rights and wrongs: The global politics of population control and contraceptive choice.* New York: Harper and Row.

Holmes, Helen, Betty Hoskins, and Michael Gross, eds. 1980. *Birth control and controlling birth: Women-centered perspectives.* Clifton, N.J.: Humana Press.

Illich, Ivan. 1976. *Medical nemesis: The expropriation of health.* New York: Pantheon.

IWHC (International Women's Health Coalition) and The Population Council. 1986. *The contraceptive development process and quality of care in reproductive health services.* Rapporteurs' Report of a Meeting. Sponsored by the IWHC and the PC. New York, October 8–9, 1986.

LaCheen, Cary. 1986. Population control and the pharmaceutical industry. In *Adverse effects,* ed. Kathleen McDonnell, 89–136. Toronto: Women's Press.

Mass, Bonnie. 1980. An historical sketch of the American population control movement. In *Imperialism, health and medicine,* ed. Vicente Navarro, 179–202. Farmingdale, N.Y.: Baywood.

Merchant, Carolyn. 1983. *The death of nature: Women, ecology and the scientific revolution.* San Francisco: Harper and Row.

Mintz, Morton. 1985. *At any cost: corporate greed, women and the Dalkon Shield.* New York: Pantheon.

Mokhiber, Russell. 1986. Criminals by any other name. *Washington Monthly,* 17, no. 1 (January): 40–44.

National Women's Health Network. 1986. In court and out of control. *The Network News,* 11, no. 1 (January/February): 3.

Paxman, John, and Rebecca Cook. 1979. Law and planned parenthood. In *Birth control: An international assessment,* ed. Malcolm Potts and Pouru Bhiwandiwala, 227–54. Baltimore: University Park Press.

Petchesky, Rosalind Pollack. 1984. *Abortion and women's choice: The state, sexuality and reproductive freedom.* New York: Longman.

Pincus, Gregory. 1965. *The control of fertility.* New York: Academic Press.

Population Council. 1983. *1983 Annual Report.* New York.

—————. 1986. *Norplant worldwide.* No. 4. New York.

Population Reports. 1980. *Social marketing: Does it work?* Population Information Program, series J, no. 21 (January). Baltimore: Johns Hopkins.

—————. 1982. *Oral contraceptives in the 1980s.* Population Information Program, series A, no. 6 (May/June). Baltimore: Johns Hopkins.

—————. 1983. *Injectables and implants.* Population Information Program, series K, no. 2 (May). Baltimore: Johns Hopkins.

Potts, Malcolm. 1981. Why the world is not getting the contraception it needs. *People* 8, no. 4: 28. New York: International Planned Parenthood Foundation.

Rakusen, Jill. 1981. Depo-Provera: The extent of the problem. In *Women, health and reproduction,* ed. Helen Roberts, 75–108. Boston: Routledge and Kegan Paul.

Savara, Mira. 1983. Report of a workshop on women, health and reproduction. In *Third world, second sex,* ed. Miranda Davies, 220–27. London: Zed Press.

Scully, Diana, and Pauline Bart. 1978. A funny thing happened on the way to the orifice: Women in gynecology textbooks. In *The cultural crisis of modern medicine*, ed. John Ehrenreich. New York: Monthly Review Press.

Seaman, Barbara. 1979. *The doctor's case against the pill*. Rev. ed. New York: Dell Publishing.

Silverman, Milton, Philip Lee, and Mia Lydecker. 1982. *Prescriptions for death: The drugging of the third world*. Berkeley: University of California Press.

Tudiver, Sari. 1986. The strength of links: International health networks in the eighties. In *Adverse effects*, ed. Kathleen McDonnell, 187–214. Toronto: Women's Press.

U.S. Office of Technology Assessment. 1982. *World population and fertility planning technologies: The next twenty years*. Washington, D.C.: Government Printing Office.

War On Want. 1984. *Norethisterone oenanthate: The other injectable contraceptive*. London: War on Want.

WHO (World Health Organization). 1982a. Facts about injectable contraceptives. *Bulletin WHO*, 60, no. 2: 199–210.

————. 1982b. *Injectable hormonal contraceptives: Technical and safety aspects*. WHO Offset Publication no. 65. Geneva.

Wolf, Margery. 1985. *Revolution postponed: Women in contemporary China*. Stanford: Stanford University Press.

Zola, Irving. 1972. Medicine as an institution of social control. *Sociological Review*, 20:487–504.

Reproductive Technology: Perspectives and Implications for Low-Income Women and Women of Color

Laurie Nsiah-Jefferson and Elaine J. Hall

The recent development of new reproductive technologies has dramatically altered the experience of conceiving, carrying to term, and giving birth. At first glance the new reproductive technologies seem to offer women greatly expanded choices regarding whether they conceive, how they conceive, and how healthy a child they produce. Technologically sophisticated alternatives are now available that enable the infertile to produce a child who is genetically their own. A variety of prenatal screening procedures that provide information on the physical and mental health of the fetus may become the basis for a decision to terminate or to continue the pregnancy. But choice is not the only issue. While increased reproductive options do now exist, a full evaluation of the new reproductive technologies should include the individual negative consequences and the economic costs of creating real access to these technologies. Moreover, a closer look reveals that the social definitions of reproductive functions—as problems that need medical attention or as nonissues—may be applied to particular groups of women differently, depending on class, race, and culture.

Even though the impact of the new reproductive technology on an individual may be positive and desirable, the impact for society in general is mixed at best, and for certain groups such as low-income women and women of color the effects may often be negative. According to Andrews (1987), the availability of prenatal diagnosis with the subsequent possibility of abortion may place added social pressure on couples to use these technologies. This pressure may be intensified if the parents are thought not to have the resources to raise a handicapped child. Several authors (Andrews 1987; Callahan 1973) foresee a possible devaluation and stigmatization of people who have genetic defects. Because the availability of prenatal knowledge of genetic "problems" assumes these conditions can be avoided, the growth of prenatal screening technology could foster an environment in which society no longer felt responsible for disabled individuals.

Another negative impact of the new reproductive technologies is the way they frame the questions we ask about reproductive issues.

Especially troublesome is the assumption that private individuals are responsible for "solving" genetic problems. Andrews (1987) argues that the new reproductive technologies focus upon genetic causes while deemphasizing environmental causes of illness. Rothman (1986) criticizes the effect of procedures such as amniocentesis, which "privatize" a public health problem. Rothman believes that in a health system in which pregnant women routinely undergo prenatal diagnosis and are encouraged to abort all "defective" fetuses, less emphasis could be placed on research into the causes and treatment of genetic disorders.

Although these general implications of the new reproductive technology affect all women and all parents to some degree, the particular form such effects take and their salience will vary with class position and racial or ethnic identity. The issues for reproductive choice, based on race and class distinctions, are not always identical, though they often overlap in practice. In this chapter we will discuss three general issues especially relevant to low-income women and women of color when they consider and/or use some form of the new reproductive technologies.

First, low-income women are often dependent upon governmental funding of prenatal and contraceptive procedures because they lack medical coverage through employment-based insurance programs and cannot pay privately. This not only limits access, but also subjects the recipients to additional eligibility requirements and shapes availability according to the political biases or agendas underlying social policy, programs, and funding. Therefore, the issue of access to the new reproductive technology is crucial: Do funding policies provide equal access to the new reproductive technologies for low-income women? What barriers exist for utilizing the technologies that are funded? What are the implications of obtaining prenatal care through publicly controlled programs?

A second issue particularly relevant to women of color is the decision-making process involved in genetic counseling. Because white Anglos dominate the health care system, this interaction frequently involves differences in cultural backgrounds of the client and the counselor or physician. The meanings attached to the various experiences involved in genetic counseling are therefore problematic. Whether the process of genetic counseling is itself desirable or intrusive, whether a particular physical or mental condition is a disability or just a difference, whether the probability of a child having a genetic condition triggers treatment or pressure for abortion, and what type of "treatment" is considered necessary or appropriate—these are all questions for which meanings and values may vary according to the social class and racial/ethnic culture of the individuals involved. Given the power differences inherent in the interaction between an "expert" profes-sional provider and a client requesting service, conflicts that arise from cultural difference often revolve around the issues of informed consent and confidentiality.

A third issue is the social definition of infertility as a "problem" that needs medical and technological "solutions." We argue in this chapter that members of minority communities have an equal and even greater need for programs to treat infertility, but that these needs have not been defined as a legitimate concern and that treatments are gen-erally not available to low-income women, who are disproportionately nonwhite. Going beyond this clear mismatch between the needs and services available, the third issue for low-income women and women of color comes down to the social construction of infertility as a "social problem." Why have the infertility problems of minority communities been ignored? What are the implications for the daily life and social status of low-income women and women of color?

Prenatal Screening: Barriers to Access

Do low-income and minority women have equal access to prenatal di-agnostic procedures and counseling? The goal of equal access is par-ticularly important because statistics have shown that nonwhite women have a significantly higher probability of complications during preg-nancy and labor (Placek et al. 1984). To assess access to prenatal diagnosis and screening procedures, we must look at both the availa-bility of services, which is an issue of funding, and the existence of barriers that may restrict utilization of the available services.

Federal funding for prenatal screening is distributed at the state level through three programs: Medicaid, Maternal and Child Health Programs, and Community or Migrant Health Centers (Gold et al. 1987). Medicaid consists of reimbursement to participating private phy-sicians, hospitals, clinics, laboratories, pharmacies, and other provid-ers of health care for designated services, while the other two programs consist of public funding via clinics; we will first discuss availability of prenatal screening techniques funded through Medicaid and then turn to public clinics. In addition, it should be noted that prenatal programs may be offered in some state-sponsored hospitals and through public health–initiated grants.

Medicaid

The Medicaid program, Title XIX of the Social Security Act (42 U.S. 1396 *et seq.*), is the nation's major vehicle for financing health care for low-income persons. Financed jointly by the federal government and the states, Medicaid's primary purpose has always been to pay for health care for persons who receive cash assistance under Aid to Families with Dependent Children (AFDC) or Supplemental Security Income (SSI). Medicaid is administered within broad federal guidelines, but individual states decide the categories of persons eligible, income eligibility levels, and the services covered. Therefore the medical services available to low-income persons vary from state to state (Gold et al. 1987).

The six prenatal screening and treatment procedures covered by Medicaid are listed in table 1. The most widely used prenatal screening procedure, amniocentesis, involves inserting a needle through the abdomen of a pregnant woman into the uterus to remove a small amount of amniotic fluid which is tested to determine fetal abnormalities. Ultrasound screening determines fetal position and may identify certain defects. A fetal oxytocin stress test is performed to assess the condition of the fetus under the stress of uterine contractions which are brought about by administering oxytocin. Nonstress testing is a form of fetal monitoring in which electrodes monitor fetal movement and heart rate. Alpha feto-protein tests are performed to detect genetic abnormalities from a blood sample. When a woman with Rh negative blood aborts a fetus or gives birth to an Rh positive infant, one or more RhoGAM shots are indicated to prevent the formation of antibodies that could lead to a subsequent miscarriage, stillbirth, or abortion (Gold et al. 1987).

As shown in table 1, the majority of states provide Medicaid reimbursement for these six procedures. As a general rule, all the component procedures required in a particular screening technique are funded, but two states provide only "partial" coverage of amniocentesis. Connecticut and Kansas reimburse physician's fees for amniocentesis but fail to fund the laboratory fees for examining the amniotic fluids (Gold et al. 1987); thus amniocentesis may not truly be available to low-income women in these two states.

Most states reimburse for prenatal diagnostic services, but Medicaid will not reimburse the full cost of these procedures and the amount reimbursed varies from state to state (Greenstein 1987). It is important to remember that prenatal screening procedures are generally very expensive. For example, estimates of the costs of amniocentesis range from $600 to $1,500 depending upon the institution and the condition tested for (Arkansas Genetic Program 1987). However, the mean reimbursement for amniocentesis by Medicaid in 1985 was $64, although payments ranged from $15 to $450 (Greenstein 1987).[1] The partial reimbursement policies of the Medicaid programs restrict the number of physicians who are willing to provide health services to low-income clients. Therefore, low-income women who live in a state where a particular prenatal screening procedure is covered by Medicaid may still find it extremely difficult to find a physician who will provide the service.

Even if they find a private physician willing to accept Medicaid,

TABLE 1. Medicaid Funding of Prenatal Screening and Treatment Procedures in Forty-eight States in 1985

| Type of Procedure | Number of States Funding Procedure[a] | | Qualifying Restrictions[b] |
	Full	Partial/None	
Amniocentesis	48	Partial: 2 Connecticut Kansas	One state imposes an unspecified type of restriction.
Ultrasound	48	0	New Hampshire requires prior authorization. Georgia, Minnesota, and Texas have a combination of age and type of medical complication restriction.
Stress testing	46	None: 2 Oklahoma Rhode Island	No restrictions
Nonstress testing	44	None: 4 Louisiana Oklahoma Pennsylvania Rhode Island	Number of previous tests restriction in New Jersey, Tennessee, Texas, West Virginia
Alpha feto-protein	45	None: 3 California Connecticut Pennsylvania	No restrictions
RhoGAM treatment	42	None: 5 Arkansas California Delaware Florida Michigan	New Hampshire requires prior authorization. Kentucky and Minnesota require further documentation with the claim form.

Source: Gold et al. The Financing of Maternity Care in the United States, 1987.

[a]Full coverage consists of both physician and laboratory fees. Partial coverage does not include laboratory fees.

[b]Qualifying restrictions consist of any of the following: prior authorization, age of the woman, type of medical complication, number of previous tests, or further documentation. At times, the available data may not specify the type of restriction applied in a particular state.

poor women are often faced with qualifying restrictions that act as barriers to obtaining quality prenatal care. Although this varies from state to state and according to the particular screening procedure, some states do stipulate restrictions based on prior authorization by a physician, age of the woman, type of medical complication, and number of tests previously completed. For example, a low-income woman can obtain ultrasound screening via Medicaid funding in all states except California. However, in New Hampshire she is subject to prior authorization, and in three states (Georgia, Minnesota, and Texas) she is subject to restrictions by age and the particular medical complication prompting the ultrasound procedure (Gold et al. 1987). Some states may cover a particular procedure, but reimburse only in those cases in which the procedure is defined as medically necessary. Some states define "medically necessary"; other states leave the definition of medical necessity to the discretion of the physician. The variability in the definition means that some low-income women may not be able to obtain a particular screening technique in the area in which they live, even though the procedure is funded in their state and they qualify for it in a neighboring state that defines "medical necessity" in a different way.

The lower rate of Medicaid reimbursement and the restrictions on the provision of services are part of a two-tiered medical system that influences access and quality of care for poor women. Although some restrictions may be medically appropriate (such as age of the woman) and others may protect poor women and women of color from unwarranted overuse of prenatal screening procedures, overall the implications for equal access to high quality health services are negative. Even when prenatal screening is actually available in a meaningful sense, poor women have less control over the quality of care they receive because only some physicians and clinics choose to participate. Thus the ability of Medicaid patients to obtain prenatal screening is markedly different from that of white middle-class women whose health insurance programs cover such screening.

Funding through Clinics

The Maternal and Child Health Program (MCH) has very broad goals, including the promotion of maternal and child health through the provision of basic prenatal care and the provision of specialized care to children with handicapping conditions. When Congress enacted the MCH block grant in 1981, prenatal care and genetic services were two of the programs covered (Gold et al. 1987, 204). Because the block grant is state administered, the emphasis placed on maternity versus other kinds of care varies greatly from state to state (Gold et al. 1987).

Community Health Centers (CHCs) and Migrant Health Centers (MHCs) provide a broad range of primary care services to medically underserved, disadvantaged populations. Over 560 agencies in urban and rural areas of forty-nine states receive federal funds (Gold et al. 1987). Two-thirds of the clients belong to minority groups and six out of ten have incomes below the federal poverty level. An additional 25 percent have incomes between 100 and 200 percent of the federal poverty level (National Clearing House for Primary Care Information 1986). Prenatal and screening services are included in the authorizing legislation that defines the primary health services that must be provided by CHCs/MHCs.

The funding of prenatal screening techniques through clinics reveals two patterns that hamper equal access for low-income women. First, prenatal screening procedures in general are available in fewer states through health clinics in comparison to Medicaid funding. Only one technique, RhoGAM treatment, is funded at a comparable level with Medicaid; RhoGAM treatment is funded by 89 percent of the states through Maternal and Child Health Programs but by only 76 percent of the states through Community and Migrant Health Centers (Gold et al. 1987). More commonly, fewer states fund clinics to perform specific prenatal screening techniques than provide coverage through Medicaid. For example, while 92 percent of the forty-eight contiguous states fund nonstress testing techniques through Medicaid, only 81 percent fund the same technique through Maternal and Child Health Programs and a mere 41 percent of the states fund nonstress testing through Community and Migrant Health Centers (Gold et al. 1987).

The second pattern is the difference in coverage between the two clinic programs. Overall, fewer states fund prenatal screening techniques through Community and Migrant Health clinics than through Maternal and Child Health clinics. For example, 75 percent of the states fund amniocentesis in Maternal and Child Health Programs but only 20 perceent of the states fund it in Community and Migrant Health Centers (Gold et al. 1987). Low-income women or women of color who use these clinics obviously have less access to the prenatal screening techniques than women who qualify for Medicaid, and much less than women who have other forms of third-party coverage.

Access to prenatal screening via the clinic system is more than a matter of the procedures funded by each state because some clients will be asked to pay a small fee for the available procedure. In forty-two states, clients who receive Medicaid or whose income is at poverty level generally qualify for free screening by the procedures funded in that state and available in that clinic (Gold et al. 1987). However, poor clients above the poverty level may be asked to pay a fee, depending on the level of family income and the eligibility requirements established in that state (Gold et al. 1987). From the clients' point of view, having to pay even a small fee, which competes with their already scarce resources, means that obtaining prenatal screening may no longer be a viable option.

The waiting period to get into general prenatal care is another aspect of the Maternal and Child Health Program that influences the feasibility of obtaining prenatal screening. The average waiting period for new patients is about three weeks, but the length varies from state to state. In six states the average waiting period was one week or less, but in twelve states it was four weeks or longer. The average waiting period in Vermont was fourteen weeks, clearly precluding early entry into prenatal care (Gold et al. 1987). A long waiting period limits the practicality of utilizing certain prenatal procedures, and this is compounded if low-income women seek prenatal care late in their pregnancies. Even when a woman does enter care in time for a test, counseling and screening procedures may then have to be conducted in such haste that absorbing all the information may be very difficult. This increases the likelihood that women will make unwise decisions.

In addition to erratic funding and the waiting period, other barriers may restrict access to quality prenatal services. Some low-income women may not be able to utilize services that are funded in their state because the prenatal services are unevenly distributed in the state and are targeted, for example, to urban women. Research shows that women are more likely to use amniocentesis if they live in metropolitan rather than rural areas and if they have higher education levels. These findings hold true regardless of race (Marion et al. 1980; Gold et al. 1987), but black women residing in the rural South may have especially limited access to prenatal screening, if any is available at all.

In contrast, some studies show that women who live in rural areas and who are less educated are more likely to be subjected to prenatal screening using X-rays (Gold et al. 1987; Hamilton et al. 1984; Kleinman et al. 1983). Although exposure to X-rays during pregnancy has a negative effect on early fetal development, "it has been estimated that one-third could have had an ultrasound procedure instead for the same purposes (determining fetal position, fetal age, and multiple pregnancy)" (Gold et al. 1987, 12). The higher rate of X-ray screening techniques for rural women and more poorly educated women may be produced by several factors—ultrasound technology and personnel may not be available, clients may be less informed about the danger of X-rays to fetal health, or physicians may simply have less regard for their health. Regardless of the cause, the more frequent use of X-ray screening produces negative consequences for these populations (Gold et al. 1987; Kleinman et al. 1983).

In summary the funding of prenatal screening techniques, particularly through Medicaid, initially appears to be adequate. However, our analysis shows that many barriers to equal access exist for poor women, and this has a disproportionate impact on women of color. Some barriers such as "partial" coverage for amniocentesis and qualifying restrictions are built into the funding policy itself. Other barriers such as the waiting periods required in most clinics or the concentration of clinics in metropolitan areas arise from the administration of health services. Regardless of their source, poor women and women of color face numerous barriers to equal access to prenatal screening and quality prenatal care.

A particular example of illogical public policy is the limited access to abortion. While many poor women have access to some form of prenatal screening, very few have access to a funded abortion should they decide to terminate the pregnancy. Thus, for low-income women, prenatal screening technologies are much less able to contribute to their reproductive choice, not only because the availability of screening is determined by governmental funding policies but because the options for response are deliberately limited by law. The Hyde Amendment, passed in 1977, prohibits federal funding of an abortion except in cases of danger to the mother's life, even though the right to choose abortion is the law of the land.

A woman dependent upon Medicaid, MCHP, CHCs, or MHCs may be able to learn about the physical condition of her fetus but may be unable to afford an abortion, the only "treatment" alternative in most cases. Abortion following prenatal diagnosis is available through Medicaid in only sixteen states (Gold et al. 1987). Many women do not have private health insurance: in 1983, 14 percent of whites, 21.8 percent of blacks, and 29.1 percent of Hispanics were not covered by health insurance of any kind (*New York Times* 1985). For women who do not have access to governmentally funded services and do not have private health insurance, the combined cost of amniocentesis and a possible abortion can be prohibitive, especially since second trimester abortions after amniocentesis are not routinely offered in many locations, require hospitalization, and are consequently expensive.

The limited availability of abortion is especially illogical as in some instances the courts have defined the provision of information about termination of pregnancy as a necessary part of good medical care. But while the courts penalize physicians for not informing couples at risk of having children with genetic disorders of their abortion options, the states themselves deny low-income women the actual option of abortion (Bowman 1977). Unless public monies are sanctioned for abortion due to genetic disorders, many persons who cannot pay for a subsequent abortion may find programs to detect genetic disease pointless and refuse to participate.

Cultural Factors Affecting the Decision-Making Process

The screening technique is part of a larger genetic counseling process which ideally educates the person being counseled about possible etiology, prognosis, management, recurrence, risks, options, and resources relating to genetic diseases (Vargas and Wilkerson 1987). In the process of genetic counseling, the client and counselor develop a plan of prenatal care that encompasses whether or not to use a screening technique, which technique to use, and what options are desirable given the results of the screening. As with any decision-making process, the meanings attached to whatever is being communicated (the "results" of the screening and the options available) depend upon the individuals involved and their sociocultural environments (Sue 1987). When the topics being discussed are reproduction and possible abortion, the individual's core values, which are often unexamined or taken for granted, are likely to be tapped.

When the counselor and the client hold different class and racial/ethnic positions in society, the interaction is likely to exhibit differences in power and even attempts at social control. Low-income women and women of color, coming from communities whose worldviews often differ from the worldviews of majority communities and the medical profession, may experience a greater disjunction between their views and the views of the counselors than, say, white middleclass women. Luker (1984), for example, documents the impact of different class-based worldviews on reproductive issues in her study of prochoice and antichoice abortion activists, and Hall and Ferree (1986) discuss the different structures of abortion attitudes by race. In this section, we describe the historical background of population control as the context in which the reproductive decisions of poor women and women of color are made, examine three ways in which conflicting worldviews may be manifested, and discuss problems of informed consent and confidentiality that arise.

The new prenatal technologies frame the entire issue of reproduction for all women in terms of the dominant worldview. These technologies embody a definition of a reproductive problem which focuses on the fetus almost to the exclusion of the mother. Rothman (1986) and Petchesky (1987) graphically depict the way ultrasound procedures foster the definition of the mother as a "habitat" for the fetus which becomes a "man in space" entity falsely assumed to be capable of independent existence. Stanworth refers to the "eclipsing of the pregnant woman's part in childbearing" (1987, 26) evident in the language used to name the new conceptive technologies. The phrase *test-tube baby* ignores the nurturing womb, the term *artificial insemination* disguises the "normal" process of conception, pregnancy and birth once sperm are present, and *surrogacy* discredits the act of pregnancy as part of mothering.

But another aspect of the dominant worldview is the historical association between eugenics and most social policy programs addressing the reproductive activities of poor women and women of color. Davis (1983) and Gordon (1977 and 1982) document how the contraceptive movement shifted from birth control (understood as women's choice) to population control for state purposes in the nineteenth century. Initially advocated by feminists, socialists, and even black radicals, the birth control movement was an attempt to provide women with more reproductive choices. However, by the 1930s, the ". . . birth control movement was increasingly absorbed into programs aimed not at self-determination but at social control by the elite" (Gordon 1982, 47). Policies were promoted to maintain the dominance of the native-born white population while restricting the reproductive activities of other segments such as immigrants, blacks, and native Americans. Davis notes the political tone of the population control movement when she states,

> class-bias and racism crept into the birth control movement when it was still in its infancy. More and more, it was assumed within birth control circles that poor women, Black and immigrant alike, have a "moral obligation to restrict the size of their families." What was demanded as a "right" for the privileged came to be interpreted as a "duty" for the poor (Davis 1983, 210).

This "duty" of the poor to have fewer children who might possibly need welfare and other governmental services has become an underlying theme of federally funded programs. One of the most blatant expressions of the population control thesis is the involuntary sterilization of women of color. Dreifus (1977) documents how some medical residents developed their surgical skills by performing tubal ligations on Hispanic women who were uninformed or misinformed of the operation they were undergoing. Davis (1983) describes several cases in which black teenagers were sterilized through various governmental agencies, including Department of Health, Education and Welfare–funded birth control clinics. Native American women have also been sterilized at high rates; one out of every four women giving birth in the Indian Health Services Hospital in Claremore, Oklahoma, was subsequently sterilized (Davis 1983). Current figures for Puerto Rican women indicate that over 35 percent have been sterilized (Davis 1983).

Given the increasing feasibility of "selecting good genes," those who are concerned about the new reproductive technology should also be concerned that we may be entering a new eugenic era (Bowman 1977). As in the 1920s, an enthusiasm for using a person's genetic makeup to make judgments about his or her social worth once again has surfaced. Decisions on who has access to the new technologies will continue to be influenced by age and race as well as more subjective factors. Subtle and not so subtle pressures will be put on women who are being counseled depending upon their socioeconomic status.

The reproductive technologies administered through federally funded programs are perceived by poor women and women of color within this tradition of eugenics and population control. The meanings and values associated with having children and abortion are often played out between a white, educated genetic counselor and a poor black or Hispanic client against a historical background of distrust, control, and unequal power.

Within this historical context, three dimensions of conflict in worldview are likely to occur for low-income and minority women. First, in many cultures people see themselves as having little control over their fate or feel as though they should not interfere with the will of God. For example, many Southeast Asians believe that amniocentesis interferes with natural selection of the population that is considered sacred (Asian Pacific Health News 1986). Devout Roman Catholics often view disability as God's will. Instead of assuming all cultures share the same attitudes, it is important to recognize cultural diversity, even within the seeming unity of the predominant Catholic Latino culture (see, e.g., Almquist 1984). Given the uniqueness of their historical treatment by governmentally funded health services, it is likely that Cuban, Chicana, and Puerto Rican women have different attitudes towards reproductive technology.

Second, different individuals and cultural groups have differing perceptions of the levels of disability they can cope with and what it might be like to live with a disability. In her in-depth study of poor women and women of color in genetic counseling sessions, Rapp observed a Puerto Rican single mother who chose to continue pregnancy after a prenatal diagnosis of Kleinfelter's disease, a genetic abnormality that results from an extra female chromosome. The woman said of her now four-year-old son: "He's normal, he growing up normal, as long as there is nothing wrong that shows, he isn't blind or deaf or crippled, he's normal" (Rapp 1987). In contrast, a professional couple faced with information that their child would be born with Kleinfelter's syndrome told Rapp that "If he was gonna be slow, if he wasn't gonna have a shot at being president, that's not the baby we want" (Rapp 1987, 12).

Third, culture will affect ideas about how to interact with authority figures and who should be included in the decision-making process within the family structure. Harwood (1981) finds that some Puerto Rican patients are unwilling to show they did not understand or agree with an authority figure such as a physician. The medical model assumes the individual patient is the paramount decision maker for testing and treatment. But for many women of color, other family members, even extended family members, may be of prime significance in the decision-making process (Harwood 1981). These and other dimensions of the worldview will heavily influence the perception of the appropriateness of abortion under specific circumstances.

Problems can and do occur in the communication process between the genetic counselor and the client because the ethics, language, attitudes, religious beliefs, and ethnicity of both the counselor and client come into play (Vargas and Wilkerson 1987). When the client's financial situation and education level unduly influence the counselor's style and emphasis, the counseling process can become directive and judgmental. For instance, Rapp interviewed a genetic counselor who said "It is often hard for a counselor to be value free. Oh, I know I'm supposed to be value free, but when you see a welfare mother having a third baby with a man who is not gonna support her, and the fetus has sickle-cell anemia, it's hard not to steer her toward an abortion. What does she need this added problem for, I'm thinking" (Rapp 1987).

Informed Consent

The legal principle that competent adult patients should have the right to decide what is to become of their bodies is firmly grounded in case law and state statutes (Andrews 1984). Patient decision making is protected under the doctrine of informed consent which requires that patient's authorization for the diagnostic or treatment option be ". . . intentional, substantially non-controlled and based on substantial understanding" (Faden et al. 1986, 56). Informed consent is impaired when clients are not given information (see Farfel and Holtzman 1984 regarding such situations with sickle-cell anemia), or when the information given is not understandable or is interpreted through different cultural filters.

Cultural factors can hamper informed consent on at least three levels. First, certain medical information may not be salient within the sociocultural context of low-income clients. For example, Rapp discovered that there was no recognition of and no Creole word for Down's syndrome among recent Haitian immigrants (Rapp 1987). Second, some low-income clients can not understand the medical terminology being used or interpret the medical information being given. Genetic counseling often relies upon ratios or odds to define possible risks, e.g., the results of screening techniques are couched as a one in two hundred chance of having a child with a particular condition. Whether a risk of one in two hundred is perceived as acceptable or not varies with the client's class and racial status as well as with previous exposure to people with this condition.

Third, the client may prioritize the medical problems differently from the physician or genetic counselor. For example, a mother of a Down syndrome baby told a genetic counselor, "My kid's got a heart problem, my kid's gonna be slow. First let me deal with that, love him for that, then I'll check out this Down's syndrome thing" (Rapp 1987, 13). To the physician, the heart problem and retardation are merely symptoms of the Down's syndrome; to the mother the "syndrome" is irrelevant compared to the specific needs of her child.

Confidentiality

Confidentiality in the prenatal screening process is an extremely important issue for people of color who have experienced adverse consequences when intimate information is revealed to third parties. Prenatal screening increases the amount and type of information included in medical files which, if revealed, could harm the reputation of individuals, increase family conflict, or restrict education or employment opportunities (Winslade 1982). Negative consequences have been documented for sickle-cell trait carriers when information was made available to third parties; employers refused to hire, promote, or even retain identified workers (Hubbard and Henifin 1984) and insurance companies refused health and life insurance coverage or inflated the cost of coverage even though sickle-cell trait has not been linked to shortened life spans (Hubbard and Henifin 1984).

When certain social groups are defined as "deviant," there is a heightened possibility of confidentiality being abused. Low-income people may more frequently be found in three such "deviant" groups, namely, unwed mothers, adolescent parents, and people who have a high risk of contracting AIDS. Unwed adolescent women fear the knowledge of their sexual activity and/or pregnancy will be revealed to their parents, and unwed adult male partners fear that their identity and whereabouts will be revealed to public officials who are mandated to collect child support (Bowman 1977). In addition, the woman herself may avoid seeking prenatal services if she fears she will be required to involve her male partner in genetic screening. Including AIDS screening in general prenatal services, as recommended by the Centers for Disease Control (CDC), may prevent some women in high-risk groups from seeking prenatal care in the first place because they fear abuses of confidentiality.

Infertility and Alternative Modes of Reproduction

In this chapter, infertility is defined as the inability to conceive over a period of twelve months or more of unprotected intercourse; impaired fecundity refers to both infertility and inability to carry a pregnancy to term. In response to the problem of infertility, the medical profession has focused on high-tech modes of reproduction. Most of these infertility procedures are extremely costly and have a disappointingly low success rate (see Corea 1985, 179–80). Nevertheless, significant research funding and enthusiasm are geared toward helping a small number of women conceive and bear healthy babies in this way. The infertility of these women has been defined as a "social problem" significant enough to warrant the expenditure of extensive technological resources. But is the infertility of members of minority communities also defined as a social problem? Or do the fertility and fecundity problems of minority communities involve a different set of meanings and values?

By emphasizing expensive and often unsuccessful reproductive technologies, the priorities of the medical and scientific community deemphasize other basic societal and medical problems that have a more substantial impact on women's ability to bear healthy children. Many of these problems could be addressed without recourse to new reproductive technologies. For example, improved education, health care, nutrition, and working conditions could dramatically enhance the ability of poor women and women of color to bear healthy children. But these problems receive far fewer dollars from researchers and social policy makers. In addition, because high-tech reproduction provides a solution only at the individual level, such resource allocation in effect devalues the structural and societal causes of fertility/infertility.

Infertility in the Minority Community

Infertility rates clearly vary by race and income group. Married black women have an infertility rate one and one-half times higher than that of married white women (Mosher and Pratt 1982, 3). The difference by race may be even higher because underreporting of infertility is minimal among married white women but substantial among married black women (Henshaw and Orr 1987). The rate of impaired fecundity is also higher: in 1981 the fetal mortality rate for blacks was approximately 1.5 times the rate for whites (U.S. Department of Health and Human Services 1985).

Many factors contribute to the higher rate of infertility among minority couples. Structural antecedents of infertility in nonwhite women include genetic conditions such as sickle-cell anemia; general health status, which may be affected, for example, by nutritional deficiencies; and alcohol or drug abuse (U.S. Department of Health and Human Services 1985). Other reasons for high infertility among poor women and women of color include a differential rate of exposure to damaging medical or environmental conditions: sterilization abuse (Childbearing Rights to Information Project 1982), unnecessary hysterectomies (CDC 1983), and unsafe or experimental birth control methods, especially intrauterine devices (IUDs) (Corea 1985). Poor people and people of color are also more likely to be exposed to hazardous working conditions which can produce miscarriages and infertility (Mullings 1984).

The functioning of these factors producing infertility and their implications for low-income women and women of color can be illustrated with pelvic inflammatory diseases (PID). One study found that the rates of pelvic inflammatory disease for nonwhite women are twice the rates among white women (U.S. Department of Health and Human Services 1985). Poor women of color are more likely to be exposed to the causes of PID—untreated gonorrhea, chlamydia bacteria, and IUDs. Several studies document the linkage between PID and infertility. Doyal (1987) reports that tubal damage occurs in 12 percent of the women who experience one attack of PID, 40 percent of the women who experience two attacks, and 80 percent of the women who have three or more attacks of PID.

Because infertility as a medical condition exists at a higher rate in the minority community than in the population at large, one important question is whether the existence of this medical need is defined as a social problem for these communities and addressed by a treatment program. Are technologies and medical treatments that address infertility actually available to low-income women and women of color?

Access Barriers to the New Modes of Reproduction

Access to the new modes of reproduction is an issue for all women due to the expense of these procedures. For example, each invitro fertilization procedure costs from $3,500 to $5,000 per attempt and most couples make several attempts before achieving pregnancy,[2] even though few ever bear a child (Lorber and Green 1987; Laborie 1987). Because private insurers rarely cover such procedures, the new reproductive technologies are often beyond the reach of even middle-class women (Corea 1986). The needs of poor and minority women for infertility services receive virtually no attention in the for-profit health care system of the United States.

Although family planning services are mandated to provide services to women and their families to aid conception as well as to prevent it (U.S. Department of Health and Human Services 1980), governmental concerns are primarily focused upon reducing fertility of minority and low-income people rather than improving it. Medicaid reimbursement for fertility services is available to no more than one-third of the poor women who need these services (Henshaw and Orr 1987). Henshaw also found that among those in need, black women are less likely than nonblacks, and low-income women are less likely than higher-income women to have obtained services.

Nonfinancial barriers that restrict access to the new modes of reproduction focus upon the characteristics of the clients. Most invitro clinics are highly selective about their clients, accepting only married, heterosexual women with adequate resources (Corea 1985, 145). Imposing this particular definition of an "appropriate" client has a differential effect on poor and minority women. For example, in 1985 over half (57.3 percent) of black women were not married (U.S. Bureau of Census 1987). To allow providers to decide who is a "deserving and appropriate client" (Corea 1986) is a dangerous practice. As Margaret Somerville writes, "We must be aware of the potential for dangerous precedents that we open up when we start to regulate such matters of reproduction and parenting. What is regarded as deviance can depend simply on what the decision-maker sees as desirable or undesirable traits, characteristics, or conduct" (Somerville 1982, 123).

A further implication is that poor women and women of color are highly vulnerable to "consenting" to experimental procedures in order to gain access to infertility services when governmental funding is so restricted and definitions of the "appropriate" client so firmly entrenched. It is imperative that poor women and women of color not be given access only to become the subjects of experiments, and that technological developments not be tested on poor women and women of color without their genuine consent (see Corea 1985, 166–68 regarding the lack of informed consent for invitro fertilization procedures).

The impact of this restricted access to infertility services is heightened for many poor and minority women due to the cultural meanings attached to having children and being a mother. Motherhood and family life are highly valued in most working class and minority communities (Billingsly 1968; Rapp 1982; McAdoo 1985). Therefore, losing the option of procreating and parenting can be devastating. Infertility may be especially problematic for some men in cultures where masculinity is at least partially based on the ability to father children (Billingsly 1968; Rapp 1982; McAdoo 1985; Baca Zinn and Eitzen 1987; Griswold del Castillo 1984; Ramirez and Arce 1981). While "informal adoption" among members of the extended family is prevalent in many cultures, formal adoption agencies often exclude people of color or may impose many socioeconomic barriers. Even minority people who believe in legal adoption may be wary of the bureaucratic structure of the adoption process.[3]

This summary of the needs of low-income women and women of color for infertility services and barriers to access reveals familiar and expected patterns—low-income women and women of color have at least as great a need for the new conceptive technologies but less access to them, and the significance of these barriers is heightened by the cultural meanings attached to mothering and bearing children for many of these women and families. Although we do not wish to devalue in any way the impact of these patterns on the lives of low-income women and women of color, we wish to address how these patterns as a whole reflect the more general issue of the social construction of fertility/infertility as a social problem requiring a "medical solution."

Perhaps even more than prenatal screening, technologies addressing infertility appear, at least initially, to dovetail with our ideologies of motherhood. In its most prevalent form, the ideology of motherhood defines the bearing (and rearing) of children as the primary function and most rewarding experience of all women. At first glance, technologies addressing infertility appear to answer the presumed "desperation of infertility," as Pfeffer (1987) calls the medical characterization of the issue. Given these assumptions, however, the access patterns summarized above appear "illogical"—the availability of few resources and the limitations of these resources to "suitable couples" can not be explained by the much broader need for the services nor by the allegedly universal significance of motherhood. Even more illogical is failure to direct resources at preventing various causes of infertility.

How then can we understand the definition of infertility as a medical and/or social problem that promotes high-tech programs of limited success and these "illogical" patterns of access? Like the medical profession's efforts to control abortion during the 1800s (Luker 1984), Pfeffer (1987) attributes the physicians' endorsement of infertility technologies in England to the increased professional status and income these technologies provide to a segment of the medical community that has previously had low status in medicine. This explanation is consistent with the new experts' focus on treating only the physical aspects of fertility (see Doyal, 1987, for a critique), the disinterest in prevention of infertility, and the predominance of ability to pay as the key to access.

Additionally, however, population control groups have historically tended to define the problem of infertility as the absence of white babies for married couples who are able to pay for them. If reproductive technologies are instead understood as a means to *birth* control— that is, increasing women's choices about when and how many children they have—the absence of concern about infertility among low-income women and women of color is itself a serious social and political problem. Resources to prevent and treat infertility in nonwhite and poor women are a necessary part of a reproductive policy that genuinely increases all women's choices.

Conclusions and Recommendations

Our analysis has shown that although most of the prenatal screening techniques may be partially funded and available, poor women and women of color do not have equal social access to them. Even worse is poor women's relative lack of conceptive technologies in comparison to affluent women. To provide all women with the option of using these reproductive technologies, to make it a personal or familial choice to utilize these forms of care, we urge that all women have financial, geographic, and social access to prenatal diagnostic and conceptive

procedures. Funding is the key but not the only ingredient in this recommendation; the availability and purpose of these technologies should
be publicized and the existing qualifying restrictions should be evaluated and removed if they function as barriers to access. Funding should
extend to more than the poorest women who qualify for Medicaid; the
state and community should be the funders of last resort for the near-
poor who are not covered by Medicaid or private insurance and who
do not have access to public clinics.

Once poor women and women of color are involved in genetic
counseling, our analysis has shown that a variety of cultural factors
disrupt the communication and education process. These disruptions
appear to reinforce the dominant worldview of medical intervention in
women's reproductive experience. Therefore, we recommend that informed consent forms be required and written in simple, understandable terms, and in a language appropriate to the community in which
they are distributed. Test results, particularly those involving sensitive
areas, should be confidential and not part of the patient's medical
record. Legal provisions guaranteeing confidentiality should be
strengthened.

Furthermore, the negative influence of cultural factors in the counseling process should be specifically addressed. First, minority genetic
counselors should be recruited. Black, Hispanic, and Asian health
professionals, including social workers, physicians, counselors, and
nurses, should be encouraged to learn genetic counseling in order to
increase the availability of counselors who are familiar with a client's
culture, religion, and language, and who share their attitudes toward
death, disease, abortion, and disability. Second, graduate genetic counseling curricula should include classes on counseling culturally diverse
populations, and graduates of past programs should be informed of the
availability of continuing education. Where such courses are not available, they should be instituted. Licensing agencies and institutions
should emphasize the need for such courses. And lastly, representatives
of the minority groups to be served should be involved in the design,
development, and operation of genetic programs from the onset.

Our analysis has shown that the major problem here is the medical
and social construction of infertility. The first effect of this construction
is that in the view of the majority population, infertility is a "nonissue"
for low-income women and women of color. Promoting this construction of infertility is the popular perception that poor women do not
deserve help in having babies because they are already "too fertile";
hence the unpopularity and/or impracticality of supporting programs
to help women on welfare to have more children. However, the more

important effect of this construction is the focus upon high-tech "treatments" for a selective number and type of individual women instead of the allocation of resources to the structural causes of infertility which would benefit a larger number of women and, more specifically, low-income women and women of color. Funding and public policy attention should be redirected from high-technology reproductive procedures to the prevention of infant mortality, to the provision of better nutrition, and to other health services. Specifically, health education programs and services geared toward good follow-up care after abortion and childbirth, toward prompt treatment of sexually transmitted diseases and PID, and toward the ending of contraceptive and sterilization abuse will do much to improve the reproductive health and increase the reproductive options for poor women and women of color.

Finally, we urge that the health and reproductive concerns of women of color be put at the center of feminist analysis. This recommendation has been made by others, who note specific benefits for feminist theory and practice by looking at gender, race, and class as interlocking systems of oppression (e.g., hooks 1984, Andersen 1988, Hill-Collins 1986). In particular, this perspective helps all women to see reproductive health technologies and the health care system as part of an entire social system, and not as isolated phenomena.

The basic purpose of reproductive health technologies ought to be to enable a woman to deliver a healthy baby when she wants to do so. Between this "theory" and the actual "practice" of the system is an enormous gap. From the perspective of women of color, all barriers to the reproductive technologies now available must be removed to provide real options and to meet the needs of individual women. But only by questioning our faith in technological progress, by illuminating the larger framework of medical care and reproduction, can we meet the collective needs of poor women or women of color. Placing their needs and experiences at the center of our analysis of reproductive technologies elucidates the operation of ideological as well as the structural factors in health care delivery. We can be more critical of how the ideology of motherhood and the drive to have "a child of one's own" are used to justify expensive and exclusive technologies when we are more aware of how that ideology is *not* applied to poor women, who also need better public health measures, access to the conventional technologies of prenatal care, and protection from sterilization abuse and other medically or environmentally induced forms of infertility.

In sum, if we begin from the perspective of women of color or low income, we see reproductive health technology as just one small piece of a health care system that is neither structurally nor ideologically prepared to meet all women's needs. Changing this will require more than creating access to any particular technology or developing new technology, because even the most useful technology is only a means, not an end in itself. The social, economic, medical, and legal context in which women's reproductive health concerns are acknowledged or ignored is important for *all* women, and the perspective of women of color and low income may help us to recognize this essential truth.

N O T E S

1. This survey information is based on a response from thirty states.
2. Personal communication with spokesperson of the American Fertility Society in Birmingham, Alabama, January, 1988.
3. Personal communication with Devera Foreman, a member of Philadelphia Black Psychologists, 1986.

B I B L I O G R A P H Y

Almquist, Elizabeth. 1984. Race and ethnicity in the lives of minority women. In *Women: a feminist perspective,* ed. Jo Freeman, 423–53. Palo Alto: Mayfield.
Andersen, Margaret. 1988. Moving our minds: Studying women of color and reconstructing sociology. *Teaching Sociology* 16, no. 2: 123–32.
Andrews, Lori. 1987. *Medical genetics: a legal frontier.* Chicago: American Bar Association.
Arkansas Genetic Program. 1987. *Amniocentesis.* Pamphlet sponsored by the Arkansas Center for Medical Science. Little Rock, Ark.
Asian Pacific Health News. 1985. *Asian Health Project.* Los Angeles.
Baca Zinn, Maxine, and D. Stanley Eitzen. 1987. *Diversity in American families.* New York: Harper and Row.
Billingsley, Andrew. 1968. *Black families in white America.* Englewood Cliffs, N.J.: Prentice-Hall.
Bowman, James E. 1983. Is a national program to prevent sickle cell disease possible? *American Journal of Pediatric Hematology/Oncology* 5, no. 4: 367–72.
Callahan, Daniel. 1973. The meaning and significance of genetic disease: Philosophical Perspectives. In *Ethical issues in human genetics: Genetic counseling and the use of genetic knowledge,* ed. Bruce Hilton, Daniel Callahan, M. Harris, P. Condliffe, and B. Berkley, 83–88. New York: Plenum Press.
Centers for Disease Control. 1983. Surgical sterilization surveillance: Tubal sterilization and hysterectomy in women aged 15–44, summary 1979–1980. Atlanta, Ga.

Childbearing Rights Information Project. 1982. *For ourselves, our families, and future: The struggle for childbearing rights.* Boston: Red Sun Press.
Corea, Gena. 1985. *The mother machine.* New York: Harper and Row.
Davis, Angela. 1983. *Women, race and class.* New York: Random House.
Doyal, Lesley. 1987. Infertility—a life sentence? Women and the national health service. In *Reproductive technologies: gender, motherhood, and medicine,* ed. Michelle Stanworth, 174–90. Minneapolis: University of Minnesota Press.
Dreifus, Claudia. 1977. Sterilizing the poor. In *Seizing our bodies: The politics of women's health,* ed. Claudia Dreifus, 105–21. New York: Random House.
Faden, Ruth, and Tom Beauchamp with Nancy King. 1986. *A history and theory of informed consent.* New York: Oxford University Press.
Farfel, Mark, and Neil Holtzman. 1984. Education, consent and counseling in sickle cell screening programs: Report of a survey. *American Journal of Public Health* 74, no. 4: 373–75.
Gold, Rachel, Kenny Benson, Maria Asta, and Susheeia Singh. 1987. *The financing of maternity care in the United States.* New York: Alan Guttmacher Institute.
Gordon, Linda. 1977. *Woman's body, woman's right.* Harmondsworth, England: Penguin.
———. 1982. Why nineteenth-century feminists did not support "birth control" and twentieth-century feminists do: Feminism, reproduction, and the family. In *Rethinking the family: Some feminist questions,* ed. Barrie Thorne with Marilyn Yalom, 40–54. New York: Longman.
Greenstein, Robert. 1987. Summary of conference proceedings. Paper presented at a conference entitled The challenge to provide genetic services: reimbursement for medical genetic services. Boston, Mass.
Griswold del Castillo, Richard. 1984. *La familia: Chicano families in the urban southwest, 1984 to present.* South Bend, Ind.: University of Notre Dame Press.
Hall, Elaine J., and Myra Marx Ferree. 1986. Race differences in abortion attitudes. *Public Opinion Quarterly* 50, no. 2: 193–207.
Hamilton, Peggy, Paul L. Roney, Kenneth Keppel, and Paul Placek. 1984. Radiation procedures performed on U.S. women during pregnancy: Findings from two 1980 surveys. *Public Health Reports* 99, no. 2: 146–51.
Harwood, Alan. 1981. *Ethnicity and medical care.* Cambridge: Harvard University Press.
Henshaw, Stanley, and Margaret T. Orr. 1987. The need and unmet need for fertility services in the United States. *Family Planning Perspectives* 19, no. 4: 180–83, 186.
Hill-Collins, Patricia. 1986. Learning from the outsider within: The sociological significance of black feminist thought. *Social Problems* 33, no. 5: 514–32.
hooks, bell. 1984. *Feminist theory from margin to center.* Boston: South End Press.
Hubbard, Ruth, and Mary Sue Henifin. 1984. Genetic screening of prospective parents and of workers. In *Biomedical Ethics Reviews,* ed. James M. Humber and Robert Almeder, 92–100. Clifton, N.J.: Humana Press.

Kleinman, Joel C., Margaret Cooke, Steven Machlin, and Samuel Kessel. 1983. Variations and use of obstetric technology. *Health: United States, 1983.* Washington, D.C.: Government Printing Office.

Laborie, Francoise. 1987. Some information about the development of reproductive technologies in France. Paper presented at the Third International Interdisciplinary Congress of Women, Dublin.

Lorber, Judith, and Dorothy Green. 1987. Couples' experiences with *in-vitro* fertilization: a follow-up study. Paper presented at the Third International Interdisciplinary Congress of Women, Dublin.

Luker, Kristin. 1984. *Abortion and the politics of motherhood.* Berkeley: University of California Press.

Marion, Janet P., Gulzar Kassman, Paul M. Fernhoff, Karlene Brantley, Linda Carroll, June Zacharias, Luella Klein, Jean H. Priest, and Louis Elsas II. 1980. Acceptance of amniocentesis by low-income patients in an urban hospital. *American Journal of Obstetrics and Gynecology* 138, no. 1: 11–15.

McAdoo, Harriet Pipes. 1985. Black mothers and the extended family support network. In *The Black woman,* ed. La Frances Rodgers-Rose, 125–44. Beverly Hills: Sage.

Mosher, William D., and William F. Pratt. 1982. Reproductive impairments among married couples. *Vital and Health Statistics.* U.S. National Center for Health Statistics. Series 23, no. 11. Washington, D.C.: Government Printing Office.

Mullings, Leith. 1984. Minority women, work and health. In *Double exposure: Women's health hazards on the job and at home,* ed. Wendy Chavkin, 121–38. New York: New Feminist Library.

National Clearing House for Primary Care Information. 1986. Community health centers: a quality system for the changing health care market. Pamphlet. McLean, Va.

New York Times. 1985. Fifteen percent of Americans found to lack health insurance. February 18, A13.

Petchesky, Rosalind. 1987. Foetal images: the power of visual culture in the politics of abortion. In *Reproductive technologies: Gender, motherhood, and medicine,* ed. Michelle Stanworth, 57–80. Minneapolis: University of Minnesota Press.

Pfeffer, Naomi. 1987. Artificial insemination, in-vitro fertilization and the stigma of infertility. In *Reproductive technologies: Gender, motherhood, and medicine,* ed. Michelle Stanworth, 81–97. Minneapolis: University of Minnesota Press.

Placek, Paul. 1984. Electronic fetal monitoring in relation to cesarean section delivery of live-birth and stillbirths in the U.S., 1980. *Public Health Reports* 99, no. 2: 173–83.

Ramirez, Oscar, and Carlos H. Arce. 1981. The contemporary Chicano family: An empirically based review. In *Explorations in Chicano Psychology,* ed. Augustine Baron Jr., 3–28. New York: Praeger.

Rapp, Rayna. 1982. Family and class in contemporary America: Notes toward an understanding of ideology. In *Rethinking the family: Some feminist questions,* ed. by Barrie Thorne with Marilyn Yalom, 168–87. New York: Longman.

———. 1987. Moral pioneers: Women, men and fetuses on a frontier of reproductive technology. Lecture delivered in Storrs, Connecticut.

Rothman, Barbara Katz. 1986. *The tentative pregnancy.* New York: Viking.

Somerville, Margaret A. 1982. Birth technology, parenting and "deviance." *International Journal of Law and Psychiatry* 5, no. 2: 123–53.

Stanworth, Michelle. 1987. Reproductive technologies and the deconstruction of motherhood. In *Reproductive technologies: Gender, motherhood, and medicine,* ed. by Michelle Stanworth, 10–36. Minneapolis: University of Minnesota Press.

Sue, Derald. 1981. *Counseling the culturally different: Theory and practice.* New York: John Wiley and Sons.

U.S. Bureau of the Census. 1987. *Statistical Abstract of the United States, 1987,* 38. Washington, D.C.: Government Printing Office.

U.S. Department of Health and Human Services. Public Health Services. 1980. *Promoting health/preventing disease: objectives for the nation.* Washington, D.C.: Government Printing Office.

U.S. Department of Health and Human Services. Public Health Services. 1985. Health status of minorities and low-income groups. *American statistical index.* HRSA HRS-P-DV-85-1. Washington, D.C.: Government Printing Office.

Vargas, Maria, and Lorna Wilkerson. 1987. Defining our cultures and bridging the gap. In *Strategies in genetic counseling: Religious, cultural and ethnic influences on the counseling process,* ed. Patricia Magyari, Natalie Paul, and Barbara Bieseker. March of Dimes/Birth Defects Foundation Original Article Series, 23, no. 6: 167–87. New York: Allen R. Liss.

Winslade, William J. 1982. Confidentiality of medical records: An overview of concepts and legal practices. *Journal of Legal Medicine* 3, no. 4: 497–533.

Technology in Childbirth: Effects on Postpartum Moods

Lynne C. Garner and Richard C. Tessler

As the reliance on technological interventions in health care becomes more ubiquitous, there is an increased need to understand their wide-ranging impact. Exploring the relationship between obstetrical technology and postpartum moods serves as an important case study for several reasons. First, unlike rarer forms of medical technology such as in vitro fertilization and hormone replacement therapy, obstetrical technology is used by the vast majority of American women. Only 10 percent of women over 44 are childless (U.S. Bureau of the Census 1982), and the use of obstetrical technology is widespread. Second, by most estimates postpartum blues affect the majority of childbearing women (Entwisle and Doering 1981). Finally, as we will show in a later section of this paper, the loss of personal control, a frequent by-product of the new birth technologies, may influence the incidence of postpartum moods.

Considered for many years to be a hormonal phenomenon, postpartum moods are increasingly linked to modern obstetrical technologies. The present chapter reports new data about this linkage. Our major premise is that technological interventions in hospital births lead to women's perceptions of loss of control and to disturbances of mood during the postpartum period. As background to the study, we first trace the history of the medicalization of childbirth in America, and then review some prior studies of moods in the puerperium, the period during and just after a woman gives birth.

Technology and Childbirth in America

Before childbirth became a medical event, it was attended by lay midwives in the homes of birthing women. Childbirth was viewed as a natural physiological process; one with risks, certainly, but normal nonetheless. In addition to the midwife, the women who were closest to the birthing women were also in attendance. Wertz and Wertz (1979) characterize this type of birth as "social childbirth." Gradually during the nineteenth century and into the twentieth, male physicians became increasingly involved and they brought with them new birth technologies.

119

The first and most important technical innovation was forceps. Because they were used by physicians and not by midwives, their use increased physicians' status as birth attendants and began to transform attitudes about birth: instead of a natural process it became one requiring specialized intervention. By the latter part of the nineteenth century, physicians had become the attendant of choice for most upper- and middle-class women. New procedures in gynecological surgery, the first use of anesthesia during delivery in 1847 and of twilight sleep in 1914, and the use of ergot to stimulate uterine contractions all enhanced the status of birth assisted by physicians (Litoff 1978).

By the 1930s and the 1940s midwives were becoming increasingly rare. In 1948, there were 14.3 lay midwives per 100,000 population; in 1973, there were only 1.1, and the majority of them were in five southeastern states (Rosengren 1980).

The evolution of physician-attended birth paralleled the increased use of hospitals as the birth setting. The use of sterile conditions, the professionalization of nursing, and the increased involvement with medical schools made hospitals an appropriate setting for the new concept of childbirth and the new interventionist approach to birthing (Starr 1982). Furthermore, it was more efficient to have patients come to the doctor, rather than to have the doctor come to the patients. Women, particularly those from the upper and middle class, also played a role in the movement to hospital births (Leavitt 1984). By the middle of the twentieth century, it was clear that the jurisdiction of medicine had expanded into the area of childbirth, and that in this sense childbirth had been "medicalized" (Conrad and Schneider 1980).

Prior Studies of Disturbance in Postpartum Moods

The studies of moods in the early postpartum are, for the most part, studies of the syndrome called postpartum blues. An understanding of the syndrome is complicated by the various names associated with the subject of women's moods shortly following birth. Postpartum blues, also called maternity blues or four-day blues, is considered by many people both in and out of the medical profession to be a normal and fleeting reaction to childbirth. The incidence of postpartum blues has been estimated at between 34 and 83 percent of all women who give birth, with most estimates approximating 80 percent (Entwisle and Doering 1981; Dalton 1971).

Postpartum blues needs to be distinguished from postpartum depression, which occurs over a number of weeks or even months after delivery. Dalton (1971) estimates that the incidence of postpartum depression is 7 to 10 percent of all birthing women, whereas Paykel et al. (1980) suggest that the number may be closer to 20 percent. Because of their far greater prevalence, access for study, and possibly greater sensitivity to environmental contingencies, postpartum blues and moods, not depression, are the focus of this paper.

The symptoms of postpartum blues are most often described as sudden episodes of crying, feeling depressed and in low spirits, being particularly vulnerable to criticism, and being mildly confused as to everyday events (Yalom et al. 1968). These symptoms typically occur after birth. Perhaps because of this close temporal link between birth and postpartum moods, the most frequently cited explanation for these moods has been biological. Accordingly, many observers including physicians believe that the cause of depressed moods shortly after birth lies in the sudden change in hormonal levels following delivery. To test this hypothesis, most studies attempt to correlate hormonal levels with postpartum moods. But the results in support of this hypothesis have been mixed at best (Cleary 1981).

One of the more frequently cited studies linking hormones to blues is by Yalom et al. (1986). In their sample of thirty-nine women, nine women who have had one child and thirty women with more than one child, the majority of women reported crying episodes that lasted at least five minutes during their first ten postpartum days. For some, the crying spells lasted for hours. Greater dysphoria (anxiety, depression, and restlessness) was also reported in the first ten postpartum days than during late pregnancy, or in the eighth month after birth. Women with higher depression and crying scores tended to have had their first period at a younger age, have more menstrual difficulty and longer length of menstrual flow, few children, and a longer interval since last pregnancy.

Findings associating hormones with postpartum moods were also reported by Stein et al. (1976) in a study of eighteen women. Self-ratings of tearfulness, depression, anxiety, loss of appetite, and insomnia seven to eight days postpartum were positively related to levels of hormones in the blood. In another study of 100 women seven to ten days after birth, one-half were diagnosed as having the "blues" (Pitt 1973). Of the women who choose to breast-feed their babies, more in the "blues" group were having difficulty nursing than the "nonblues" breast-feeders. Pitt thus concludes that the changes in progesterone and estrogen levels during postpartum may be significant in explaining both the blues and problems with breast-feeding. However, Pitt fails to account for the fact that social and psychological factors, including factors related to the management of the delivery, may be the cause of a greater percentage of the "blues" women experiencing difficulty breast-feeding.

Other studies have focused on the link between moods around the time of birth and other biological factors. Heitler (1976) measured both blues and more serious levels of depression in ninety-one women and found that the combined effect of loss of sleep, the duration of labor, delivery stress, and physical discomfort was significantly correlated with postpartum blues. In a similar vein, Pitt (1977) states that perineal soreness, often exacerbated by an episiotomy, may contribute to postpartum blues.

In the studies mentioned above, as with most research on moods after childbirth, there has been little systematic attention to the effects of technology on postpartum moods. Few studies consider the birth experience in their analyses, and they often fail to make note of the actual variation in the management of labor and delivery. Births by caesarean section are sometimes excluded from study because they are not "normal" births, and investigators routinely fail to report whether chemically induced or stimulated deliveries were included in the sample or to separate out such cases in the analysis. Studies also fail to take account of hormones administered after delivery to stem bleeding or suppress lactation. Not only is the variation in obstetrical procedures ignored, but there is also little attention given to women's attitudes and subjective responses to birth under these varying technological conditions.

The tendency to ignore technology as a variable in childbirth is unfortunate because studies that do measure it report frequent use. Arms (1979) found that 45 percent of the deliveries in her data were stimulated and 12 percent were induced by hormones. Oakley's (1980) data show that close to one-quarter of the sample, 22 percent in 1975 and 24 percent in 1976, had induced labors. In the Entwisle and Doering (1981) sample, 48 percent of the women had their membranes artificially ruptured.

The current research builds on the studies by Oakley (1980) and Entwisle and Doering (1981), which are among the first to consider nonbiological (social) factors. Oakley found that blues and depression were positively associated with the use of technological interventions in the management of labor and delivery. In particular, the use of epidural anesthesia, instrument delivery, and the woman's report of dissatisfaction with second-stage labor were associated with the blues, while having a medium or high degree of technological intervention, feeling little control during labor, and dissatisfaction with birth management were associated with depression. In Entwisle and Doering's

(1981) study of 120 primiparous couples, only 19 percent of the women reported no episodes of postpartum blues. Although they note a link between obstetrical interventions and the severity of the depression, these investigators concluded that "dissatisfaction of the mother with the quality of the birth experience is a less likely cause of the depression than the physical demands of caring for a new baby" (Entwisle and Doering 1981, 132). The use of obstetrical intervention is viewed by these authors as leading to a slower and more painful recovery that, in turn, makes the physical demands of mothering more difficult.

The purpose of the present study was to follow up on the association between obstetrical practices and postpartum moods articulated in the two studies reviewed above. In doing so, links between technology, birth experience, perceived loss of control, and disturbance in postpartum moods are explored. In addition, we sought to expand on the literature by examining factors affecting uplifted as well as depressed moods in the period around birth. We do this through inclusion of a bipolar measure. In general, our objective is to offer an alternative to the hormonal explanation based on an analysis of the possible negative effects of obstetrical inter-ention and failure to include the birthing woman in decision making.

Research Methods

Sample and Design

Data were collected longitudinally so that moods after birth could be differentiated from moods both before birth and in later postpartum. Each respondent was interviewed three times: three weeks before the expected due date, one week after birth, and one month after birth. These data were gathered between October, 1984 and June, 1985.

The data were collected via telephone interviews, which proved to be a flexible method for establishing and maintaining contact with the respondent before and after birth. Many of the women appeared to appreciate the attention and concern implied by the research questions.

The respondents were drawn from prenatal classes and physicians associated with three hospitals in southern Vermont and northwestern Massachusetts. Excluded from participation were women who were younger than 18 or older than 40, and women who received or whose infant received extraordinary medical treatment (e.g., extended hospital stay due to infection, transporting to neonatal intensive care unit in another hospital) during their postpartum.

One hundred forty-two women agreed to participate in the study. Of these, fifty-four were not actually included for several reasons. The largest number of the nonrespondents, thirty-one, had already given birth by the time they were called for the prenatal interview. In addition, twelve women could not be contacted by telephone. Seven women decided they did not want to participate in the study when called for the first interview. Four women completed the first interview but were excluded from further participation. Specifically, two suffered severe medical problems following birth; one woman who responded early in her pregnancy was no longer pregnant when called for the first interview; and one woman was not included in the sample because her baby was stillborn. In all, eighty-eight women comprised the final sample and each of these women completed the series of three interviews.

Measurement

In all three interviews the women were asked about their moods. The Bradburn mood affect scale, a bipolar scale designed for the general population, was used to measure both positive and negative emotion. The ten-item scale included questions such as: "During the past week did you ever feel proud because someone had complimented you on something you had done?" and "During the past week did you ever feel bored?" In addition to the Bradburn scale, questions about the frequency of occurrence of the classic symptoms of postpartum blues were also asked at each interview. The blues symptoms that were assessed were crying, feeling depressed, feeling particularly upset by someone finding fault with something you did, and being mildly confused about everyday things.

In addition to the mood questions, the prenatal interview assessed women's desire to participate in decisions surrounding the birth. Respondents were asked how important it was for them to be involved in making decisions about the use of ten obstetrical procedures such as the electronic fetal monitor, having a companion present during a planned caesarean, and being able to try different body positions during labor and delivery. Questions about the nature and intensity of stresses in the lives of these women were also included in the prenatal interview. To measure stress, respondents were asked how often they felt pressured by situations both related and unrelated to pregnancy and birth, such as doing household tasks, and handling household finances. Social and demographic background information was also obtained in the first interview.

The one-week postpartum (Time 2) interview repeated the measures of mood and blues symptoms. In addition, it asked about the kinds of obstetric technologies used in the birth and the women's role in each decision. First we asked about the use of the obstetrical interventions. For example, respondents were asked: "What type of delivery did you have: planned caesarean, unplanned caesarean, vaginal with forceps, or vaginal with no forceps?" Then we asked: "How much would you say that you were involved in the decision to have that kind of delivery? Would you say it was entirely your doctor's decision, mostly your doctor's decision, that you shared equally in making the decision, or it was mostly your decision?"

Mood, blues symptoms, and stress were assessed once again during the one-month postpartum interview (Time 3). Information on medical complications during pregnancy and birth such as toxemia, diabetes, and fetal heart distress was also collected at this time.

Results and Discussion

Characteristics of the Births

The sample for this study can be described as consisting predominantly of women pregnant for the first time (70 percent), with some college education (26 percent) or a college degree (34 percent), who were employed (62 percent), married (93 percent), and in their twenties (63 percent) or thirties (33 percent). All respondents were white. The majority (71 percent) of the women reported that their pregnancy was planned. With these characteristics, this group of women is not representative of birthing women in general, particularly with respect to race and educational level, and these differences may limit the ability to generalize about the findings.

The birth management practices for our sample were quite varied. Table 1 represents these results. The majority of the births began with a spontaneous labor, although 16 percent of the women reported an induced labor. Approximately one-third of the sample had a surgical or instrumental delivery. Sixty-six percent had a vaginal delivery with no forceps.

The average number of obstetrical procedures used during the births was two, with a range of zero to seven. Electronic fetal monitors were the most frequent (58 percent) intervention used. The second most frequent (51 percent) kind of intervention was drugs for pain during labor and delivery.

The degree to which the practitioner or the birthing woman was

126   Healing Technology

TABLE 1.   Birth Management Practices

	N	Percentage
Type of delivery		
Planned caesarean	4	3
Unplanned caesarean	13	15
Vaginal with forceps	13	15
Vaginal with no forceps	55	66
Induced labor	14	16
Drugs for pain		
Analgesic	24	27
Spinal block	2	2
Pudendal block	15	18
Epidural block	8	9
Other regional anesthetic	5	6
Can't remember what was used	3	3
No drugs used	43	49
Drugs to stimulate contractions	16	18
Electronic fetal heart monitor	51	58
Companion in delivery room	78	89
Did not stay in bed during first-stage labor	32	36
Used position other than on back during second-stage labor	49	56
Days in hospital after birth		
1 day or less	10	11
2 days	20	23
3 days	22	28
4 days	18	21
5 days	11	12
6 days or more	4	4

responsible for decisions made about obstetrical practices varied according to the procedures. Evidently, certain aspects of birthing are negotiable while others are decided upon solely by the practitioner. Decisions about the use of electronic fetal monitors and drugs to stimulate uterine contractions are made, most often, solely by the doctor. Not a single woman reported that either of these decisions was made mostly by her. By contrast, the use of drugs to alleviate pain, the position used during labor and delivery, and the length of the postpartum hospital stay are determined to a large degree by the woman. Decisions concerning the type of delivery and whether labor should be induced appear to be shared more or less equally. In many instances what actually occurred stands in marked contrast to the ratings made in the prenatal interview of how important it was to be involved in obstetrical decisions. Table 2 compares woman's prenatal desire for inclusion in decision making, as she expressed it before the birth, with the results of her one-week postpartum report about actual involvement. Only having a companion in the delivery room shows little disparity. Ninety-three percent indicated in the prenatal interview that being involved in that decision was important to them, and almost 90 percent reported after the birth that they had indeed been involved in this decision.

However, the other procedures show considerable disparity between prenatal and postchildbirth reports. All women said they wanted to be involved in the decision about body position during labor and delivery, but only 69 percent reported control over choice of body position during labor. Even fewer, 59 percent, reported control over that decision during delivery. There was also a large diffference between Time 1 and Time 2 reports on decision making about use of drugs for pain. Ninety-four percent said they wanted to be involved in that decision, but only 64 percent said the decision had been either shared or mainly their own. The greatest difference was in the use of electronic fetal monitors, where 83 percent said at the prenatal interview that it was important for them to be involved, but subsequently only 7 percent said the decision was either shared or mostly made by them.

Two general observations can be made about these data. First, the form of technology being decided upon is a major factor in the degree of practitioner hegemony over decision making. The more sophisticated the technology in question, the less likely the woman is to participate in decisions affecting its use. Second, there exists in most cases a notable difference between prenatal expectations of involvement in decision making and postpartum reports of what actually transpired.

TABLE 2.   Desired versus Actual Participation in Decision Making about Obstetrical Procedures, in Percentage

Percentage Reporting	Important to Be Involved in Decision (prenatal)	Shared or Mostly Respondent Decisions (postnatal)	Both Wanting and Being Involved (congruence)
Drugs for pain	94	64	68
Position for labor[a]	100	69	69
Position for delivery	100	59	59
Electronic fetal monitor	83	7	8
Companion in delivery room	93	90	97

[a]The question in prenatal interview was worded "body position for labor and delivery."

128   Healing Technology

Moods and Blues in the Puerperium

The present study attempted to monitor trends over time in mood shortly before and after birth. Included were questions inquiring about the specific symptoms of postpartum blues. These symptoms are frequently noted in the clinical literature and described by Yalom et al. (1968) as crying, feeling mildly depressed or in low spirits, feeling particularly vulnerable to criticism, and being mildly confused as to everyday things. Because these items are not synonymous with a major depressive disorder, they are more appropriately called "blues" rather than depression.

On the assumption that the four blues symptoms could be treated as a cluster of symptoms, we constructed an index of postpartum blues by adding up scores on each of the four items and using a common metric. The result was interesting. As table 3 shows (see row 1), there were no significant differences in the means of the postpartum blues index comparing Time 1 (prenatal), Time 2 (one week postpartum), and Time 3 (one month postpartum). That is, when their responses were treated as a symptom cluster, the women reported feeling approximately the same shortly before birth, at one week, and at one month postpartum. This similarity was of course contrary to expectation, as the clinical literature led us to expect an increase in the blues after birth. In retrospect, our finding should not be surprising. Many

TABLE 3. Late Pregnancy and Postpartum Moods[a]

	Three Weeks Before Birth (Time 1)		One Week After Birth (Time 2)		One Month After Birth (Time 3)	
	Mean	SD	Mean	SD	Mean	SD
Postpartum blues symptom index	9.51	3.54	9.85	3.11	9.49	2.84
Crying	1.19	1.95	1.85[b]	1.94	1.23	1.20
Low spirits	1.86	1.93	1.70	1.90	1.21	1.31
Confusion	.80	1.49	1.17	1.69	.88	1.86
Vulnerable to criticism	.77	1.60	.61	1.22	.61	1.25
Positive affect	.14	1.87	1.22[b]	2.59	.45	2.27
Negative affect	−.13	1.80	−.90[b]	1.67	−1.08	1.50

[a]For low spirits, confusion, and vulnerable to criticism, 0 = none, 4 = more than once a day; Crying = frequency times length, with higher scores denoting more frequent and longer spells. For affect: −1 = rarely, 1 = often.
[b]T-tests indicate significantly higher scores at Time 2 than at Time 1 and Time 3; $p = .001$.

women find the last weeks of pregnancy difficult due to anxiety about the upcoming birth and uncertainty about when labor will begin. Late pregnancy is also a time of growing physical discomforts.

For this reason, it is curious that postpartum blues have become the focus of attention in the clinical literature. One explanation is that mood changes are more likely to go unnoticed before birth. Except for short prenatal examinations, doctors and nurses are not available to observe pregnant women's moods and behaviors. During the postpartum stay, there is more opportunity for a woman's mood to be noticed by hospital staff and to become a subject of concern in its own right. This would explain how the phenomenon of postpartum blues or depression arose and how it, and not prenatal or perinatal blues, has become a matter of concern among practitioners.

Although the summary index failed to reveal any significant differences across time, analysis of the individual symptoms did uncover some interesting patterns. Crying, in particular, shows the predicted curvilinear pattern (see row 2, table 3). As shown, there was more crying one week after birth than in late pregnancy or at one month postpartum. In contrast, the periods before and after the birth showed no significant differences in the proportion of women feeling vulnerable to criticism or mildly confused as to everyday things.

The fourth measured postpartum blues symptom, feeling depressed or in low spirits, also produced unexpected results. On average, the birthing women reported the same level of depressed mood shortly before their birth experience as at one week postpartum. By one month postpartum, however, their depressed mood tended to lift, with the women being least likely to report feeling depressed or in low spirits at this time.

Results of the Bradburn affect scale showed that late pregnancy—not the immediate postpartum period—was the time when women reported the highest levels of negative emotion. As indicated in row 4 of table 3, there is no significant difference in the levels of negative affect one week and one month postpartum. Further examination of table 3 indicates that the women also reported their highest levels of positive emotion (e.g., feeling excited, proud, pleased) shortly after birth.

It is curious that both crying and positive affect peaked at one week postpartum. Indications are that the tears shed were not tears of joy. When asked to explain their crying in postpartum, most of the women stated that they felt overwhelmed by caring for a newborn, and in some cases other children, and also doing their household tasks. In hindsight it seems clear that feelings of both joy and depression are quite common among people experiencing many of the milestones in the life course, such as marriage, divorce, or moving to a new residence. Such events are sources of positive excitement, in addition to posing difficulties of adjustment, and it should not be surprising to discover similar paradoxes in the case of childbirth.

Interestingly, more of the respondents cited hormones or "blues" as their reason for crying *before* birth than after birth. In this way women's construction of their crying appears different from prevailing medical conceptions. Women seem ready to accept a biological explanation for their crying before giving birth, but attribute the sources of their tears after the birth to reasons that are external to them.

Predicting Early Postpartum Moods

As already reported, the women under study wanted to be in control of, or at least active participants in, the births of their children. Yet in many cases their desire for control was thwarted, as several kinds of obstetrical technology were decided upon without the woman's active participation.

In order to assess the influence of control in decision making and other factors on mood at one week postpartum, three regression equations were computed. The dependent variables selected for these equations were those mood and blues symptoms that differed after the birth when compared to before the birth. Because they changed, it is reasonable to expect that something in the birth process was responsible for their change. These three measures were levels of crying, positive affect, and an index of three negative affect items: how often the respondent felt lonely, bored, and depressed or very unhappy. The models used for each of these three measures were based on five potential predictors: the number of medical complications during pregnancy and birth, the level of stress, and mood as assessed prenatally at Time 1, and two measures of control over the birth process. Control was indicated both by the women's subjective assessments of their involvement in decisions made about obstetrical procedures, and by an objective count of the number of procedures used.

Only the model for the prediction of the negative affect index was statistically significant. In this equation, four of the five predictor variables considered had significant effects. Subjective reports of involvement in obstetrical decision making was the only factor that was not significant, although it did show a strong zero-order relationship with the number of obstetrical procedures used $(-.32)$. That is, women who had more interventions reported feeling less involved in the decision making about their use.

The number of obstetrical procedures performed does show a significant effect even after controlling for other factors. The fewer the obstetrical procedures carried out, the less the negative affect at one week postpartum. The total number of medical complications during pregnancy and birth also affected the level of negative emotion, but not in the expected direction. Women reporting more complications had less negative affect. As expected, feeling stressed by life circumstances predicts more negative affect. Finally, negative affect at Time 1 was directly related to negative affect at Time 2.

Summary and Conclusion

The purpose of this chapter was to bring technology into focus in the study of postpartum mood disturbance. Hormonal factors are undoubtedly relevant, but it is unlikely that they alone can provide a sufficient explanation. Childbirth is an event whose meaning is socially constructed, and explanation of it must also be informed by women's obstetrical experiences and involvement.

The major research question we addressed was whether postpartum blues symptoms are indeed higher in the early puerperium than might be expected. Surprisingly, only crying, one of the four measured symptoms, was higher then than during late pregnancy or at one month postpartum. As expected, the women did report more crying at one week after birth than at the other two measurement times. However, the earlier postpartum period was also a time of increased positive emotion. As measured by the Bradburn items, positive emotion was lowest in late pregnancy and highest at one week after the birth.

Negative emotion was predicted by the number of obstetrical procedures. Even when other factors were controlled, women who had a higher number of interventions during birth reported more negative emotion one week later. We interpret obstetrical technologies as impeding a woman's control, both real and perceived, over the birth of her child. Thus, the summary measure of obstetrical procedures measures the degree of active participation in the birth, with high technology begetting low participation and low perceived control. This lack of control leads to negative affect in the early puerperium. However, the summary measure of obstetrical procedures can also be interpreted another way. What, exactly, does it really measure? Aside from measuring participation in birth, it may be measuring other things as well. It is likely that women who experience fewer obstetrical procedures will, as a result, feel better physically one week later. The number of obstetrical procedures may therefore be confounded with physical well-being one week after birth, and this could explain why women exposed to less technology also experience less disturbance in mood. This explanation is consistent with that presented by Entwisle and Doering (1981). In either interpretation, technology is of causal importance. What is at issue is how its effect is generated.

Although the measure of participation in decision making did not consistently show the hypothesized effect on postpartum moods, it did reveal some interesting features of childbirth. First, there is a fairly large discrepancy between prenatal desire for participation in decision making and reports of what actually happened. Second, the degree to which the woman does contribute to the decision making, by her report, is dependent upon her age, level of education, and the number of obstetrical procedures used in the birth (Garner 1986). Third, low control in decision making is associated with a greater number of obstetrical procedures being used.

In addition, there is some evidence that reported involvement in decision making is dependent upon the nature of the intervention being negotiated. Specifically, decisions on the use of caesarean section, forceps, drugs to enhance contractions, and electronic fetal monitors were more frequently made by the physician. Whether the labor should be induced was reported, in most cases, as being a shared decision. The use of drugs for pain, the position taken during labor and delivery, having a companion in the delivery room, and the length of the postpartum hospital stay were most frequently reported as being decided by the birthing woman.

Concluding Note

The growth of technology in health care for women generally, and in childbirth in particular, is producing positive as well as negative effects. Technology makes childbirth, by some measures, safer for women and their babies. But these gains tend to be offset by a variety of negative, if unanticipated, consequences. Iatrogenic morbidity, including postpartum blues and the alienation of the woman from the birth, are among the most significant costs. Although alternative interpretations exist, it is clear that an increased use of birth technology puts women at greater risk for depressive symptoms during the early postpartum period.

It may be too early to assess recent trends in the use of birth technologies or to project into the future. It is clear, however, that hospital births have been humanized during the past decade. For example, policies about companions in labor and delivery rooms and during caesarean section have been relaxed, fewer drugs for pain are used, and maternity visiting policies in many hospitals allow more interaction among the mother, her infant, partner, and other children. Many routine prepping procedures are being waived. Many hospitals have birthing rooms and birthing chairs, and in some settings women are no longer, as a policy, being confined to bed. Even the policy of repeat caesarean section is being questioned.

These changes not withstanding, invasive procedures remain a prevailing characteristic of childbirth in the United States. Further scrutiny of obstetric technology in terms of its effects during birth as well as during the postpartum period is clearly needed.

N O T E

This paper is based on a dissertation by the first author and chaired by the second. The authors gratefully acknowledge contributions by Naomi Gerstel, Gene Fisher, and Catherine Riessman, who all served on the dissertation committee.

B I B L I O G R A P H Y

Arms, Suzanne. 1979. *Immaculate deception.* New York: Bantam Books.
Cleary, Paul. 1983. Proposal for research on postpartum depression. Harvard Medical School, Cambridge, Mass.
Conrad, Peter, and Joseph W. Schneider. 1980. Looking at levels of medicalization. *Social Science in Medicine* 14A:75–79.
Dalton, Katarina. 1971. Prospective study into puerperial depression. *British Journal of Psychiatry* 118, no. 547: 689–92.
Entwisle, Doris R., and Susan Doering. 1981. *The first birth: A family turning point.* Baltimore: Johns Hopkins University Press.
Garner, Lynne C. 1986. Control in childbirth: A study of postpartum moods. Ph.D. diss. University of Massachusetts, Amherst.
Heitler, Susan. 1976. Postpartum depression: A multidimensional study. *Dissertation Abstracts International* 36, 11B: 5792–93.
Leavitt, Judith. 1984. Science enters the birthing room. *Journal of American History* 70 (September): 281–304.
Litoff, Judith Barrett. 1978. *American midwives: 1860 to the present.* Westport, Conn.: Greenwood Press.
Nelson, Peggy. 1982. Class differences in the preparation for childbirth. *Journal of Health and Social Behavior* 23, no. 4: 339–52.

Oakley, Ann. 1980. *Women confined: Toward a sociology of childbirth.* New York: Schocken Books.

Paykel, E. S., E. M. Emms, and E. S. Rassaby. 1980. Life events and social supports in puerperial depression. *British Journal of Psychiatry* 136 (April): 339–46.

Pitt, Bruce. 1973. Maternity blues. *British Journal of Psychiatry* 122, no. 569: 431–33.

————. 1977. Psychological aspects of pregnancy. *Midwife, Health Visitor and Community Nurse* 13 (May): 137–39.

Rosengren, William. 1980. *The sociology of medicine: diversity, conflict and change.* New York: Harper and Row.

Starr, Paul. 1982. *The social transformation of American medicine.* New York: Basic Books.

Stein, George, Frank Milton, and Peggy Babbington. 1976. The relationship between mood disturbances and free and total plasma tryptophan in postpartum women. *British Medical Journal* 6033 (August): 457.

U.S. Bureau of the Census. 1982. *Fertility of American women: June 1980— Advance Report.* Washington, D.C.: Government Printing Office.

Wertz, Richard W., and Dorothy C. Wertz. 1979. *Lying-in: A history of childbirth in America.* New York: Schocken Books.

Yalom, Irvin D., Donald T. Lunde, Rudolf H. Moose, and David A. Hamberg. 1968. Postpartum blues syndrome: A description of related variables. *Archives of General Psychiatry* 18, no. 1: 16–22.

Should Pregnancies Be Sustained in Brain-Dead Women?: A Philosophical Discussion of Postmortem Pregnancy

Julien S. Murphy

> Life keeps me alive; all its tubes
> and wires are connected to me and give support
> in ways that life determines for my needs.
> On a bed of earth, in house, its calendars
> and clocks are programmed to me: the various airs
> of mornings, evenings, noontimes, in and out.
> —William Bronk, "Life Supports"

As the current abortion debates indicate, the relationship between a woman and her fetus in pregnancy has become far more than a biological matter. It is one of the most complex social, legal, and ethical controversies of the twentieth century.[1] Opinions vary widely on the rights and responsibilities of women in pregnancy, as the frequent criticisms of *Roe v. Wade* show. Moreover, the continual innovations in reproductive technology present, almost daily, new possibilities that may alter the very meaning of *pregnancy*. One irony of our century may be that, although we are biologically dependent on pregnancy for the survival of our species, we could end the century lacking agreement on such formerly basic matters as what pregnancy is, what one is pregnant with, and who or what is pregnant. Amid the flurry of high-tech possibilities (embryo transfer, donor eggs, frozen embryos), a little-mentioned low-tech procedure, seldom applicable, may tilt the meaning of pregnancy in the most unfamiliar and perhaps dangerous direction: the use of *postmortem maternal ventilation* (PMV) to sustain pregnancy in brain-dead women.[2] PMV marks a shift in the use of respiratory systems away from use on patients who might otherwise recover to those whose lives will thereafter be terminated. Like much of low technology, PMV is cost-effective. It requires standard hospital life-support equipment and decreases the need for high-cost prenatal technology.

Postmortem maternal ventilation is the term I have selected to refer to the practice of applying ventilation (i.e., a life-support machine) to a brain-dead pregnant patient to sustain the maternal vital functions

135

necessary for continued fetal development. If PMV is successful, the subsequent postmortem caesarean section results in a live birth. I will refer to the brain-dead pregnant patient as a *pregnant cadaver* and when PMV is in progress, as a *ventilated pregnant cadaver*. Both terms stress the fact that the body to which PMV is being applied is a dead body since it has been judged brain-dead, fulfilling the medical and legal criteria for determining the person dead. The Uniform Determination of Death Act approved in 1980 and adopted in twenty-three states includes brain death in its definition of death:

> An individual who has sustained either (1) irreversible cessation of circulatory and respiratory functions, or (2) irreversible cessation of all functions of the entire brain, including the brain stem, is dead. A determination of death must be made in accordance with accepted medical standards. (*Uniform Laws Annotated* 1988, 293)

A ventilated cadaver may simulate the state of being "alive" by retaining a fleshy skin color, by being warm to the touch, and by lacking the coloration and stiffness of a dead body. Since its vital circulatory and respiratory processes have irreversibly failed, however, it is not a live body. Whereas other brain-dead bodies are usually removed from life support systems and interred, or are used for organ transplants or medical research before interment, the pregnant cadaver presents a unique case, for a healthy pregnancy can continue to thrive in a ventilated pregnant cadaver.

The philosophical significance of PMV is the challenge it poses to these assumptions, which I will argue, are basic to pregnancy: *that a woman must be alive to be pregnant* and *that the mother in pregnancy must be a person*. The use of PMV depends on a refusal to think that the pregnancy must end with the death of the mother and an assumption that a mother, when alive, adds nothing essential to her pregnancy. The challenge to both of these formerly taken-for-granted beliefs is unsettling. Common-sense attitudes conceal the deeply rooted philosophical issues inherent in PMV: either people are quickly pleased at the unexpected prospect of fetal survival and favor PMV or they find PMV grotesquely necrophilic and undesirable. Proponents are fascinated with the possibility of continuing pregnancy in a body after death or are concerned with maintaining fetal life, either because they may believe that a fetus always has a right to life or because the fetus is favored out of love for the mother, as a way in which some part of her can live on beyond her death.

While sociologists might look for a correlation between views on

PMV and views on either abortion or euthanasia, the philosopher's task is to evaluate the implications of the practice of PMV for the social community and to ask how PMV might affect the discourse about pregnancy, especially assumptions about pregnancy and social policy. Despite the appeal that PMV may have to medical practitioners and interested parties, serious ethical objections can be raised about its underlying implications. Feminists and those concerned with the value priorities of medical technology can find strong grounds from which to argue against PMV even though the choice not to use PMV may result in the death of an otherwise healthy fetus.

This discussion will oppose PMV on the moral grounds that there is a feminist definition of pregnancy and that this definition precludes even the deliberate choice of PMV. The feminist view of pregnancy advanced here asserts two fundamental requirements: first, that *human consciousness is necessary to pregnancy.* Pregnancy ought to include the conscious state of being pregnant. A woman need not be conscious all the time (i.e., in sleep, blackouts, light comas) but she must at least have the capacity for consciousness in order for her activity of "being pregnant" to be properly a human activity. Second, *pregnancy ought to result from a choice a woman makes to be pregnant.* The choice to be pregnant is essentially a woman's choice, as it is her body that sustains the pregnancy. One who is pregnant ought to be one who is choosing pregnancy as an existential project. A woman may not have deliberately chosen to become pregnant (i.e., conception could result from a contraceptive failure), but if she remains pregnant it should be the result of her conscious choice of pregnancy as an activity.

While other medical practices that seek to separate pregnancy from maternal consciousness outside of women's bodies (i.e., experimentation on pregnancy in vitro) may be objectionable on other grounds, in this paper I will argue that in vivo pregnancies, those occurring in women's bodies, require the possibility of maternal consciousness if the pregnancy is to uphold respect for women as persons. In fact, the practice of PMV undermines women as persons precisely because the female role in reproduction occurs in a nonperson form of a woman. I argue that a careful examination of the practice of PMV along with the medical, philosophical, and legal problems inherent in this new obstetric practice will reveal an eliminative view of pregnancy. Any mandatory PMV policy can be seen as directly violating women's reproductive freedoms and brain-dead patients' right to privacy. Any voluntary PMV policy must assume that PMV is similar to organ donation, that the allocation of medical resources for PMV is justifiable by community health needs, and that the practice of PMV is not detrimental to persons. All three of these assumptions can be shown to be problematic. I will conclude that the practice of PMV should not continue unless such issues are resolved.

The Practice of Postmortem Maternal Ventilation

Difficult ethical issues arise in considering whether or not pregnancy should be sustained in nonconscious female bodies, where the woman may either be reversibly comatose or even brain dead. While pregnancy has been sustained in comatose women for as long as twenty-eight weeks (See table 1, case 2), life support was not required for these patients and they were by no means dead.[3] In fact, in case two, the child was born by a vaginal delivery even though the mother remained comatose. Whether or not pregnancy should be sustained in comatose women is a difficult issue as all but those in an irreversible comatose state are technically alive and no "extraordinary means" are needed to sustain bodily life. Admittedly, the stage of pregnancy as well as the stage of coma may be difficult to discern in comatose pregnant women. Whatever decision is made about sustaining pregnancy in comatose cases, it must be remembered that as long as the woman can survive without life support she is medically defined as alive.

The practice of PMV, however, continues pregnancy in patients classified as dead. PMV practices apply life support to brain-dead comatose patients whose bodies have not been otherwise severely damaged. The definition of brain death is a recent development in medicine. It developed as a result of the need to distinguish other comatose patients from those irreversibly comatose patients on life support who have no central nervous system activity. This distinction aids physicians in determining when life support is futile and should be ended. It is particularly suitable for determining the point at which organs can be removed from a brain-dead donor. A team of researchers at the Harvard Medical School in 1965 established a set of criteria for determining the state of irreversible coma, establishing it as a definitive way to determine brain death in a patient and judge the patient as "dead." The team claimed "that responsible medical opinion is ready to adopt new criteria for pronouncing death to have occurred in an individual sustaining irreversible coma as a result of permanent brain damage" (Harvard Ad Hoc Committee 1968).

The Harvard Brain-Death Criteria which are used in PMV as well as organ transplant cases consist of four components: (1) unreceptivity and unresponsivity, (2) lack of movements or breathing, (3) absence of reflexes, and (4) flat electroencephalogram (Harvard Ad Hoc Commit-

TABLE 1. U.S. Cases of Sustaining Pregnancies in Comatose Women

Place and Date	Age of Woman (years)	Cause of Maternal Coma	Onset of Coma[a]	Length of Coma at Birth (in weeks)	Maternal Death[b]	Live Birth	Birth Weight (oz.)	Court Battle for Abortion	Court Ruling
S. Dakota, 1977	30	Brain injury from car accident	6	27	Yes	Yes vaginal delivery	58	None	
Florida, Feb.-Aug. 1984	16	Brain injury from car accident	12	24	c	Yes c-sect.	c	None	
New York, March 1985	21	Anticancer drug mistakenly injected into spinal column	25	1	c	Yes c-sect.	34	None	
Connecticut, January 1986	24	Oxygen loss in attempted hanging	9	15	Yes	No		Yes	Sustain Pregnancy

[a]gestational age in weeks
[b]maternal death following the birth
[c]information unknown

tee 1968). In PMV cases, the Harvard Criteria are slightly altered. Normally, the respirator is turned off for three-minute intervals to see if the patient can breathe spontaneously. This usual test is not performed to prevent possible fetal damage. According to the Harvard team, the patient should be declared dead *before* the respirator is turned off, to provide legal protection for physicians. Hence if life support is continued after the test confirms brain death, then life support is being applied to a dead body. It is also recommended that, in order to avoid a conflict of interests, the physician making the diagnosis of brain death should not also be involved in subsequent transplant efforts using organs from the same patient. It is unclear whether this restriction is included in the application of the Harvard Criteria to PMV cases.

The instances of brain death during pregnancy in the United States are quite rare. Even more unusual are pregnancies in brain-dead women in which neither the mother's internal organs nor the fetus is damaged. Yet at least seven cases suitable for PMV practices have been reported in the United States since 1976 (table 2), and the known instances may increase with the apparent tendency to bring such cases into court in recent years.[4]

Only one of the seven publicized PMV cases (Buffalo, 1981) has been written up in the medical journals by the medical team (Dillon et al. 1982). Writing about the Buffalo case, they describe a young epileptic woman, who shortly after hospital admission, suffered irreversible neurological deterioration—slurred speech, ataxic gait, respiratory collapse. Despite ventilation and intubation, the woman, while twenty-five weeks pregnant, began to die: "her pupils were fixed and dilated," and two days later "her reflexes were absent; and all sedation and anti-seizure medications were withdrawn" (Dillon et al. 1982, 1090). But as long as the mother's body was artificially aerified and fed, it remained capable of sustaining the fetus. The mother herself "had no spontaneous respirations; all limbs were flaccid; deep-tendon reflexes were absent throughout. The eyes were fixed in the midline. . . ." and "she was unresponsive to deep pain." The fetus, however, continued to thrive: "the fetal heart rate was audible and ranged between 140 and 160 beats per minute after the mother was diagnosed as brain-dead" (1089–91). PMV enabled the pregnancy to continue until the twenty-sixth week when the onset of fetal distress indicated cessation of PMV and a birth by caesarean section. Not only was the Buffalo case successful, but it was offered as grounds to recommend life-support measures in appropriate brain-dead pregnancies (Dillon et al. 1982, 1090). The authors' recommendation states:

TABLE 2. U.S. Cases of PMV Pregnancies

Place and Date	Age of Woman (years)	Cause of Maternal Brain Death	Onset of PMV[a]	End of PMV[a]	Reason for Ending PMV	Live Birth	Birth Weight (oz.)	Court Battle over PMV	Court Ruling
Colorado, Dec. 1976	b	b	b	b	Futile	No	b	No	None
Brooklyn, N.Y., Dec. 1977	27	Coma	16	17	Maternal heart attack	No	b	No	None
Buffalo, N.Y., Jan. 1981	24	Encephalitis	25	26	Maternal instability	Yes	32	No	None
San Francisco, Calif., March 1983	b	Seizure	22	31	Fetal maturity	Yes	48	No	None
Roanoke, Vir., July 1983	b	b	c	c	b	Yes	59	No	None
Santa Clara, Calif., July 1986	34	Brain tumor	24	31	Fetal maturity	Yes	69	Yes	Sustain pregnancy
Augusta, Geo., Aug. 1986	25	Drug overdose	17	24	b	No	17	Yes	Sustain pregnancy

[a]gestational age in weeks
[b]information unknown
[c]84 days of PMV

Having established a diagnosis of brain-death in a patient with a potentially viable fetus (24–27 weeks' gestation), we recommend that vigorous
maternal support and fetal monitoring be instituted. . . . Our experience
indicates that after 24 weeks' gestation, each extra week in utero increases
the chances for fetal survival. (1090)

The goal of PMV is to sustain the fetus in its mother's ventilated
cadaver until the fetus can survive on its own. Whereas abortion discussions emphasize fetal viability (the earliest point in fetal development in which the fetus would be likely to survive birth), PMV aims
to sustain the fetus in utero until fetal pulmonary maturity, the point
somewhat beyond viability at which it is likely that the fetal respiratory
system is fully developed. The odds of a live birth increase dramatically
as fetal development approaches fetal pulmonary maturity. The onset
of PMV has begun as early as the sixteenth week of gestation (case 2)
and as late as the twenty-fifth week (case 3). In the Buffalo case, life
support was applied latest in pregnancy of all seven cases. Nevertheless, its eight days of ventilation did not set the record for the longest
use of PMV. Since then, three cases have exceeded that duration:
(case 4) with sixty-three days of ventilation, (case 6) with fifty-three
days of ventilation, and (case 5) with eighty-four days of ventilation.
The trend to maintain ventilation in pregnant cadavers for a matter of
weeks or even months makes Dillon's suggested management of PMV
pregnancies conservative. The two limiting factors for determining the
duration of PMV are indications of maternal instability and indications
of fetal distress. Barring these, the fetus can be sustained in utero after
maternal brain death for long periods.

Sustaining pregnancy in a ventilated cadaver is no easy matter.
The Buffalo team recognized that "the medical problems encountered
in attempting this are profound and time-consuming but not insur-
mountable" (Dillon et al. 1982, 1091). For instance, the fetus must
receive nourishment through the cadaver, so the cadaver must be given
intravenous infusions of nutrients as well as antibiotics to prevent infection; the respirator must be continually adjusted; and the body temperature of the cadaver must be regulated by applying warm or cooled
blankets. And PMV is not merely a matter of applying machines to a
pregnant cadaver, but involves medical staff in daily services to the
cadaver. In case 4, environmental stimulation for the fetus was supplied
by nurses who "stroked the mother's abdomen and murmured soothing
words," and played music on a tape recorder near the bed (*Newsweek*
1983). The vital role that nurses play in the care of ventilated pregnant
cadavers calls forth a complex range of attitudes. Some nurses believe
the mother is actually a live person and value their role in the preg-

nancy, while other nurses see the mother as dead and find it difficult to provide the necessary services. A wide range of attitudes from approval to disgust also mark the legal controversy surrounding PMV.

The Legal Controversy Over PMV

Along with medical difficulties that arise in ventilating a pregnant cadaver, conceptual difficulties are inherent in the very nature of the practice. To begin with, confusion exists about how the ventilated cadaver is to be regarded, what rights if any it has, and whether any possible rights of the cadaver could outweigh claims of fetal rights. The confusion is found in Dillon et al., who diagnosed their patient as brain dead and yet referred to it not as a cadaver but as "a fatally ill pregnant woman whose vital functions have been preserved" (1089). They speak of their attempts "to prolong maternal life in the face of brain death" (1089). But as Siegler and Wikler note in their preface to the Dillon et al. report "one cannot prolong life in a dead body" (1982, 1101). Dillon et al. refer to the maintenance of "somatic life" in their patient (1982, 1089). However, if one grants somatic life in a ventilated cadaver, it is artificially sustained somatic life and not spontaneous somatic life as in a patient in a vegetative state. And if somatic life essentially means the ability of an organism to sustain itself spontaneously, then it is inappropriate to grant somatic life to ventilated cadavers. Even with a general acceptance of brain-death criteria among physicians, evidence suggests that many doctors would not turn off the respirators of patients who satisfied the Harvard Criteria for Brain Death (Pinkus 1984). Siegler and Wikler claim that "clinicians who find it congenial to speak of brain-dead patients as 'terminally ill' (and the like) do not, on our interpretation, really view the bodies of these patients as dead" (1982, 1101).

Amidst the conceptual disagreement about the status of brain-dead patients in general, little clear-cut legal ground exists to guide physicians through the perplexing ethical issues of PMV. Since PMV is a new practice and since brain death occurred quite unexpectedly in the cited cases, there was no opportunity to obtain consent from the women prior to death. In the Buffalo case not even paternal consent was obtained for PMV. Also there was no clear legal authority for researchers to keep a pregnant cadaver on life support for the sake of the fetus. The authors acknowledged that they chose "to sin bravely," by proceeding with PMV (Dillon et al. 1982, 1091). Apparently their intent was to provide the best care possible for the fetus. Their decision presupposes that PMV for the sake of fetal survival outweighed all

other possible considerations. The nature of this controversial decision
is indicated by court battles over the use and continuation of PMV in
two of the seven cases. In fact, without patient consent the legal grounds
are not clear for postmortem caesarean sections in unventilated cases
even when they would be routine in late trimester pregnancies. As one
physician advised his colleagues in a medical journal:

> . . . (failing consent) perform the procedure [postmortem caesarean sec-
> tion] even without consent because (*a*) even if you are sued, the likelihood
> of being found liable is slim (no one has so far), and (*b*) the courts may
> well hold next that you MAY be sued, if you FAIL to perform the section,
> by the legal representatives of the child (and that case may be yours).
> (Arthur 1978, 179)

In PMV cases, it can be claimed either that the mother has no
interests because she is dead, and hence the protection of fetal life
warrants PMV, or that the mother's death should be respected and not
artificially postponed, so PMV should be prohibited. On both sides,
there may be benevolent wishes—those of well-meaning relatives who
want the fetus to survive, and those of well-meaning relatives who want
no further treatment applied to a mother who is clinically dead. The
claim that the mother's interests die with her is commonly held. Siegler and Wikler, for instance, argue that as the mother in the Buffalo
case gave no prior request prohibiting PMV and as the physicians were
unable to restore the mother to health or consciousness, "the mother's
interests, apart from earlier desires to bear a healthy child, were not
at issue. Further treatment could be considered neither beneficial nor
harmful" (1982, 1101).

In both legal battles over PMV, (cases 6 and 7), the court ruled for
the continuation of life support. In case 6 the brain-dead patient's parents protested life support while the father of the fetus, supported by
the court, demanded it. The intentions of the father in supporting PMV
appeared to be based on his love for his brain-dead fiancée and his
desire for their child, for after the successful PMV birth, the father told
the press, "I'm very happy about the outcome for Michele (the baby),
but I'm still grieving a little bit. Michele's birth today makes things a
little easier. When I looked into her eyes, I could see the extension
from Odette into her" (Associated Press 1986b, 1).

In the second legal battle over PMV (case 7), the brain-dead patient's husband was not the father of the fetus and the two men disagreed about PMV. Her husband protested life support while, once
again, it was the father of the fetus who demanded it. This case pre-

sented an interesting legal conflict of rights, for the patient's husband presumably had the right to consent concerning medical treatment for his spouse, but would have no paternity rights over the fetus. The biological father might have paternity rights over the fetus but no right to consent for the brain-dead patient. The lawyer for the biological father, along with lawyers representing the fetus and the hospital argued for continuation of PMV as a right-to-life issue. It was claimed that discontinuing maternal life support was tantamount to feticide under Georgia law, which prohibits killing a fetus that is capable of movement (quickening), and that the mother's right to privacy, upheld by *Roe,* ended with her brain death, and hence "the state may intervene. . . . The state has an interest in the protection of human life" (Associated Press 1986a, Georgia Superior Court 1986). While the state attorney asked for a dismissal of the case, finding it outside of the court's jurisdiction because the fetus could not survive outside the womb, the court did not dismiss the case, but ordered in favor of PMV. Despite the court ruling, the life support was prematurely ended due to maternal instability. The fetus died.

The court rulings in PMV cases have been consistently in favor of continuing ventilation on pregnant cadavers. Such rulings assume either that the brain-dead mother no longer has rights or that her rights are not sufficient to outweigh those of the fetus. What is most alarming in the legal controversy over PMV is the failure to recognize the mother's right to a speedy death. In particular, it is important to examine the parameters of reproductive freedom to show that they include women's right to die.

PMV: An Eliminative View of Pregnancy

At one level, PMV seems to show that no matter how valuable higher brain functions might be within our society, they are not required in the third trimester of pregnancy. In fact, at the very stage in fetal development when the fetus is becoming neurologically advanced, it appears that it can be sustained in a body lacking all neurological activity. This point is not astounding from a medical standpoint, for it has been known that brain-dead patients on life support could maintain respiratory, circulatory, and digestive functions, and even generate new tissue. But, from an ethical point of view, the practice of PMV suggests that its proponents do not believe that maternal brain activity *ought* to be a requirement for pregnancy. Such a belief suggests an eliminative view of pregnancy. Eliminative views subtract or leave out one or more otherwise essential requirements of a definition. An eliminative view of pregnancy eliminates consciousness from the essential requirements for pregnancy, reducing women from "pregnant persons" to "pregnant bodies." The use of PMV suggests that pregnancy is a mindless act, and that what women themselves, as conscious beings, contribute to their pregnancies in the third trimester is not essential to the moral community. To imagine a dead woman's body as "artificially" pregnant is to claim that a woman's connection to her pregnancy is neither vital nor necessary, since PMV finishes a woman's pregnancy in her aerated and intubated remains. Once again, the point is not that the pregnancy is "artificial" or "unnatural" but that the cadaver is used to extort in death the female work of reproduction unfinished in life. Would we think nothing of mechanically ventilating and automating the bodies of brain-dead workers for the purpose of extracting additional labor from them? Both acts would eliminate consciousness as a necessary requirement for extracting work from human bodies and diminish the status of persons in the moral community by using human bodies for labor after their human life had ceased. The danger of eliminative views of human activities, such as pregnancy, is that they further diminish the human community by granting no special status to dead bodies as opposed to living ones. One difficulty in combating an eliminative view of pregnancy, such as that found in PMV, is that the right to privacy, which has been the framework for respecting human beings in matters of reproduction and health, is itself under attack, and not an obvious right as critics of *Roe* point out.

PMV, *Roe,* and Reproductive Freedom

The initiation of PMV is an instance of how the relationship between a woman and her fetus is interpreted from a sexist point of view. It poses a serious challenge to the right to abortion by obscuring even further the relationship between a pregnant woman and her fetus. The obscuring of the relationship between a pregnant woman and her fetus begins with conservative interpretations of the Supreme Court decision, *Roe v. Wade* (1973). The Supreme Court, when deciding in favor of Roe, granted women the right to abortion in early trimester pregnancies while leaving to each state the possibility of refusing abortion to women in third trimester pregnancies, the trimester most suitable for PMV, provided a state could show a "compelling interest" in fetal life. Conservatives interpret *Roe* as validating fetal life from the point of fetal viability. *Roe* defines fetal viability as the capacity for meaningful life outside the mother's womb even if it requires technological assistance for an ex utero fetus. One could argue that there is only a slight difference between life support for a twenty-seven week infant and life support for a maternal cadaver twenty-seven weeks' pregnant. Yet to blur the distinction is to undermine the assumption behind abortion rights, namely, that reproductive freedom must include the right not to be pregnant against one's will. For women, PMV raises the dangerous possibility that it could be claimed that *every* brain-dead pregnant woman with a healthy fetus *ought* to be ventilated. PMV could become mandatory for all suitable cases, particularly those in the third trimester, requiring of women that they finish their pregnancies even beyond the point of their own deaths. Just as women resorted to back-street abortions before *Roe,* relatives and friends of brain-dead pregnant women might need to resort to "back-street burials" or seek out physicians who might agree to claim that PMV would be "unfeasible" in particular cases.

If the practice of PMV were to become not only a medical option for physicians but a legal requirement in all appropriate cases, women would be forced into pregnancy beyond the point of their deaths, and it would be much harder to convince people that women should not be pregnant against their will in life. Clearly there are moral grounds to argue against mandatory PMV. *Roe* does not imply that (live) women are "natural" life support machines for the fetus, nor does *Roe* always require women to remain pregnant even in the third trimester. Hence, *Roe* is a decision that supports women's reproductive freedom, specifically the freedom to terminate pregnancy.

PMV, on the other hand, plays havoc with women's freedom in pregnancy by allowing for the condition of pregnancy without a woman's capacity for choice. A woman's will, her desire, is nonexistent in her ventilated pregnant cadaver. Even more oppressive than the most restrictive state abortion regulations, PMV practices are using women's bodies without their prior consent solely for the maintenance of pregnancies. Women's bodies, in the practice of PMV, are exclusively means to ends. In PMV practices, the body of a brain-dead pregnant woman continues to labor under the functions of an artificially sustained pregnancy despite the fact that the woman, qua woman, no longer exists.

Roe reaffirmed the necessary connection between a right to one's body and a right to terminate pregnancy through its appeal to the right of privacy. The right to privacy had successfully been used prior to *Roe* to guarantee the right for adult bedroom pornography and contraception. But the Court's understanding of privacy has not granted women full protection in pregnancy. By granting the possibility of states claiming a compelling interest in viable fetuses, *Roe* has implied that women's bodies in pregnancy both are and are not their own, declaring the right to privacy a contingent right for pregnant women:

> The right to privacy, whether it be founded in the 14th Amendment's concept of personal liberty and restrictions upon state action, as we feel it is, or as the District Court determined, in the 9th Amendment's reservation of rights to the people, is broad enough to encompass a woman's decision whether or not to terminate her pregnancy. (*Roe v. Wade* 1973)

And yet, *Roe* also says:

> The pregnant woman cannot be isolated in her privacy. She carries an embryo, and later, a fetus. . . . The woman's privacy is no longer sole and any right of privacy she possesses must be measured accordingly. (*Roe v. Wade* 1973)

Hence, it is suggested by the Court that the right to privacy, which guarantees persons the "right to be let alone," is a right for the pregnant woman in early trimester pregnancies, but a right that can become increasingly contingent as her pregnancy develops, if a state chooses to claim a compelling interest. The longer a woman remains pregnant, the less right to her body she may be seen to have. Limitations on the right to privacy for pregnant women undermine the basis for reproductive freedoms including the freedom to not be pregnant when dead.

Reproductive freedom means the freedom to engage in or refrain from acts of reproduction. Human reproduction ought to be based upon free acts of consenting adults. An act of "consent" is one in which the agent of the act does not feel motivated primarily by coercion, but rather enters the act willingly and of her own accord. Coercion can happen to an individual as well as on a social level. A person could feel coerced into an action if another individual through threat of physical or psychological force demands performance of the action. In such a case, the act will have been done at the expense of her liberty. Coercion at the social level happens when a person finds a particular action appealing only in virtue of a complex social context of major incentives and penalties linked with a particular scheme of choices. Of course, it can be argued that no choice is totally free of cultural values. But the crucial issue is whether or not reproductive freedom ought to be a basic freedom in human societies, deeply rooted in the very foundation of rights that makes individual liberties possible. I would argue that reproductive freedom is basic to a system of rights in human communities, as evidenced by public outrage at instances of reproductive coercion, such as forced sterilization of workers. If the right to reproduce is judged to be integral to one's freedom and basic sense of dignity as a human being, then similarly, the right not to reproduce must be equally vital. Nothing should take precedence over a woman's right to engage in or terminate her pregnancy freely. Acts of either the legal system or individuals that threaten women with restrictions on their liberties in reproduction are tantamount to acts of coercion. Any mandatory PMV policy would similarly be coercive for women in pregnancy, for it would take away a woman's liberty not to be pregnant after she had ceased to exist.

PMV and Cadaver Rights

PMV raises the issue of the rights of persons after the clinical diagnosis of death. Do dead bodies have rights? Specifically, can a cadaver be harmed and if so, does the act of ventilation bring about harm to that cadaver? Or do dead bodies have a right to privacy that would exclude the possibility of PMV?

Clearly, brain-dead bodies do have some rights: the right not to be exploited, invaded, mutilated, mishandled. It is illegal to willfully, recklessly, or negligently mutilate a body after death. But are laws prohibiting cadaver abuse meant to protect the cadaver itself, the deceased person, the friends and family of the deceased, or the moral community as such? It seems that the capacity to be harmed requires the capacity to suffer, either physically by feeling pain, or emotionally by realizing the wrong that has been committed. Hence, since a cadaver has no central nervous system activity and is incapable of consciousness, it cannot be harmed. Only the living can be harmed. Cadaver abuse is an act of harm inflicted on the living. This view is consistent with legal assumptions inherent in Abuse of Corpse Laws. There is liability for cadaver abuse to relatives who are entitled to damages because they have the obligation to bury the cadaver and are seen to suffer "mental anguish," which means "grievous injury to their feelings" from cadaver abuse. The fact that it is the relatives who are able to collect damages for abuse to a cadaver evidences the assumption that harm to a cadaver is harm to those who hold the memory of the deceased in high regard. But what if relatives do not claim to suffer mental anguish from a case of cadaver abuse. Has harm occurred? Nonrelatives, even strangers, might be capable of being harmed by cadaver abuse in the sense that abusive treatment of any human cadaver has implications for the regard for persons in general within the community. How we treat our dead can be seen as a reflection of our regard for the living. If PMV harms, it harms the moral community as well as those directly associated with the deceased.

Does a right to privacy preclude the possibility of PMV? If we assume, along with the Harvard team, that brain death and an irreversibly comatose state are equivalent and result in the diagnosis of death, then, along with the Supreme Court of New Jersey in the Karen Quinlan case, we can grant brain-dead bodies a right to privacy. It was assumed that Karen Quinlan was an irreversibly comatose patient, completely dependent on life support. In the Quinlan case, the Supreme Court of New Jersey granted Quinlan's legal guardian the right to stop life support on privacy grounds, finding that ventilation, intubation, drugs, and constant medical care, which Quinlan required, constituted extreme bodily invasion, particularly since Quinlan could never recover consciousness:

> We think that the State's interest *contra* weakens and the individual's right to privacy grows as the degree of bodily invasion increases and the prognosis dims. Ultimately there comes a point at which the individual's rights overcome the State interest. (*Atlantic Reporter* 1976)

The Quinlan case showed that the right to privacy included the right not to have one's body unduly maintained by life-support machines. The privacy that was protected could be seen as belonging to a body capable of being judged dead. After the court ruling, the respirator was turned off and Quinlan, surprisingly, was able to breathe spontaneously and lived for several years after the court ruling. Yet, the importance of the Quinlan case was that when the court assumed she was irreversibly comatose (brain dead), she was granted a right to privacy. In cases of ventilated brain-dead cadavers, the same invasive treatment is required as was required for Quinlan. Do the philosophical differences between a brain-dead patient and a pregnant brain-dead patient warrant that the same treatment not be regarded as invasive in the latter? Does pregnancy in death, as well as possibly in life, diminish women's right to privacy?

The potential conflict between a pregnant woman's right to privacy and a state's right to protect an interest in fetal life occurs in PMV cases as well as abortion cases. At least one court battle over PMV (case 7) illustrates the confusion of attributing a privacy right to a ventilated cadaver. In the hearing for continuation of PMV, the hospital lawyer claimed that "Mrs. Piazzi is dead. . . . She has no more right of privacy," while hospital officials who were advocates of PMV appealed to Mrs. Piazzi's right to privacy as grounds for the refusal of details about the time and manner of childbirth (Associated Press 1986a). Does PMV violate a dead woman's right to privacy? In the case of ventilated bodies diagnosed as brain dead, it seems that a right to privacy can be understood to include the right to a bodily death. Every body that cannot be returned to a state of consciousness or at least spontaneous respiration would therefore have a right to be allowed to die, which includes the right not to have the process of dying interrupted. Ventilated brain-dead cases have a right to privacy, for though they are classified as "dead patients" they have not been granted the right to a full bodily death. Ventilated bodies have the processes of death postponed. Although it makes sense for the right to privacy to end with death, full bodily death has not occurred in PMV cases.

The major difference between PMV and the Quinlan case is that PMV offers a benefit: the possibility that the fetus might survive. A feminist view opposing PMV must show that the harm of PMV to women and the moral community in general outweighs the benefits of a possible live birth. I have already argued that PMV can be seen as harming the moral community and violating the brain-dead patient's right to privacy. I further contend that it is inappropriate to require the bodies of women to remain pregnant in death but not in life, unless a dead body has some reproductive obligation that a live body does not have. Do cadavers have reproductive obligations? Clearly not, since an obligation requires an agent capable of fulfilling the obligation by performing an act. As a cadaver is incapable of being the agent of an act, a cadaver cannot be seen to have any obligations. Others may have obligations vis à vis the cadaver, for instance the obligation to bury it, but the cadaver itself is incapable of being obligated or responsible for anything. Someone might claim that the woman herself is obligated from life, to have her pregnancy continued beyond the point of her brain death. Such a view might point to other obligations in life that are interrupted by one's death, for instance a parent's death interrupts the parent's abilities to fulfill obligations toward her children. Death always interrupts one's financial obligations. But it has been argued that PMV cannot help meet a woman's obligation to continue her pregnancy because she ought not be obligated to be pregnant. And if a cadaver has no reproductive obligations, then it cannot have reproductive rights. In fact, cadavers are excluded from reproductive rights precisely because they are cadavers. Reproductive freedom is properly attributed to people, not cadavers. PMV violates the reproductive freedom of women. The strongest opponents of this view would argue that PMV would create no harm to the moral community if it were based on consent and seen as an instance of organ donation, but this results from conceptual confusion about the nature of consent, organ donations, and pregnancy.

PMV and Individual Consent

Would PMV be riddled with problems if it were not mandatory, but based on consent? Like much reproductive technology, PMV is expensive, has a high failure rate, and undermines women by emphasizing pregnancy as a woman's highest fulfillment. Nevertheless, some women might want the chance to participate in PMV for individual reasons— to have an heir, to leave their spouses with a last child, to have their deaths afford something positive, to have their own processes of death delayed. It is feasible that some women might choose PMV, prior to brain death, as the possibility of PMV becomes more widely known. Physicians might even decide to discuss PMV routinely with every pregnant woman in order to be informed of her wishes in the unusual event of sudden brain death.

If consent were the essential moral requirement for PMV, whose consent is necessary? The woman's own? In which case there ought to be PMV consent forms available in every obstetric practice. Should the biological father have a right to consent to PMV? If so, how would a conflict between the mother's and the father's wishes be resolved? Should the mother's wishes take precedence because it is her body? Or should the father's wishes take precedence because he has paternal responsibilities if the fetus were to be born alive? A woman's interest in terminating the pregnancy ought to outweigh the interests of her sexual partner with respect to PMV, for I believe that it would be inconsistent with the abortion right to assume that a father has rights to an in utero fetus if the mother is dead, but not if she is alive.

If PMV were based on consent, there would always be cases in which consent was unclear, as well as current cases in which consent was not given because no one envisioned that a particular pregnant case might be appropriate for ventilation. Is it plausible for physicians to assume that because, in all seven PMV cases cited, the women had not terminated their pregnancies before the onset of brain death, they would have wanted their pregnancies continued beyond their brain deaths? Clearly, one cannot infer that any intention in life applies as well to intentions in death. For instance, if my neighbor donates blood regularly in blood-drives, I cannot automatically infer that it would be his intention to make a large donation of his blood upon his death. There might be reasons for donating blood in life that would not be valid in death. For instance, suppose my neighbor was an active blood donor primarily because he liked chatting with the nurses at the blood-mobile. This motive would not be served by donating blood after his death. Similarly, if a woman has not terminated her pregnancy before suffering brain death it cannot be inferred that she would desire her pregnancy to continue beyond the point of her brain death. For instance, lacking a partner, she may not want to bring a child into the world with no one designated to care for it, or she may not want her body to be seen by others and artificially sustained after her brain death.

As one cannot infer consent to be pregnant in death from consent to be pregnant in life, a physician cannot properly infer that a woman would have wanted PMV simply from the fact that she had not aborted earlier in pregnancy. Such an inference would confuse the intent to sustain one's pregnancy in life with the intent to have one's pregnancy artificially sustained in one's ventilated corpse. The two intentions are quite distinct, as are a conscious body and a brain-dead body. Moreover, the fact that a woman is pregnant now does not mean it is her intent to remain pregnant in the future. Hence, physicians must consider the possibility that a pregnant brain-dead woman is not necessarily a woman who desires her pregnancy to continue. Of course, it could be argued that it would violate a woman's wishes to infer that she doesn't want the pregnancy continued. However, as PMV requires the active maintenance of life in a cadaver, and as we do not routinely apply active measures when no consent is given, it would be inappropriate to apply active "extraordinary" measures automatically in pregnant cases. Though a physician's duty is to save lives, this is not a duty without limitations. A physician is not expected, for instance, to use cadavers as incubators for the nurturing of previable life, anymore than the physician is expected to find tissue mediums where aborted fetuses might possibly be sustained. After all, the physician's patient is the woman, not the fetus, and the physician owes her patient a speedy and dignified death. She is obligated to treat the fetus as a vital part of her patient's body, providing sound medical advice and obstetric care, but it would be exploitive of the pregnant woman for a physician to elevate fetal interests over the welfare of the mother herself.

The right to consent to PMV ought to include the right to refuse PMV. Living wills, typically used to indicate a patient's wishes in cases of terminal illness, might contain requests regarding PMV. Currently, there are living will acts in thirty-five states. But living wills tend to favor the fetus and not the pregnant woman. Twenty-seven acts include a pregnancy clause that forbids implementation if the patient is pregnant (MacAvoy-Snitzer 1987). In order for women to be able to prohibit PMV in a living will, pregnancy clauses would need to be invalidated.

It has been assumed that consent might make PMV morally permissible, but consent alone does not make an act morally permissible. PMV would not be morally permissible if the violations of rights outweigh the benefits of possible live birth. PMV violates women's reproductive freedoms by failing to treat the bodies of brain-dead women as ends in themselves. There is a need for maternal brain death to be a clear and steady marker beyond which a woman and her body should no longer be pregnant. Otherwise, the distinction between the dead and the living disintegrates. For if pregnant cadavers ought to be used for reproductive work, then *any* cadaver might be seen as obligated to partake of service in sustaining human life. Not only could we find ourselves in intensive care wards full of plugged-in cadavers functioning as uteri, kidney machines, transplant banks, and tissue suppliers, but the implications of attributing obligations to cadavers would include a deterioration in the status of the right to one's body and the regard we might have for each person as an end in herself.

One could imagine a woman's request for PMV as a way in which she regarded herself as an end. She might desire PMV in order to actualize her life and plead with her physician before the onset of brain death, "Keep my baby alive. Do all you can to save this pregnancy. The birth of my child matters to me more than anything I have ever done in my whole life." Even though this wish might reflect the patriarchal socialization of women for motherhood, nonetheless, it demonstrates that pregnancy has become a very meaningful choice for the woman herself within her unique life situation. Still, the harm to fundamental personal freedoms can be judged more significant than the harm of denying an individual's wish for PMV. For neither moral decisions nor technological practices can be isolated from the context of social and political meanings that structure reality.

PMV as Organ Donation

It might be argued that PMV ought to be seen as an instance of a woman donating her cadaver to be used for sustaining the fetus, and hence analogous to the practice of donating organs for human transplants or donating one's entire body to medical research. Exploring PMV as an instance of organ donation reveals a significant aspect of the ontological relationship between a woman and her fetus in pregnancy. Whether one donates a ventilated cadaver for research, or a ventilated pregnant cadaver for fetal support, a positive end results. Since cadaver donations for both research and transplants are legal in all fifty states under the Uniform Donor Act, it might be claimed that PMV also ought to be legal, for it is simply another case of donating one's cadaver for use by the living (Schwartz 1985).

But differences in intent and end result indicate an ontological difference between cadaver donations and PMV. Only PMV uses a cadaver for maintaining another (living) body, the fetus, which would not otherwise qualify as a transplant recipient. The pregnant cadaver is not transplanted into the fetus, like an organ donation, nor does it require the surgical connection between the donor and the recipient, for the fetus has been in utero since conception. Most importantly, PMV greatly alters the ontological relationship between a woman and her fetus in pregnancy. In pregnancies in living women, the fetus is biologically contingent on the woman's body. In PMV the woman's body is contingent on the fetus—somatic life will be sustained in the woman's body only as long as the fetus is present and thriving. Once the fetus is born, life support on the woman's body is ended, natural bodily death is allowed to occur, and the woman's remains are interred. If PMV is to be seen as merely another case covered by the Uniform Donor Act, it must be argued that the PMV cadaver is analogous to donated cadaver organs, yet the analogy breaks down because the ontological relationship between the donated organ and the human recipient undergoes no reversal. Further, the organ recipient is not using the donated organ while it is still a part of the donor. Nor does the transplant recipient use the donor's body to grow its own new organs. The fact is, the pregnant body has never been disconnected from the fetus after conception, unlike other donations. Live pregnancies similarly are not donor/recipient relationships. A pregnant woman is not "donating" her body temporarily for the maintenance of the fetus. Rather, pregnant women are autonomous beings engaged in a variety of projects, not the least of which is the project of growing a fetus. Hence, neither in life nor in death can pregnancy be seen as an instance of organ donation. Organ donation is a false analogy for PMV, for pregnancy, as always, is a special case. A pregnant body affords no suitable analogies. What is needed is clarification of what pregnancy is and discussion about the parameters of pregnancy that make it a human endeavor. Were PMV to become standard obstetric practice, it would suggest that the moral community values fetal survival more than the privacy rights of pregnant persons.

Pregnancy Rights

Ours is a century in which reproductive technology is increasingly expanding alternatives to traditional reproductive practices. Yet the technology is too often placed in the control of medical professionals, which supercedes women's control over their pregnancies. PMV is another procedure that threatens to separate pregnancy from women's control while altering the social meaning of pregnancy (Lenow 1983, Johnsen 1986). Neither *Roe,* the right to privacy, nor the Uniform Donor Act is able to subsume the issues of PMV. Even an appeal to cadaver rights provides no basis for the prohibition of PMV as long as it can be claimed that the pregnant cadaver is a "special case." Clearly, without a definition of pregnancy, human rights can be seen as inapplicable to women in pregnancy, leading to such preposterous claims as the belief that pregnant women are entitled to less control over their bodies, less protection from bodily mutilation in noncognitive states, less of a right to immediate bodily death, less of a right to privacy, less of a right to have their cadavers protected from exploitative medical uses. Rather than sorting out women's rights in pregnancy by direct application of basic human rights to the "special case" of pregnancy, a definition of pregnancy should be established at the outset and women's rights in pregnancy derived from this definition. Needless to say, feminists must take an active role in establishing any definition of pregnancy to be used to determine women's legal rights.

If we understand the mother/fetus relationship in pregnancy as determined solely by the mother, who is the only autonomous party in the relationship, and who sustains the relationship only insofar as she regards it as a meaningful project resulting from her own free choice, then the practice of PMV would be impermissible. PMV fundamentally alters the mother/fetus relationship in pregnancy by making the mother contingent on the fetus and severing pregnancy from human consciousness. PMV poses a serious threat to abortion rights by sustaining pregnancy in a female cadaver without prior consent.

Serious objections have been raised about PMV within a patriarchal society. However, at least two kinds of objections to PMV could be raised even in an egalitarian society. First, PMV might still have serious implications for reproductive freedom. One would need to consider whether or not PMV necessarily presupposes an eliminative view of pregnancy. If so, then PMV would be undesirable. Of course if the egalitarian society had a high infertility rate and if brain death in pregnancy became quite common, then the society might be in dire need of live births and a limited use of PMV might be justifiable. Assuming that this extreme situation does not exist, an egalitarian society would need to consider whether or not PMV would be a fair use of medical technology. In the United States, PMV perpetuates the unequal allocation of scarce medical resources. PMV requires that technology, staff, and medical resources be used not for the treatment of human beings but for the sake of saving previable fetuses. Moreover, PMV is an arbitrary use of medicine. It is used to maintain a few previable pregnancies in cadavers (some of whom were from working class and black families) while thousands of pregnant women, often in the same city in which the practice of PMV occurred, lack a minimal level of prenatal care. Isn't it alarming that the country with the greatest number of publicized PMV cases is also the country that ranks seventeenth in low infant mortality rates in the West? The individual benefits of PMV cannot outweigh such an allocation of medical resources. There are better ways to use and distribute our technological resources that would effectively serve the common good. A poet writes

> We study the wrong subject in the maze
> of inquiry, we took a false corner. The ways
> we came to there are known and plotted but we end,
> still, at a blind wall.
>
> William Bronk, "The False Corner"

Like other new possibilities for pregnancy, PMV perpetuates the desire to control life and deny death. PMV, like modern medicine in general, is based on an assumption of metaphysical dualism: that the body can be perceived and managed by seeing it as separate from human consciousness. Higher human activities such as consciousness, cognition, and imagination are devalued. We cannot diminish the value of human pregnancy without diminishing the value of being human. PMV is but one instance of such an attempt, an instance of one of the limitless uses for cadavers and technology. Yet the measure of our social community lies not in the number of its technological exploits, but in the ends we strive for. The most fundamental human end is the valuation of human consciousness. Postmortem maternal ventilation, by requiring pregnancy of women after their brain deaths, fails to envision what the capacity for maternal consciousness in pregnancy should mean to a human community.

N O T E S

1. This discussion applies to U.S. pregnancies. For European discussion of PMV see Metter and Estel (1972) and Pietchowiak (1984). The legal ambiguities of *Roe v. Wade* are further explored in Rhoden (1986), Rice (1983), and Martyn (1981–82).
2. For analysis of the exploitation of women in embryo transfer research see my article (1984). For discussion of the legal issues in reproductive technology see Smith (1985). For analysis of the effects of reproductive technology on abortion rights, see my article (1986).
3. The table is by no means a complete registry of cases. (1) Sampson (1979), (2) Associated Press (1984), (3) Sampson (1979), (4) Associated Press (1987a,b).
4. The table is by no means a complete registry of cases. (1) and (2) Meyer (1977), (3) Associated Press (1982), (4) Associated Press (1983a,b), (5) As-

sociated Press (1983c), (6) Associated Press (1986b), (7) Associated Press (1986a,c,d).

REFERENCES

Ad Hoc Committee of the Harvard Medical School to Examine the Definition of Brain-Death, 1968. A definition of irreversible coma. *Journal of the American Medical Association* 205, no. 6: 337–40.

Arthur, Robert K. 1978. Postmortem caesarean section. *American Journal of Obstetrics and Gynecology* 132, no. 2: 175–79.

Associated Press. 1982. Doctors report birth of baby in 1981 to brain-dead woman. *New York Times,* September 5, 1982.

———. 1983a. Life from death. *New York Times,* October 16, 1983.

———. 1983b. Woman legally dead gives birth to a boy. *New York Times,* March 31, 1983.

———. 1983c. Brain-dead mother dies. *New York Times,* July 7, 1983.

———. 1984. Healthy baby delivered from mother in coma. *New York Times,* August 21, 1984.

———. 1986a. Ruling by a court keeps fetus alive: Man who claims fatherhood wins fight for life support for brain-dead woman. *New York Times,* July 26, 1986.

———. 1986b. Baby born to dead woman. *Portland Press Herald* (Portland, Maine), July 31, 1986.

———. 1986c. Baby is weak after birth to brain-dead woman. *New York Times,* August 16, 1986.

———. 1986d. Baby in court battle dies after one day. *New York Times,* August 17, 1986.

———. 1987a. Mother chooses for comatose daughter, fetus. *Hartford Courant.* March 19, 1987.

———. 1987b. Comatose woman's fetus is focus of dispute. *New York Times,* March 8, 1987.

Atlantic Reporter. 1976. "In the matter of Karen Quinlan, an alleged incompetent," Supreme Court of New Jersey, 2D, 355:647, March 31, 1976.

Bronk, William. 1982. Life supports and the false corner. In *Life Supports.* San Francisco: North Point Press.

Dillon, William P., Richard V. Lee, Sharon Buckwald, Michael Tronolone, and Ronald J. Foote. 1982. Life support and maternal brain death during pregnancy. *Journal of the American Medical Association* 248, no. 9: 1089–91.

Johnsen, Dawn E. 1986. The creation of fetal rights: Conflicts with women's constitutional rights to liberty, privacy, and equal protection. *Yale Law Journal* 95, no. 599: 21–47.

Lenow, Jeffrey L. 1983. The fetus as patient: Emerging rights as a person? *American Journal of Law and Medicine* 9, no. 1: 1–29.

MacAvoy-Snitzer, Janice. 1987. Pregnancy clauses in living will statutes. *Columbia Law Review* 87:1,280–1,300.

Martyn, Ken. 1981–82. Technological advances and Roe v. Wade: The need to rethink abortion law. *UCLA Law Review* 29, nos. 5,6: 1,194–1,215.

Meyer, Lawrence. 1977. Two lives involved: "Brain-dead" mother kept alive in effort to save four month fetus. *Washington Post,* December 2, 1977.

Metter, D., and C. Estel. 1972. Arztliche und rechtliche probleme der sectio in mortua et in moribunda (Medical and legal problems of death and dying). *Zeitschrift fur arztliche Fortbildung* 66, no.6: 351–53.

Murphy, Julien S. 1984. Egg-farming and women's future. In *Test-Tube Women,* ed. R. Arditti, R. Klein, and S. Minden, 66–75. New York: Routledge and Kegan Paul.

———. 1986. Abortion rights and fetal termination. *Journal of Social Philosophy* 17, no. 1: 11–16.

Newsweek. 1983. Out of death, a new life comes. April 11, 1983.

Piechowiak, J. 1984. Der mutterliche hirntod am ende des zweiten trimenons. *Rundschau Med. Praxis* 73, no. 12: 361–62.

Pinkus, Rosa Lynn. 1984. Families, brain death, and traditional medical excellence. *Journal of Neurosurgery* 60:1,192–94.

Rice, Julie E. 1983. Fetal rights: Defining "persons" under 42 U.S.C. 1983. *University of Illinois Law Review,* no 1: 347–66.

Rhoden, Nancy K. 1986. Trimesters and technology: Revamping Roe v. Wade. *Yale Law Journal* 95, no. 4: 739–97.

Roe v. Wade, 410 US 113 (1973).

Sampson, Milo B., and Loren P. Petersen. 1979. Post-traumatic coma during pregnancy. *Obstetrics and Gynecology* 53, no. 3: 2–3.

Schwartz, Howard S. 1985. Bioethical and legal considerations in increasing the supply of transplantable organs: from UAGA to "Baby Fae." *American Journal of Law and Medicine* 10, no. 4: 397–437.

Siegler, Mark, and Daniel Wikler. 1982. Brain death and live birth. *Journal of the American Medical Association* 248, no. 9: 1101.

Smith, George P., II. 1985. Australia's frozen "orphan" embryos: A medical, legal and ethical dilemma. *Journal of Family Law* 24, no. 1: 27–58.

Uniform Laws Annotated. 1988. Uniform determination of death act. Supplement. 12:293–96. St. Paul: West Publishing.

University Health Services v. Piazzi. 1986. Document no. CV86-RCCV-464, Georgia Superior Court, August 4, 1986.

**Part 2
Health Care Technologies:
Political and Ethical Considerations**

Introduction

Glenda D. Price

In the two decades between 1966 and 1986 the U.S. health care system experienced greater growth than at any other time in history. The health care workforce swelled from 446,000 to 1.165 million, with total health care expenditures growing from $42 billion to $320 billion. Concurrently the use of technology increased tremendously. Extensive research in space technology and spillover from this research into the health care field, together with vast governmental and private sector investment in new technology, contributed to this growth. Miniaturized circuitry, lasers, computer monitoring, synthetic fabrics, and slow-release medications are all examples of space research achievements that have been introduced into health care. Furthermore, investments in technology have led to automated chemistry analyzers, heart-lung machines, infusion pumps, monoclonal antibodies, laser surgery, and transcutaneous medication patches, now common tools of the health practitioner.

However, the money and time devoted to producing new devices and techniques has not been matched by investments in evaluating their usefulness or appropriateness. Rapid expansion of the number and types of laboratory tests, diagnostic procedures and therapeutic regimes has made it difficult for both practitioners and the public to decide when particular technologies actually contribute to improvements in well-being. A variety of institutional and interpersonal pressures encourage health care providers to turn to technology, even when the quality of care is not improved by its use; these pressures include the status and income that tests and procedures can generate, the need to practice "defensive medicine," the compulsion to be complete by ruling out even the remotest possible diagnosis, the desire to show that something is being done, and the wish to communicate concern by doing all that is feasible. The potential for employing a new technology has grown exponentially while the ability to judge when these innovations are useful as well as the concern for the political and ethical implications have lagged perceptibly behind. Perhaps due to the growth of health care and health care technology, health issues are increasingly the subject of both political and ethical debates. Political and ethical ramifications of health care technologies and their effect on women's health are the two themes of this part of the book.

The first theme is the politics of health care. The fact that health care is a large and continually growing industry necessarily brings it into the arena of politics in the conventional sense. It involves the courts, the legislature, and the federal bureaucracy of the executive branch in mandating, limiting, subsidizing, and scrutinizing health care decision making at all levels. The industry interacts with government in setting many of the conditions of health policy, funding, licensure, and reimbursement that are central to the industry. The available technology, actual and potential markets, and the economic and regulatory climate in which it operates are all factors in which government plays a leading role. Government is the object as well as the subject of political action. Insofar as consumers want to have a significant impact on the type or quality of care that is offered, bringing pressure upon the institutions of government can be an important route to changes in health care priorities or practices. The women's health, wellness, and hospice movements all serve as catalysts for change through political activity, along with more traditional pressure groups such as the pharmaceutical and instrument manufacturing industries and the various health professions organizations. The politics of health care has become as important as the existence of care.

However, neither government regulation and subsidy, no matter how extensive, nor other forms of political activity will be able to determine appropriate care at the individual level. The fact that some of the most significant decisions about the uses of technology in health care will have to be made at the individual level seems at first to remove them from the realm of politics. But the feminist slogan "the personal is political" may serve to remind us that politics is not merely the actions of state, federal, and local government. Politics is the study of power relations, and power is manifested in a variety of forms in interpersonal and institutional relations at all levels. The political considerations evident in the chapters of Part 2 range from the governmental and institutional level (Ratcliff; Whatley and Worcester) to the power dimension in interpersonal relations between provider and client (Wertz and Fletcher; Bell; Lind).

The second major theme of these chapters is the ethics of health care. Questions of ethics are becoming increasingly complex as technological advances are changing the nature of the interaction between patients/clients and health care providers. Ethical principles come more in conflict with each other as the lines become blurred between the individual's responsibility for personal health care and the responsibility of the providers to use their expertise to benefit the client. The historic admonition to do no harm and the professional's need to conserve life may present a conflict of rights. It is no longer clear when actions designed to preserve life cause psychological and emotional harm, nor is it any longer sufficient to focus on the physical care an individual requires; consideration must also be given to social, personal, and generally human needs.

Political and ethical issues are clearly intertwined. A short personal story that I believe to be typical of the interaction between the health care system and family members of patients may illustrate these dynamics. When my stepfather at age sixty-three went to the hospital with shortness of breath, chest pain, and a severe headache, his EKG showed mild changes and blood chemistry results reflected "normal values." He was admitted "for observation." Although my mother accompanied him to the hospital and was present throughout the examination and admission process, her repeated questioning of hospital personnel elicited only replies of "don't worry." She left the hospital uncertain of her husband's diagnosis or prognosis. His condition deteriorated rapidly with kidney failure and coma occurring within twenty-four hours. Without contacting my mother, the physician initiated intensive therapy including IVs, a respirator, catheterization, and cardiac monitors. Although a considerable amount of technology was used to maintain his life, he died after twenty-two days. Throughout this time my mother was told what was being done, but at no time was she asked to help decide on the care that her husband was to receive. And at no time was she given sufficient information to understand the magnitude of his illness or the probability of his recovery.

Many people can tell a similar story, especially when the patient's next of kin is female, elderly, or both. Even when the care is technologically correct, it may not be the "best" care, or even ethical care. In this case the patient and his family lost their autonomy, too little information was provided to the next of kin to constitute informed consent, and too little interaction occurred to ensure that the system did no harm. Had the situation been reversed, with my mother the patient and her husband the concerned family member, it is less likely that he would have been merely told not to worry. Men are seldom patronized by physicians in the same way as women.

This story illustrates three ethical themes that emerge as central elements throughout this part: Patient autonomy, informed consent, and nonmalfeasance. Giving patients the power and authority to participate in, or indeed decide upon, the care they receive; providing sufficient information at an appropriate level to allow individuals to accept or to reject specific technologies; and acknowledging the right of a client to personally determine what constitutes harm—all these are explored here as fundamental issues of ethical care. At the same time the basic power dynamics in the situation become clear. Too often the health care system takes over, develops a momentum of its own, and fails to include the patient and family in the process.

Kathryn Ratcliff begins Part 2 with her discussion of the powerful influences that have fostered the growth of technology in today's health care system. She explains how a bias toward technology is developed in medical school education, supported by governmental policy and procedure, and greatly reinforced by the profit motive. The expansion of the for-profit sector of health care has accelerated these trends, and a feminist analysis of these tendencies suggests how the troika of profits, control, and expanded reliance on technology in health care can be especially dangerous for women. Federal agencies as the major regulators of technology and the primary third-party reimbursers of services exert their own political force as well as being subject to the political influences of others. Ratcliff's analysis indicates why the government's assessment programs have been ineffective in restraining the use of dangerous and ineffective technologies in women's health care.

The ethical issues introduced by Ratcliff are thus clearly intertwined with political ones. She points to profits and power as influencing the physician's use of technology to shape patient care, to identify and treat disorders about which the patient may be unconcerned, and to diagnose problems unrelated to the individual's primary needs. Patients are given little real opportunity to participate in the decisions about diagnostic and therapeutic procedures offered. Furthermore, Ratcliff shows that consideration of the ethical implications of technology takes a backseat to pressures for "technological progress." She points out the inclination to view technology as scientific and therefore objective, with no need to consider the human aspects of its use. Because something is scientifically possible, it must automatically be good; the benefit of the doubt goes to new technologies and the costs fall on groups exposed to dangerous and undertested practices until the harm becomes evident in their lives.

While Ratcliff's focus is societal, Mariamne Whatley and Nancy Worcester explore some of the political and ethical implications of health care at an organizational and individual level. The role of the for-profit sector and insurance companies in defining the standards of care and access to services have shaped the delivery of health services to women. The women's health movement has been a major critic of the rampant use of technologies of dubious value. Feminist pressures have been effective in increasing care oriented toward health promotion and disease prevention, participatory decision making, and alternative approaches to traditional care. But as Whatley and Worcester show in their chapter, the movement is vulnerable to co-optation by market forces that use consumer concern with health to sell procedures to women that may not contribute to their well-being.

Using bone mass measurement and mammography as two examples of technology, Whatley and Worcester examine the degree to which the principles of the women's health movement have been maintained. Has the momentum of the movement brought about fundamental change in the health system, or has the health care system used the women's health movement for its own gain? Whatley and Worcester suggest that the reliability and effectiveness of the technologies have been "over-sold" to women. They make an important distinction between detection and prevention, and question the significance of early detection when, as in the case of osteoporosis, there is little evidence of beneficial effect except on the manufacturers' balance sheet.

In their discussion of osteoporosis and breast cancer screening Whatley and Worcester also explore ethical issues of autonomy and informed consent. They show how marketers prey upon the fears, and when fear is used to induce a woman to request screening, her autonomy has been reduced. Women are not informed of the difficulties of comparing radiographs of bone density or the differences between available technologies. The value of baseline mammograms is often misunderstood; the sensitivity and specificity of these techniques are not always explained; and women often consent to technologies that they know little about.

While both Ratcliff and Whatley and Worcester focus on contending political forces in the United States, Dorothy Wertz and John Fletcher direct concern toward the political and social climate affecting decision making within one professional arena internationally. Studying medical geneticists from eighteen countries, they explore the influence of culture, gender, and professional role on the geneticists' preferred courses of action with regard to ten ethical situations. In countries with different cultural values, counselors exercise their power as experts to shape the clients' decision making in particular directions. For instance in the German Democratic Republic and Hungary, where the health care systems are under greatest government control, the tendency is toward the most directive counseling. However, it is interesting to note that the cultural tendency in Japan to obey authority did not influence the geneticists toward directive approaches. In the United States, where patient autonomy is highly valued, counselors emphasized nondirective advice, even when the patient sought prenatal diagnosis solely for sex selection. As in India, counselors in the United States were willing to refer patients for abortion if the fetus was the "wrong" sex, ducking the ethical issue for themselves by emphasizing the client's right to decide. The political climate and individual decision making are clearly linked for both the genetic counselors and their clients, and the consequences of their choices also have political ramifications.

The issues of client autonomy and informed consent are also addressed directly by Wertz and Fletcher. The question of a woman's right to request prenatal screening in the absence of age or medical indications for such screening was one of ten questions posed in their survey. A significant difference was found on this question among geneticists from various countries, with those from the United States emphasizing most client autonomy. American women genetic counselors were especially likely to put their emphasis on autonomy and freedom of choice, reflecting the language in which reproductive issues have primarily been discussed in this country. However, another question in the Wertz and Fletcher survey focused on the alternatives presented about new or controversial reproductive technologies and many American geneticists, as well as those of other nationalities, indicated that they would not present certain options. How well can client autonomy be respected when providers would fail to share all known information? On the other hand, offering information could be doing harm, especially if it creates expectations in the parent that could become a self-fulfilling prophecy for the child.

The issue of nonmalfeasance also surfaces in Wertz and Fletcher's discussion of responses to a question on full disclosure of information in a false paternity situation. The husband's right to know and the geneticists' mandate to do no harm are in conflict; however, 96 percent of the respondents indicated that they would protect the confidentiality of the woman. It would appear that the principle of nonmalfeasance was a higher priority for this group of geneticists, male and female alike, in this situation.

Ethics and political issues arise for consumers as well as practitioners. In the following paper Susan Bell uses the story of one woman to demonstrate how the acceptance of her situation led her to become politically active in the women's health movement. When "Sarah" became an active participant in DES Action, a women's health organization, in order to share information and change government policy on diethylstilbesterol (DES), she found that her politics gave her a framework for interpreting personal experience and medical advice more productively. Through intensive linguistic analysis of interviews with "Sarah," Bell shows us the emotional changes that underlie one individual's transition from denial on a personal level to action on a political level, and clarifies how social movement politics can transform individuals as well as social systems. Building on the work of Elliot Mishler, Bell advances the position that an individual must be ready to listen to the "voice" of her lifeworld and not simply the "voice" of medicine. The context in which the voice is heard will determine the level of understanding and the readiness for information. Unless an individual is receptive to both the voice of medicine and the voice of her lifeworld (social context) she will be unable to make informed decisions and function as an autonomous individual. Neither voice will penetrate until an individual is ready to listen. The ability of individual women to make ethically responsible and informed choices is not fostered either in or outside the health care system. But Bell suggests that an active women's health movement can be an important resource for individual women to draw on in developing their ability to evaluate and choose.

In the final chapter in Part 2, Alice Lind clarifies the hospice concept and explains how it differs from traditional medicine in ways that are consistent with feminist goals and ethics. A political theme is evident in this paper in her discussion of the locus of power in the two settings. The motivation for technology use shifts from maintaining life to easing dying, the balance of power moves from the health care provider to the client, and the change of location from hospitals to home brings different priorities and decision makers into sight. Lind's reflection on her own experience of care-giving in hospital intensive care units and in hospice suggests how the change in power relations can be positive not only for the patient but for the provider. The feminist perspective on power—that it increases when it is shared, rather than requiring a zero-sum conflict over control—is borne out within the supportive setting provided by hospice. However, Lind also points out how few dying patients experience hospice care and she argues for efforts to change the health care system as a whole.

The basic philosophical foundation of hospice contributes to more ethical care. Informed consent, nonmalfeasance, and client autonomy are fostered by empowering individuals to take control of their care and determine the manner of their death. Hospice challenges providers to "be with" not to "do to" their clients. For example, Lind recalls that in seven years as an intensive care unit (ICU) nurse she doesn't remember ever actually seeing a patient die. She was always focused on the monitors, the IVs—the technology, not the patient. In hospice Lind learned to "be with" the client and recognized that it is the person that matters.

As a group, these papers indicate how the type and quality of health care, access to care, use of technologies, and type of provider available to us are determined as much by politics as by need. Moreover, the relationship between patient and provider in making decisions about the use of particular technologies in specific instances also has an important ethical dimension as power differences allow certain values and priorities in care-giving to dominate others. These papers enhance our awareness of the need for continuing political involvement not only as a means to ensure the type of system that serves the needs of the client, but also as a form of personal empowerment that may help the client to understand better what her own needs are.

Collectively these chapters focus our thinking not only on the politics of technology in women's health care and the ethical problems that certain technologies produce, but also on the intricate links between political and ethical issues at many different levels. The government's role in funding and regulating both health care and technology creates not only political pressures but also opportunities for change in the system as a whole. Markets for new technologies such as mammograms can be politically expanded or restricted, and the women's health movement faces ethical dilemmas in lobbying for availability and choice in situations in which information necessary for real consent is lacking. Where health professionals have the power to give or to withhold information, the values by which they make decisions about the good or harm that information will do are shaped by the language of political discourse within their culture. Individual patients also bring their own political and personal expectations to bear on interactions with health care providers, and need to be empowered not only to ask questions but to be able to hear and respond to the answers if genuinely informed consent is to become possible. The political movement that is making hospice care feasible is also changing the structure of ethical choices for practitioners. Once the needs of the patient for a "good" death become more salient than the beeping, blinking monitors' demands for attention, care-givers will become aware of the harm they inadvertently have been doing, and will be forced to make choices based on this new information.

In sum, these chapters argue for the value of information as a political resource and prerequisite for ethical choice. But they do not pretend that information can or will always be used by either patients or practitioners in an empowering or even ethically responsible way. They recognize that women have had less power to determine the way technology is used in health care settings, and that women have consequently suffered harm; but they do not argue that women automatically have a more ethical viewpoint. Nonetheless, they suggest ways in which a feminist analysis of the politics and ethics of health care technologies could be of great value in creating a safer, more equitable, and more humane health care system.

Health Technologies for Women:
Whose Health? Whose Technology?

Kathryn Strother Ratcliff

Today controversy surrounds the broad range of health technologies for women that have been aggressively marketed and broadly utilized in recent years despite potential hazards and uncertain benefits. Many women, and in some instances their children, have suffered major health problems as a direct result of the use of these technologies which include drugs, surgery, and other treatments for birth control (the Dalkon Shield), pregnancy (diethylstilbesterol [DES]), childbirth (electronic fetal monitoring [EFM] and caesarean sections), cancer (radical mastectomy and hysterectomy), emotional problems (prescription drugs), menopause and aging (estrogen replacement therapy) (Corea 1985; Kasper 1985; Koumjian 1981; McCrea 1983; Mintz 1985; Orenberg 1981; Perry and Dawson 1986; Ruzek 1986, 187; Vance and Millington 1986; Weiss 1983). Many technologies can have beneficial results: they may be safer procedures, they may allow earlier detection, and they may provide for better health. However, the cases of harmful outcomes are nonetheless instructive because they push us to look at the larger social context and pose some hard questions. What roles have scientists, physicians, and the health care system as a whole played in the spread of hazardous technologies? Could these hazards have been avoided, and if so, how? Why has health care technology stimulated such outrage among feminists and other women?

To address these questions, this chapter discusses the financial incentives and educational structure of the health care system that has fostered the growth of technologically intensive practices at the expense of a primary concern for health, and considers how women and the health of women have been particularly affected by these influences. I argue first that the U.S. health care system is characterized by a strong "technological favoritism," i.e., it is heavily biased in favor of the use of technology to solve or to prevent medical problems; and second, there are strongly gendered values in both western technology and western medical practice that make this technological favoritism particularly problematic for women.

Feminist research in health care has documented the extent to which new technologies threaten the health and well-being of women, but to understand why this occurs we must combine elements of the feminist critique with an analysis of other social forces that have been reshaping the health care system. While considerable research on the restructuring of American health care in the past two decades exists (Relman 1980; Starr 1982; Gray 1983), little of this work acknowledges or investigates the differential impact of technological favoritism on women.

The feminist critique of health care has been wide ranging but two broad areas of criticism are particularly relevant. First, feminist scholars have documented the male-dominated character of western medicine and argued that male domination means that technology will be used in the medical system to reinforce the subordinate role of women. These analyses trace the evolution of a system of health care in which the high-ranking health care providers are male (Wertz and Wertz 1979; Ehrenreich and English 1972; Gordon 1976), they document these men's contributions to the medicalization of natural processes occurring in women (Ehrenreich and English 1973; McCrea 1983; Reissman 1983), and they argue that both are linked to a patriarchal system.

A second area of feminist concern has been the analysis of the history of science and technology. They suggest that western science and technology embody stereotypically male values such as control, distance, power, objectivity, and domination and that these values promote invasive solutions to problems. Analyses of influential early writings in science and technology, for example, note how these writings incorporated sexual metaphors endowing science and technology with typical male traits while portraying the objects of science and technology as female. Renaissance philosophers revered nature or mother earth, and their writings evidence a moral mandate to protect her from the greed and lust of those who would "mine her womb" (Merchant 1980). But the scientific revolution changed the role of science and technology from protector to dominator of nature. Bacon and other prominent scientists promised science and technology would not "merely exert gentle guidance over nature's course; they have the power to conquer and subdue her, to shake her to her foundations" (quoted in Keller 1985, 36). The use of gendered imagery has distanced women from science and technology, but more importantly has produced a scientific and technological culture with an unbalanced value system. Western science and technology value stereotypically male traits such as subduing and controlling nature, rather than adjusting to or respecting nature. Such values encourage invasive technological solutions to problems.

But these feminist critiques should not stand alone. Technology is encouraged not only by stereotypically male values and a system in which men have greater decision-making power, but also by economic and social factors that structure care-giving. In the following discussion I will consider three influences: the growth and restructuring of for-profit health care; the education and socialization of health care providers; and the systems that assess and evaluate technology. Each of these factors has helped propel the entire health care system toward more intensive use of technology. Central to my argument is that each includes strong gender forces that make the "technological favoritism" of the system a particular problem for women.

The Growth and Restructuring of For-Profit Forces in Health Care

American medicine has long been an industry shaped by the profit and income orientations of key participants who have developed and promoted various technologies including health care devices, procedures, and pharmaceuticals (Relman 1980). In recent years major organizational changes have altered and intensified the for-profit aspect of the health care system. First, major health care institutions have adopted business orientations that stress economic returns and diminish service. Second, doctors have reorganized their practices increasingly to stress income maximization. And third, educational institutions are becoming more explicitly involved in profit-seeking activities. The growth and power of these for-profit arenas help us understand the technological favoritism now embedded in health care delivery.

The Growing Business Orientation of Health Care Institutions

Many observers note the rapid intrusion of for-profit interests in our health care delivery system (Starr 1982; Relman 1980; Gray 1986). While the change to more business- and profit-oriented managerial forms has characterized health institutions in general, this transformation has been most apparent in hospitals and clinics that are organized explicitly as "for-profit" businesses and are owned by corporations that see profit as their primary goal. Hospital chains, free-standing health centers, for-profit health maintenance organizations (HMOs), and home health chains are growing rapidly and changing the setting in which health care is delivered.

Hospital chains have become so large that they now dominate the health care market in some geographic areas. The five largest hospital management corporations in 1981 (HCA, Humana, AMI, NME, and Lifemark) had net revenues that year of over $5 billion, a five-fold increase in five years (Siegrist 1983). Their rise to prominence is recent. Most of today's largest hospital management corporations were founded only in the last twenty years (Gray 1986, 27). The new management systems they introduced into hospitals have changed how doctors and hospitals relate to each other. A recent Institute of Medicine report notes that some hospitals now offer incentive arrangements to doctors, such as reduced rates for leasing office space, in order to encourage them to make patient care decisions that benefit the institution. Consultants to hospitals recommend that the hospital administration enter into joint ventures with doctors for mutual benefit (Gray 1983, 9). A 1985 newsletter to hospital administrators showing this changed relationship between health care settings and doctors is quoted in an Institute of Medicine volume: "Too many doctors treat 'marketing' as a dirty word. Don't let them get away with it. Be direct. Ask doctors how they plan to send their kids to college" (Gray 1986, 166). Institutions influenced by such an ethos are not merely physical plants for the delivery of health care. They actively influence the health care decisions made by health care providers, encouraging the most profitable ones.

For-profit HMOs, which were virtually unheard of until the 1970s (Starr 1982; Gray 1986, 33), are now experiencing "land rush" growth (Gray 1986, 34). Similarly, free-standing health care centers, which include ambulatory surgery centers and emergency care centers (emergicenters), have evidenced dramatic growth (Starr 1982, 439). The first emergicenter opened in 1973 and by 1985, 2,600 such centers were operational. The free-standing centers are primarily for-profit endeavors (90 percent by an Institute of Medicine estimate: Gray 1986) and are increasingly linked into larger for-profit organizations. Thus chains of free-standing centers have developed, sometimes owned by corporations involved in other health care areas. A final for-profit health care area, proprietary home care, has grown dramatically in the last ten years. There were 145 agencies in 1978 and 1,569 in 1984 (Gray 1986, 35). Like the free-standing centers, many are linked to other for-profit interests. For example, major medical supply companies like Abbott Labs offer home care services in conjunction with their "high technology home care products" (Gray 1986, 35).

These corporate interests, from home health agencies to hospital chains, are often large and sometimes multinational (Ost and Antweiler 1986; Gray 1983; Starr 1982). Through their influence, over the last twenty years, managerial capitalism has been introduced into American medicine on a large scale (Starr 1982, 431). What is notable about the for-profit health care institutions is their acknowledged managerial practice of identifying and utilizing those services and products that give the greatest economic return and decreasing the intensive personal service aspects of hospital care (Siegrist 1983, 43–47). The for-profits' definition of what constitutes a "profitable mix" of services (Siegrist 1983, 48) has of course been influenced by the structure of the insurance-based reimbursement system, which is biased toward technologically intensive care rather than service (Gray 1986; Budrys 1986; Sisk, Behney, and Banta 1984; Schroeder and Showstack 1978). Within the reimbursement system, the ability to make separate charges for technologically based services, procedures, or other treatments substantially increases the utilization of technologies (Banta and Thacker 1979). For instance, hospitals have rushed to acquire new technologies, such as ultrasound to monitor pregnancies, that can be billed as separate procedures. Some have proven to be quite profitable (Luft 1983).

The growth of a business orientation in health care institutions is dramatic. At the core of the health care delivery system are settings—hospitals, HMOs, home health care agencies—that are increasingly concerned with the financial balance sheet and less concerned with maintaining individual wellness. Technology, because it has been profitable, has been encouraged in this context beyond its value to the health of the individual.

Doctors' Tendencies to Maximize Income

Just as for-profit interests shape health care institutions and encourage technology, economic interests increase the use of technologies in doctors' private practices. Doctors have not typically needed much external pressure to restructure their office practices so as to increase their use of income-producing technologies. In an era when there is little increase in the number of patients per physician, increases in income must come from higher fee bills for the patients who do come. While the potential for higher payments from basic office visits is minimal, income growth from the use of more tests or new procedures is great. There is evidence that when the patient load is low, doctors tend to respond with more treatment for each case. Thus doctors with practices in high-density physician areas show tendencies to use more tests and to hospitalize patients more frequently than doctors treating similar cases in low-density physician areas. The result is an increase in per case income (Hemenway and Fallon 1985). In primary care general internal medicine, a doctor employing sets of tests and procedures that are typically used though not demonstrably effective could nearly triple net income (Schroeder and Showstack 1978, 292).

Further, evidence exists that if doctors have the technology in their office or laboratory they will use it more than if they have to refer a patient elsewhere. Several studies show that the use of X-rays increases if the doctor owns an X-ray machine and does not need to refer to a radiologist. Other evidence indicates that the average per patient reimbursement is higher in laboratories in which the "primary physician had an ownership interest than in 'non-practice-related laboratories' " (Gray 1986, 158). Furthermore, doctors appear to operate more frequently if the patient is insured. Hysterectomies, for example, are twice as likely for insured as for uninsured women (Kasper 1985, 114). Because the reimbursement system is set up so most costs are borne by insurance companies, there are few effective market checks on the doctor. In fact, the reimbursement system that limits charges for office visits but pays for most tests and procedures that the doctor prescribes tends to act as an incentive for using technologies (Sisk, Behney, and Banta 1984, 10). Reimbursement under Medicare has also been seen as "clearly biased in favor of procedures. . . . A gynecologist would have to perform 275 office visits on elderly women each week to achieve the income earned by one cardiac surgeon doing two operations per week" (Eastaugh 1987, 58).

Because doctors do respond to economic inducements, the behavior of doctors as they become vested in for-profit health care is a matter for concern. One observer notes:

> Physician owners or shareholders in a hospital or nursing home do not realize their full income potential when the facility's beds are not fully occupied. When they can fill empty beds with their own patients, the economic incentive to inappropriate use is obvious. Likewise, a physician with a substantial financial interest in a laboratory, a CAT scanner, or a home health care service usually profits in direct relation to the number of lab tests, CAT scans, or paraprofessional services performed. (Miller 1986, 155).

The interaction between the profit orientation of the physician-provider and the for-profit setting (hospital or home-care agency) is therefore multiplied when the profit shares are directly linked. Although each sector has an economic incentive to encourage inappropriate or excessive use of technology by the other, this cycle of reinforcement is not defined as conflict of interest or a less-than-ethical inducement to lower quality of care. To the contrary, there is a respectability accompanying the use of technology because of the involvement of educational institutions in the technology enterprise.

The Linking of External For-Profit
Interests to Universities

Universities and medical schools constitute a third area of the health care system being transformed by profit seeking and the exploitation of new technologies. Just as university hospitals have altered their health care operations and put a much greater emphasis on increasing their incomes, so, too, have there been extensive efforts to tie such institutions into the entrepreneurial side of technology development.

Again, this is not totally new. Academic medical centers have been quite supportive of technological innovations in the past. They have served as test sites for such technologies (Ost and Antweiler 1986), both evaluating new ones and teaching medical students and other health care professionals in their use (Schroeder and Showstack 1979). In these academic contexts, researchers acting as individuals frequently assume active and sometimes entrepreneurial roles in the development of technologies. Some individuals profit financially from the relationship with corporations, while others benefit from the resulting publications and prominence. Many have actively promoted specific products (Waitzkin 1979, 1265).

Increasingly, medical schools and research institutions are trying to share in the technological developments of individual researchers. Thus many schools now license patents (Kenney 1986). This effort to profit from technology is also reflected in the increasing number of research universities seeking to develop "technology parks." In 1981 there were nineteen, three years later forty, and by 1986 about one hundred university-affiliated research parks (Wright 1987, 353). Universities seriously compromise their role as evaluators and critics of changing trends promoted by for-profit interests when they become partners with these corporations. In such a partnership, businesses gain respectability along with access to the latest technological developments; universities gain a vested interest in specific technological innovations and encourage their marketing and use. The academic medical centers lose their potential for objectively evaluating these new devices and procedures when they stand to gain only by their adoption.

Parks and other cooperative ventures change the relationship between for-profit interests and the practitioners who make the decisions to adopt technology. Formerly, corporate involvement in the development of technology could be characterized as an external interest de-

signing and manufacturing devices and drugs, which were then brought
to health care decision makers. In the case of pharmaceuticals, these
health care decision makers were individual doctors; for equipment,
hospital administrators and physician committees decided. Today, corporate interests not only sell technologies to for-profit hospitals and
free-standing surgical centers as potential profit-enhancing devices,
but also develop marketable health care technologies in partnership
with health care researchers in the university and the government.
These linkages increasingly encourage technology by vesting even nonprofit organizations and individuals in profit-seeking endeavors based
on new inventions.

Women and the For-Profit Growth

There are multiple economic linkages between health institutions, health
professionals, and new technologies in the health care system that have
important consequences for women. First of all, women are recognized
as a major "market" for the new technologies and efforts to improve
profits are correspondingly directed at women. Second, women are
particularly threatened by a profit-generating system that is male-dominated and frequently indifferent to the interests of women.

The extensive exposure of women to technological experimentation is in part due to women's greater use of the health care system,
especially for reproductive processes and problems. Women are a guaranteed market; the health care system can count on most women having life events that have been socially and legally defined as belonging
to the medical world. Women come to health care providers for birth
control, for health care during pregnancy and childbirth, and for regular obstetrical-gynecological checkups. Birth control, abortion, and
childbirth are all controlled by medical doctors. The likelihood that
most women will need these basic services is high in contrast to the
uncertain number of people likely to suffer any particular disease. The
relegation of life events such as childbirth or abortion to the medical
arena sets women up as an ideal market for new technologies. After
childhood many men have little involvement with the health care system until problems associated with middle age arise; women, however,
are in more sustained contact. This contact typically increases when
women are responsible for the health care of children. Given these
continuous contacts with the health care system, especially in the new
profit-oriented era of medicine, women represent the most accessible
potential market from whom income can be obtained.

The guaranteed market aspect of women's health has encouraged for-profit endeavors. Abortion is a good example. Many for-profit clinics have emerged to take advantage of the legalization of abortion. Here is an area in which ironies abound. On one hand, establishment of for-profit clinics has made abortions more available; on the other hand, doctors who perform abortions in for-profit facilities may be caught in a conflict between caring for patients and running a business. A study in Los Angeles after abortion was liberalized in the late 1960s indicated that physician entrepreneurs, namely physicians who owned and operated an abortion facility and employed at least one other doctor, shaped the development of abortion services in the area and defined the options available to women (Goldstein 1984a and 1984b). The physician entrepreneurs typically saw themselves primarily as businessmen and only secondarily as physicians. As one such doctor noted: "I'm interested in anything except medicine. I've always been in business. Before abortions I owned occupational health clinics, hospitals and many other businesses. I've always been an entrepreneur" (quoted in Goldstein 1984a, 521). The entrepreneurs viewed health care as a commodity and recognized the economic advantages in performing many abortions in an efficient manner. "You did maybe 15 to 18 an hour. . . . It was an assembly line. You couldn't slow down or take a break," noted one of the physician entrepreneurs (Goldstein 1984a). The resulting low cost for abortions drove many more traditional doctors out of the market and defined abortion as an impersonal interaction between a woman needing a health service and a man building a financial empire.

The for-profit emphasis is a special threat to women in a male-dominated decision-making system. Women are rarely in positions of power in health care corporations. The merging of this indifference to women with the active pursuit of profits has produced particularly disastrous results. The Dalkon Shield can serve as an example.

The Dalkon Shield was a birth control intrauterine device (IUD) produced by the A. H. Robins Company in the 1960s and 1970s (Mintz 1985; Perry and Dawson 1986). Company records and interviews indicate that male corporate decision makers pushed to produce the Shield quickly and at the lowest possible price. In the process they disregarded early evidence that the device was hazardous to the health of women. This indifference to the health interests of women is particularly striking as the company knew that the dangers arose from specific features designed to minimize the discomfort experienced by male partners during intercourse. The result was the widespread distribution of a product that caused grave physical harm to thousands of women (Yanoshik and Norsigian, this volume). The judge who presided over the class-action suit brought against A. H. Robins clearly noted the connections between for-profit motives and antifemale sentiments:

> Gentlemen, the results of these activities and attitudes on your part have been catastrophic. . . . None of you has faced up to the fact that more than nine thousand women have made claims that they gave up part of their womanhood so that your company might prosper. . . . I dread to think what would have been the consequences if your victims had been men rather than women, women who seem through some strange quirk of our society's mores to be expected to suffer pain, shame, and humiliation. . . . you planted in the bodies of these women instruments of death, of mutilation, of disease. . . . The only conceivable reasons you have not recalled this product are that it would hurt your balance sheet and alert women who already have been harmed that you may be liable for their injuries. You have taken the bottom line as your guiding beacon, and the low road as your route. This is corporate irresponsibility at its meanest. (Mintz 1985, 265–67)

For women technology has often reflected and reinforced the power asymmetries in health care and society. Profit as a driving force encouraged technology even if the health outcomes were dubious and, because of women's position in the health care system, frequently exposed women to technologies that were often not in the best interests of their health. As the educational and evaluation systems would be the normal sources to regulate the growth of technology, we need to examine why they do not check, but rather contribute to, the technological favoritism built into the profit-oriented delivery system itself.

The Education and Socialization of Doctors and the Context of Medical Practice

It is certainly not just economic interests that promote and sustain the increasingly technological approaches to medicine. Doctors have long looked favorably upon innovations in technology. Twenty years ago Fuchs (1968) noted the favor with which doctors greet technology when he discussed the "technological imperative" in medicine which defined the quality of care in terms of what was technologically possible. In fact, this disposition would appear to be embedded both in the training they receive and in the values common in their work contexts.

Feminists have extensively researched and criticized the training of doctors and their workplace practices. The education of specialists in obstetrics-gynecology has come under close scrutiny by feminists because women have so much contact with this speciality. Obstetrician-gynecologists are specialists who provide generalist care for women in their reproductive years. As surgical specialists, obstetrician-gynecologists tend to provide surgical solutions to problems. Obstetrician-gynecologists are, for instance, more likely to deliver by caesarean section than are generalists (Kasper 1985). The surgical mentality of obstetrician-gynecologists conflicts with the health needs of women who typically come with everyday nonsurgical problems. Because surgery is a major avenue for advancement in the profession (Guillemin 1981), "the situation is ripe for the proliferation of unnecessary operations" (Scully 1980, 139). The history of the development of obstetrics-gynecology and the care of the laboring and menopausal woman demonstrates a powerful linking of sexist views, interventionist modalities, and technology. Reviews of obstetrical texts indicate a persistently paternalistic and sometimes condescending attitude toward the female patient (Scully 1980, 107), and gynecologists have been characterized as treating women "as though they were children" (reference to Kaiser and Kaiser in Scully 1980, 19). Women's role, according to an early president of the American Gynecological Society, was to attract a husband and bear children (Summey and Hurst 1986, 109).

The paternalistic views of obstetrician-gynecologists have been coupled with a changed view of the normal processes of life. The movement of childbirth from a home-centered, normal event attended by midwives to an event requiring not only a medical setting but also extensive medical intervention (Wertz and Wertz 1979; Rothman 1982; Gordon 1976) is a clear illustration of the medicalization of women's lives. In fact, central to the development of obstetrics and gynecology as areas of specialization in medicine has been the creation of a pathogenic view of pregnancy and labor as conditions mandating such extensive medical interventions (Bogdan 1978). According to the first president of the American Gynecological Society, the childbirth experience was similar to "a woman falling on a pitchfork with a handle driven through the perineum and the child's experience of childbirth as compared to having its head caught in the door" (Summey and Hurst 1986, 138).

The medicalization of childbirth and the growing acceptance of active obstetrics (Summey and Hurst 1986, 118) encouraged the introduction of high technology medical therapies and techniques for pregnancy, labor, and childbirth. Past experience has shown many of these innovations, such as drugs intended to prevent miscarriages and sedatives used to limit pain during childbirth, are in fact hazardous. More recently, other invasive techniques, including electronic fetal monitoring, ultrasound, and caesarean section have been challenged (Banta and

Thacker 1979; Bolsen 1982; Haverkamp et al. 1978). The general pattern is that once the processes of pregnancy and childbirth became medicalized, even the discrediting of specific treatments does not slow the deployment of technology to new population groups or the development of additional ones.

Today the medicalization of women's lives continues and has been extended to menopause (McCrea 1983). Instead of being seen as a natural aging process that causes few difficulties for most women, menopause has come to be seen as a "deficiency disease" that merits technology-based medical interventions. From a clearly male perspective, menopausal women are described as suffering a "malfunction" that threatens the "feminine essence" (McCrea 1983). Since the condition has now been medicalized and identified as a problem, a search for "cures" for the malfunction is proceeding on a number of fronts that involve technological interventions.

A surgical speciality providing general care for women combined with the paternalism of the profession has exposed women to excess technology. Yet even in a system more concerned with women, the general problem of technological favoritism would be present because the care of women is embedded in a general medical education system that encourages the use of technology. The emphasis in medical training on basic science courses reflects the image that at its core medicine is a science and doctors are scientists seeking out the causes and the cures for the illnesses of individuals that they encounter. Having a particular technology shapes patient care. One physician notes: "The existence of antibiotics provides the pressure to find an infection, even if infection while perhaps present is not the patient's problem" (Cassell 1986b, 192). A bias toward action and intervention takes over (Reissman and Nathanson 1986), even when it is not appropriate to the solution of the individual's problem. The use of high-technology diagnostic procedures is one reflection of this tendency. It is common for physicians to go to great lengths to identify the precise origin of diseases such as cancer, even when such knowledge has little relevance in treatment (Cassell 1986a, 20). The prestige system in medicine further reinforces this tendency. Among doctors, prestige is associated with identifying causes and making dramatic interventions. This focus on curing the individual encourages the acceptance of diagnostic and treatment technologies. A cure orientation and acceptance of technology both focus on the individual; they locate the problem and the solution there. Such a focus and system of values discourages doctors from practicing preventive medicine (Scully 1980, 139) and from devoting their attention to public health activities. These latter activities would turn the focus away from the individual and technology.

These tendencies in modern medicine have been further encouraged by the pattern of doctors' choices for training. Due, in part, to entrance requirements (Schroeder 1985), to the organization of medical education around speciality medicine with its higher prestige and status (Aiken and Freeman 1980, 547), and to speciality residents being more profitable to hospitals (Schroeder 1985), the American medical school system and the system of residency training is producing a disproportionate number of specialists. While medical students today tend to receive their basic training at sophisticated centers that are likely to have the latest high-technology equipment and to encourage its use, they are also likely to go into speciality training because of their rising debt from medical school (Schroeder 1985). Their speciality training is then situated where the emphasis on high technology is even more intensified. One result of the overabundance of doctors with specialist training is that such specialists now provide a large share of general medical care. Trained in advanced medical technology, the specialists believe in tests and in surgical procedures and typically provide more of both (Mechanic 1978; Schroeder and Showstack 1979).

But technology is not only used by specialists; it can also create medical specialization. Schroeder and Showstack (1979) note the case of a technology (flexible fiberoptic endoscopy) which led to a speciality with its own society (American Society of Gasterointestinal Endoscopy) and its own journal (*Gasterointestinal Endoscopy*). Use of this new technology escalated rapidly, until even the president of that society questioned its uncritical acceptance in clinical settings. Similarly, in obstetrics and pediatrics, technology and specialization have clearly grown together. Obstetrics and pediatrics have been "sliced up" to parallel the increasingly fine-tuned technology controlling ever smaller slices of the birth trajectory (Strauss et al. 1985). Technological developments have also shifted the patient focus. In pregnancy and childbirth, increasingly the fetus is the patient (Murphy, in this volume; Rothman 1987, 162). The technology targets the fetus and the woman is seen "at best as a passive receptacle, and at worst a meddlesome or even dangerous third party" (Summey and Hurst 1986, 112).

Doctors are also influenced to use high technology procedures due to factors in their work context. For example, because of the perceived threat of malpractice suits as well as the growing complexity of the body of medical knowledge, doctors tend to practice "defensive medicine" which calls for more extensive diagnostic tests (Aiken and Freeman 1980, 554). The patient often undergoes a barrage of tests, many routine and most low in informational payoff (Reiser 1978, 150), primarily because the doctor is seeking documented evidence confirming the wisdom of treatment decisions that were made on the basis of limited but still sufficient information. Formal studies increasingly define the specific criteria that warrant the use of a procedure. Doctors then feel pressure to provide solid evidence that the criteria have indeed been met (Strauss et al. 1985). Many doctors and malpractice lawyers deem "hard copy" from a machine readout more "solid" than clinical judgment.

Once exposed to the hard copy information available, doctors are often drawn into repeated use. The technology captures their attention and binds physicians to a machine. The compelling nature of technological information is graphically discussed by clinicians. One, speaking of intensive care units (ICUs), says: "Call to mind an ICU with monitors blinking and beeping and remember how all eyes (even family members') go to the monitors—and away from the patient. It requires effort *not* to watch the monitors" (Cassell 1986b, 192). Referring to electronic fetal monitors, another doctor notes how monitoring has dehumanized obstetrics. "We cannot divert our eyes or ears from E[F]M's alluring LED's [light emitting diode], beeps, and stylus chattering graphs. We no longer listen to, talk with, gaze upon, or touch our patient" (Munsick 1979, 410). Some have argued that we have ended up with a health care system that values machine information more than that obtained by mere humans (Banta and Gelijns 1987). The machine, not the physician, ends up dictating the treatment (Crawshaw 1983).

The growth of technology in medical education and practice is reinforced by career ladders rewarding specialization, invasive procedures, and greater control over normal processes. Technology in the health care setting enhances the power and prestige of doctors vis à vis the patient. The growth of technology and the increasing power asymmetry in health care is a particular problem for women because of the paternalistic views within the field of obstetrics-gynecology.

The System of Technology Assessment and Evaluation

Thus far this analysis has focused on the influences pushing for the utilization of high technology in health care. The strength of these influences is apparent. The third area I identified at the outset is the system of assessment and evaluation. It is an area relatively neglected by both feminist critics of health care and by critics of the for-profit forces in medicine and technology development. It is an additional important force fostering technology and degrading health.

There exists a widespread belief in a force restraining technology—a formidable structure of assessment and evaluation that tests innovations must undergo before they pass into general use. Actually, the evaluation system is much more formidable in appearance than in reality.[1] It is, at best, a severely flawed method for determining the effectiveness and safety of health care innovations.

New technologies are supposed to be evaluated at many levels. The most basic level is represented by the direct health care provider. However, while doctors are taught to be competent users of the latest medical innovations, they are not taught to be very critical consumers or evaluators of such innovations. Their biases in favor of high technology treatments are combined with an unsophisticated training in research methodology. Their typical training in basic science, but not in statistics and research methodology, ill equips them to evaluate the often confusing and conflicting literature. Definitive easy-to-understand conclusions are rare in the published literature. In addition, the sheer volume of such publications is overwhelming (Chalmers 1974; Schroeder and Showstack 1979), often putting doctors at the mercy of industry sources for information on specific technologies (McKinlay 1981; Waldron 1977). Thus, in a study of one drug, sales representatives from pharmaceutical companies were found to be the first source of information for half of the doctors (McKinlay 1981, 384). Compared with sources of information like the *New England Journal of Medicine,* industry sources are predictably biased in favor of the technologies they are selling, with more benefits and fewer risks noted (Waldron, quoted in McKinlay 1981).

The problem of inadequate technological evaluation does not lie just with the doctors. Even the literature that has emerged on many new technologies has been less than adequately critical. Thus the doctor who does read available published research will likely find that those results tend to confirm or support the use of the technology. Clinical research evaluations of technology commonly take little account of the fact that many diseases are self-limiting in nature. Any treatment can seem to produce positive results unless adequate research controls are employed (Schroeder 1985). The enthusiasm that accompanies a new technology enhances its placebo effect and, together with poorly designed research, it can lead to results that seem impressive to unskeptical audiences. For instance, five treatments for angina pectoris, introduced in the 1950s and 1960s and now abandoned, were reported as producing 70 to 90 percent "effectiveness" in studies that used neither double blind models nor random trials. Later, more skeptical investigators assessed each of the treatment modalities and found an effectiveness of 30 to 40 percent, "which is comparable to the level of a placebo effect" (Tancredi 1982, 104).

Unfortunately, doctors and other direct health care providers are not in a position to serve as scientific evaluators and guardians in the process of technology development. Still, a good system of evaluation is conceivable. Academic research and government agencies such as the Office of Technology Assessment (OTA) could work reasonably well to protect the public. The mere existence of a regulatory system can delay the adoption of technology until better information is available. In the case of the Dalkon Shield, experts suggest that had "devices" been included under the original Food and Drug Administration (FDA) legislation the Shield would have been delayed for years or never have been marketed (Mintz 1985, 56). But at this level of the system flaws and loopholes seem to outnumber effective checks. Four major problems bias the system in favor of technology.

First, many technologies receive no evaluation whatever, are widely used prior to any systematic assessment (Banta and Behney 1981; McKinlay 1981), or are used despite negative evaluations. The electronic fetal monitor (Kunisch, in this volume), coronary care units (Waitzkin 1979), ultrasound (National Institute of Child Health and Human Development et al. 1984), IUDs (Ruzek 1980, 337), oral contraceptives (Corea 1985), and DES (Mintz 1985) are among the technologies that have been poorly, belatedly, or negatively evaluated. The negative evaluations sometimes included strong statements, yet use of the technology persisted and even increased. Thus, a government-convened conference on intensive care units concluded that "for some patients the risk of iatrogenic illness may now outweigh the benefit of ICU care" (quoted in Knaus et al. 1983, 576). And a government-convened conference on ultrasound, noting an extensive literature documenting the effects of ultrasound on biological material and the lack of studies on the physical safety of ultrasound on pregnant women, concluded that "diagnostic ultrasound may not be totally innocuous" and that if ultrasound effects occur in human development, they "may well be delayed in expression" (National Institute of Child Health and Human Development et al. 1984, 55). Yet without answers to major questions, the use of ultrasound is becoming routine.

A second problem in the evaluation system is the fact that evaluators are often interested parties. Evaluations of drugs are often based on industry-supplied data or on industry-funded research. The government often gives money to interested parties because of their knowledge of the technology. If a diagnostic or treatment tool has been developed at a particular university, then the expertise for the evaluation often rests there, too. A former head of the Office of Technology Assessment noted this bias in the selection of evaluation grant recipients and indicated such parties are clearly not the ideal ones to conduct an objective evaluation (Banta and Thacker 1979).

Third, reports evaluating health care technologies use standards and language with a built-in bias favoring technology. In terms of standards, what constitutes a finding of "harmful" or "harmless"? Often because the rates of very serious side effect are low (the side effect occurs, but not that often), because the appearance of the side effect is not immediate, or because it is influenced by other contributing factors, large differences between the treated group and the untreated one are not found. Depending on the level of statistical significance chosen and the size of the group studied, the investigator may not be able to reject the hypothesis of no difference between the two groups. It is therefore assumed that the new technology is not harmful. However, the technology has not been shown to be harmless; the study has simply failed to find it is harmful enough to be noticed given the constraints imposed on the study. The new technology is given the benefit of the doubt, just as our legal system gives the benefit of the doubt to the accused. While this is an admirable standard in criminal justice, it is a questionable standard for evaluation, given the track record of many new technologies.

The bias toward technology is enhanced by the language that is then used to discuss the relative merits of the technology. Not only has the definition of safety undergone a transformation from a dictionary definition of "free from harm" to one that means the "hazards will likely be outweighed by the benefits" (Cowan 1980, 37), the evaluation of "risks and benefits" has also been manipulated semantically. A 1984 Consensus Development Conference demonstrates this bias clearly. The report of the conference begins with a statement of the prevailing view on ultrasound:

> Lack of risk has been assumed because no adverse effects have been demonstrated clearly in humans. . . . Likewise, the efficacy of many uses of ultrasound in improving the management and outcome of pregnancy also has been assumed rather than demonstrated." (National Institute of Child Health and Human Development et al. 1984, 3)

This professional assessment of ultrasound shows a clear bias toward accepting technology. With no evidence of either risk or benefit, the professional experts tell doctors and consumers that the benefits are assumed positive and the risks are assumed nil. If this logic were reversed, the assumption would be that the benefits are nil and risks are possible. These same conference conveners posed questions to the Consensus Development Conference panel to frame their inquiry. The questions provide additional evidence of technological favoritism. When the conveners asked the panel to consider ultrasound's benefits (the outcomes), the term "outcomes" was not qualified. ("What is the evidence that ultrasound improves patient management and/or outcomes of pregnancy?") Yet, when the conveners asked the panel to consider risks, an important qualifier was added: "What are the *theoretical* risks . . .?" (National Institute of Child Health and Human Development 1984, 4. Emphasis added). The logic that makes risks for which there is suggestive evidence merely *theoretical* is a logic that is seriously flawed and favors technology.

Key federal officials have acknowledged that this bias exists. After William Ruckleshaus left the Environmental Protection Agency in 1985 he commented that the evaluation system in place clearly failed to do an aggressive job of protecting the environment. He commented that risk analysis:

> is a kind of pretense; to avoid paralysis of protective action that would result from waiting for "definitive" data, we assume we have greater knowledge than scientists actually possess and make decisions based on those assumptions. (Quoted in Hattis and Kennedy 1986, 66)

In addition to the bias in the standards and language of assessment, there is active hostility toward evaluation on the part of other key officials. Former Office of Management and Budget (OMB) head David Stockman referred to the work of the National Center for Health Care Technology and its supporters as "latter-day Luddites" (quoted in Blumenthal 1983, 606). These examples suggest that the political support for serious evaluations of technology is limited.

Fourth, the evaluation system favors technology because the evaluations are often limited in focus. Sometimes they are limited to evaluating the claims of the manufacturer. Thus, for example, diagnostic accuracy, not improved health, may become the focus of the evaluation (Banta and Thacker 1979). We may find out whether electronic fetal monitoring correctly detects fetal distress, but we don't find out whether detecting distress improves the health of women or their newborns, or if the use of the monitoring has hazardous health consequences, like increasing rates of caesarean sections. At other times social and ethical concerns are excluded as assessment focuses on safety, efficacy, or economic considerations (Fox 1986). This bias in the evaluations away from social issues is in part due to the overwhelming governmental concern that a major impact of technology is to increase health care costs (Fein 1977).

But the disproportionate attention to economic issues also reflects a bias for the supposedly more scientific, objective, or quantifiable components of evaluation. Cost-benefit analyses (CBA) or cost-effectiveness analyses (CEA) which stress economic considerations are seen as more scientific than technology assessment which by definition takes the social implications into account. Yet, CBA and CEA have major problems. One problem is that "the analytical technics may appear coldly neutral—pure science at its best. This impression is misleading. . . . Behind the arithmetic lie values" (Fein 1977, 752). The valuing of human life is a clear example. CBA rests on the assumption that pain and pleasure (cost and benefits) can be given a meaningful value. CBA has typically placed a value on human life. Because women, the elderly, and minorities are typically assessed as having less worth on the employment market, and hence are valued less in such calculations, major debates have raged. A second problem with these seemingly "scientific" analyses is the quality of the data used in arriving at the benefits and costs. Data on efficacy are often poor; epidemiological data on incidence and prevalence are lacking, although they are needed to estimate the likely case mix—sex, age, other health problems—of people using the technology and the numbers of affected individuals (Sisk, Behney, and Banta 1984). A third problem of these economically oriented analyses is that they often ignore the context in which the technology will be used. Most health care technologies have first been employed with carefully selected patient groups and administered by a select group of health care practitioners. When the technology becomes accepted, the patient group expands and may include less appropriate individuals (as when ultrasound, amniocentesis, or electronic fetal monitoring become nearly routine procedures used on many patients, not just the population they were developed for) for whom the cost-benefit picture is very different (Fein 1977). Thus CBA and CEA for all their "scientific" aura have embedded values, rest on poor data, and ignore the context of their use.

Despite these problems with a cost-effectiveness-driven evaluation, a suggestion to include social and ethical considerations in a technology assessment is immediately attacked because there is no "systematic" way to incorporate them. A focus on the social and ethical implications, it is claimed, does not produce a number that can unambiguously say "this technology should be used." The push for the quantifiable reaches its peak with a demand for a computerized system of evaluations. One discussant at an Office of Technology Assessment–sponsored conference commented:

> . . . more use of formal computer-based models for [technology assessment] purposes might be better than the present mixed studies. The formal models are explicit, allowing clarity of assumption-making and communication. They are manipulable, allowing ready substitution of different assumptions at the level of parameters or relationships. They permit complete consistency and ease of testing for alternative scenarios about the socioeconomic environment, the path of technology development itself, or the policies for technology use. . . . Today's computer hardware and modeling software technologies permit inexpensive and relatively easy-to-use approaches that I believe would enhance the practice and outcomes of technology assessment. (Roberts 1985, 676)

Such a trend would likely move us to an increasing dependence on economic rather than social or ethical considerations and would further hide the implicit assumptions behind inaccessible language and equations.

The effectiveness analyses do produce information but it is information collected within an unacceptable framework, and thus it may limit our view and restrict our choices. If we accept efficiency as a major value, we downgrade justice, equality, and fairness (Hastings Center 1980) because they are not well incorporated into these analyses. And by proceeding to evaluate technology with these models, we contribute to a momentum that moves us to disregard certain other values.

A feminist critique of the assessment of technology would place equity at the center of values to consider. Technology raises many equity issues. The introduction of health care technologies can create inequities (Aiken and Freeman 1980), or it can be used to alleviate differences. Thus, an equity framework, in contrast to a CBA, might positively evaluate a screening procedure ". . . even if it yields a low rate of return because it reaches persons whom the private sector would otherwise neglect" (Fein 1977, 753). Equity issues also arise in questions of who gets a treatment technology. For instance, in the early days of renal dialysis committees developed selection criteria. "The criteria for selection included highly value-laden information, such as age and sex; intelligence; the 'likelihood of vocational rehabilitation'; a social welfare evaluation of the patient and his or her family; demonstrated social worth of the patient; and potential social contribution if rehabilitated" (Tancredi 1982, 98). Selecting organ transplant recipients raises similar equity issues (Kutner 1987). Feminist analyses of technology stress the centrality of such equity issues. "Technology has everything to do with who benefits and who suffers, whose opportunities increase and whose decrease, who creates and who accommodates" (Bush 1983, 163). These key issues are not included in the evaluations that are limited to economic concerns.

Conclusion

Technological innovations in medicine have become sources of real and potential danger, as well as a means to improved health care for women. New technologies will likely always carry some risks, but the risks seem to have become unreasonably high in recent times. Too often technological innovation has become technological recklessness. This analysis shows that the causes of this recklessness as it affects women are multiple. First, modern medical systems have encouraged the use of technology as profit-seeking becomes increasingly important and health less so. Women are particularly threatened due to their vulnerable positions as a lucrative market for technological innovations. Second, this recklessness is fostered in a system in which dominating nature and technological tools to do so are presumed to be good. Women, a relatively powerless group whose values and interests are not well represented or widely respected in the male-dominated health care system, are exposed to technologies that enhance professional control at their expense. Finally, a system supposedly designed to protect health care consumers from risky innovations has failed both to identify the risks tied to specific technologies, to block the use of such technologies when definite risks have been identified, and to incorporate social and ethical concerns.

The many problems that accompany the modern development and utilization of technology in medicine have inspired differing responses. However, few critics argue that health consumers can do without technology entirely or that the technological level of society can be held constant. Feminist critics emphasize seeking appropriate technologies. They call for technology that both meets the real health needs of women, as well as other consumer groups, and that gives health care consumers greater control over treatment. In some areas of medicine particular efforts are underway to rectify this situation. In the area of contraceptive technology, for example, the women's health movement has pushed technologies that give women greater control while protecting their health and minimizing the intrusions of the health care system (Yanoshik and Norsigian, in this volume).

Feminist critics of modern medicine have been concerned with equity, both in power and in the availability of adequate medical care, and autonomy. Women as consumers have not had sufficient power within the medical care system to effectively represent their own interests. Attention to issues of economic equity and fair access to medical care are essential if women's rights are ever to be adequately protected in the medical care system. Since a disproportionate share of the poor are women, including young mothers, they have been especially vulnerable either to the lack of available medical care, to experimentation, or to risky treatment techniques.

Advocating economic equity and autonomy, and arguing for appropriate technology distinguish feminist critics of the medical care system from other critics who have focused on the abuses with risky technologies or the excesses of the for-profit orientation. For feminist critics, these latter problems are certainly important, but they need to be merged with the will to build a health care system that is not just safer and less expensive but one that will work particularly for women consumers, and encourage the development of appropriate technologies that are truly beneficial to all human beings.

N O T E

1. In addition to the Office of Technology Assessment (OTA), founded in 1972 as an advisory arm of Congress, the National Center for Health Care Technology (NCHCT) founded in 1978 but funded for only three years, the FDA, including the Medical Devices Program implemented in 1976, and the Office of Medical Applications of Research have all been involved in the evaluations of health care technologies.

B I B L I O G R A P H Y

Aiken, Linda, and Howard Freeman. 1980. Medical sociology and science and technology in medicine. In *A guide to the culture of science, technology and medicine,* ed. Paul T. Durbin, 527–82. New York: Free Press.
Banta, H. David, and Clyde J. Behney. 1981. Policy formulation and technology assessment. *Milbank Memorial Fund Quarterly* 59, no. 3: 445–79.
Banta, H. David, and Annetine Gelijns. 1987. Health care costs: Technology and policy. In *Health care and its costs,* ed. Carl J. Schramm, 252–74. New York: W. W. Norton and Co.
Banta, H. David, and Stephen B. Thacker. 1979. Policies toward medical technology: The case of electronic fetal monitoring. *American Journal of Public Health* 69, no. 9: 931–35.
Blumenthal, David. 1983. Federal policy toward health care technology: The case of the national center. *Milbank Memorial Fund Quarterly* 61, no. 4: 584–613.

Bogdan, Janet C. 1978. Care or cure: Childbirth practices in 19th century America. *Feminist Studies* 11: 92–99.

Bolsen, B. 1982. Question of risk still hovers over routine prenatal use of ultrasound. *Journal of American Medical Association* 247, no. 16: 2,195–97.

Budrys, Grace. 1986. Medical technology policy: Some underlying assumptions. In *Research in sociology of health care.* Volume 4: *The adoption and social consequences of medical technologies,* ed. Julius A. Roth and Sheryl B. Ruzek, 147–83. Greenwich, Conn.: JAI Press.

Bush, Corlann Gee. 1983. Women and the assessment of technology: To think, to be; to unthink, to free. In *Machina ex Dea: Feminist perspectives on technology,* ed. Joan Rothschild, 151–70. New York: Pergamon Press.

Cassell, Eric J. 1986a. Ideas in conflict: The rise and fall (and rise and fall) of new views of disease. *Daedalus* 115, no. 2: 19–42.

———. 1986b. The changing concept of the ideal physician. *Daedalus* 115, no. 2: 185–208.

Chalmers, Thomas C. 1974. The impact of controlled trials on the practice of medicine. *Mount Sinai Journal of Medicine* 41: 753–59.

Corea, Gena. 1985. *The hidden malpractice.* New York: Harper and Row.

Cowan, Belita. 1980. Ethical problems in government-funded contraceptive research. In *Birth control and controlling birth: Women-centered perspectives,* ed. Helen B. Holmes, Betty B. Hoskins, and Michael Gross, 37–46. Clifton, N.J.: Humana Press.

Crawshaw, Ralph. 1983. Technical zeal or therapeutic purpose: How to decide? *Journal of American Medical Association* 250, no. 14: 1,857–59.

Eastaugh, Steven R. 1987. *Financing health care: Economic efficiency and equity.* Dover, Mass.: Auburn House.

Ehrenreich, Barbara, and Deirdre English. 1973. *Complaints and disorders: The sexual politics of sickness.* Old Westbury, N.Y.: Feminist Press.

———. 1972. *Witches, midwives and nurses: A history of women healers.* Old Westbury, N.Y.: Feminist Press.

Fein, Rashi. 1977. But on the other hand. *New England Journal of Medicine* 296, no. 13: 751–53.

Fox, Renée C. 1986. Medicine, science and technology. In *Applications of social science to clinical medicine and health policy,* ed. Linda H. Aiken and David Mechanic, 13–30. New Brunswick, N.J.: Rutgers University Press.

Fuchs, Victor. 1968. The growing demand for medical care. *New England Journal of Medicine* 279, no. 4: 190–95.

Goldstein, Michael. 1984a. Creating and controlling a medical market: Abortion in Los Angeles after liberalization. *Social Problems* 31, no. 5 (June): 514–29.

———. 1984b. Abortion as a medical career choice: Entrepreneurs, community physicians and others. *Journal of Health and Social Behavior* 25 (June): 211–29.

Gordon, Linda. 1976. *Woman's body, woman's right: A social history of birth control in America.* New York: Grossman.

Gray, Bradford H., ed. 1986. *For profit enterprise in health care.* Washington, D.C.: National Academy Press.

————. 1983. *The new health care for profit.* Washington, D.C.: National Academy Press.

Guillemin, Jeanne. 1981. Babies by cesarean: Who chooses, who controls? *Hastings Center Report* 11 (June): 15–18.

Hastings Center. 1980. Appendix D: Values, ethics, and CBA in health care. In *The implications of cost-effectiveness analysis of medical technology: A report by the Office of Technology Assessment,* 168–82. Washington, D.C.: Government Printing Office.

Hattis, Dale, and David Kennedy. 1986. Assessing risks from health hazards: An imperfect science. *Technology Review* 89, no. 4 (May/June): 60–71.

Haverkamp, Albert D., Miriam Orleans, Sharon Langendoerfer, John McFee, James Murphy, and Horace E. Thompson. 1978. A controlled trial of the differential effects of intrapartum fetal monitoring. *American Journal of Obstetrics and Gynecology* 134, no. 4: 399–412.

Hemenway, David, and Deborah Fallon. 1985. Testing for physician induced demand with hypothetical cases. *Medical Care* 23, no. 4: 344–49.

Kasper, Anne S. 1985. Hysterectomy as social process. *Women and Health* 10, no. 1: 109–27.

Keller, Evelyn Fox. 1985. *Reflections on gender and science.* New Haven: Yale University Press.

Kenney, Martin. 1986. *Biotechnology: The university-industrial complex.* New Haven: Yale University Press.

Koumjian, Kevin. 1981. The use of Valium as social control. *Social Science and Medicine* 15E, no. 3: 245–49.

Knaus, William A., Elizabeth A. Draper, and Douglas P. Wagner. 1983. The use of intensive care: New research initiatives and their implications for national health policy. *Milbank Memorial Fund Quarterly* 61, no. 4: 561–83.

Kutner, Nancy C. 1987. Issues in the application of high cost medical technology: The case of organ transplantation. *Journal of Health and Social Behavior* 28, no. 1: 23–36.

Luft, Harold S. 1983. Economic incentives and clinical decisions. In *The new health care for profit,* ed. Bradford H. Gray, 103–23. Washington, D.C.: National Academy Press.

McCrea, Frances B. 1983. The politics of menopause: The "discovery" of a deficiency disease. *Social Problems* 31, no. 1: 111–23.

McKinlay, John B. 1981. From "promising report" to "standard procedure": Seven stages in the career of a medical innovation. *Milbank Memorial Fund Quarterly/Health and Society* 59, no. 3: 374–411.

Mechanic, David. 1978. Approaches to controlling the costs of medical care: Short range and long range alternatives. *New England Journal of Medicine* 298, no. 5: 249–54.

Merchant, Carolyn. 1980. *The death of nature: Women, ecology and the scientific revolution.* New York: Harper and Row.

Miller, Frances H. 1983. Secondary income from recommended treatment: Should fiduciary principles constrain physician behavior? In *The new health care for profit,* ed. Bradford H. Gray, 153–69. Washington, D.C.: National Academy Press.

Mintz, Morton. 1985. *At any cost: Corporate greed, women and the Dalkon Shield.* New York: Pantheon Books.

Munsick, Robert. 1979. Comment on "A controlled trial of the differential effects on interpartum fetal monitoring" by Haverkamp and others. *American Journal of Obstetrics and Gynecology* 134, no. 4: 409–11.

National Institute of Child Health and Human Development, Office of Medical Applications of Research, Division of Research Resources, and Food and Drug Administration. 1984. *Diagnostic ultrasound imaging in pregnancy. Report of a Consensus Development Conference.* Washington, D.C.: Government Printing Office.

Orenberg, Cynthia. 1981. *DES: The complete story.* New York: St. Martin's Press.

Ost, John, and Phillip Antweiler. 1986. The social impact of high cost medical technology: Issues and conflicts surrounding the decision to adopt CAT Scanners. In *Research in the sociology of health care.* Volume 4: *The Adoption and social consequences of medical technologies,* ed. Julius A. Roth and Sheryl B. Ruzek, 33–92. Greenwich, Conn.: JAI Press.

Perry, Susan, and J. Dawson. 1986. *Nightmare: Women and the Dalkon Shield.* New York: Macmillan.

Reiser, Stanley Joel. 1978. *Medicine and the reign of technology.* New York: Cambridge University Press.

Reissman, Catherine Kohler. 1983. Women and medicalization: A new perspective. *Social Policy* 14, no. 1: 3–18.

Reissman, Catherine Kohler, and Constance A. Nathanson. 1986. The management of reproduction: Social construction of risk and responsibility. In *Applications of social science to clinical medicine and health policy,* ed. Linda Aiken and David Mechanic, 251–89. New Brunswick, N.J.: Rutgers University Press.

Relman, Arnold. 1980. The new medical-industrial complex. *New England Journal of Medicine* 303, no. 17: 963–70.

Roberts, Edward B. 1985. Health information systems. *Medical Care* 23, no. 5: 672–76.

Rothman, Barbara K. 1987. Reproduction. In *Analyzing gender,* ed. Beth B. Hess and Myra Marx Ferree, 154–70. Beverly Hills: Sage.

————. 1982. *In labor: Women and power in the birthplace.* New York: Norton.

Ruzek, Sheryl Burt. 1986. Feminist visions of health: An international perspective. In *What is feminism: A reexamination,* ed. Juliett Mitchell and Ann Oakley, 184–207. New York: Pantheon.

————. 1980. Medical responses to women's health activities: Conflict, accommodation and co-optation. In *Research in the sociology of health care.* Volume 1: *Professional control of health services and challenges to such control,* ed. Julius A. Roth, 335–54. Greenwich, Conn.: JAI Press.

Schroeder, Steven A. 1985. The making of a medical generalist. *Health Affairs* 4:26–46.

Schroeder, Steven A., and Jonathan A. Showstack. 1979. The dynamics of medical technology use: Analysis and policy options. In *Medical technology: The culprit behind health care costs?* ed. S. H. Altman and R. Blendon, 178–212. Proceedings of the 1977 Sun Valley Forum on National Health. Washington, D.C.: Government Printing Office.

————. 1978. Financial incentives to perform medical procedures and laboratory tests: Illustrative models of office practice. *Medical Care* 16, no. 4: 289–98.

Scully, Diana. 1980. *Men who control women's health.* Boston: Houghton Mifflin.

Siegrist, Richard B. 1983. Wall Street and the for-profit hospital management companies. In *The new health care for profit,* ed. Bradford H. Gray, 35–50. Washington, D.C.: National Academy Press.

Sisk, Jane E., Clyde J. Behney, and H. David Banta. 1984. Evaluating the costs of medical technology. In *Research in sociology of health care.* Volume 3: *The control of costs and performance of medical services,* ed. Julius A. Roth, 9–26. Greenwich, Conn.: JAI Press.

Starr, Paul. 1982. *The social transformation of American medicine.* New York: Basic Books.

Strauss, Anselm, Shizoko Fagerhaugh, Barbara Suczek, and Carolyn Weiner. 1985. *The social organization of medical care.* Chicago: University of Chicago Press.

Summey, Pamela S., and Marsha Hurst. 1986. OB/GYN on the rise: Part I and II. *Women and Health* 11, no. 1: 133–45 and 11, no. 2: 103–22.

Tancredi, Lawrence. 1982. Social and ethical implications in technology assessment. In *Critical issues in medical technology,* ed. Barbara J. McNeil and Ernest G. Cravalho, 93–113. Boston: Auburn House.

Vance, Michael A., and William R. Millington. 1986. Principles of irrational drug therapy. *International Journal of Health Services* 16, no. 3: 355–62.

Waldron, Ingrid. 1977. Increased prescribing of Valium, Librium and other drugs: An example of the influence of economic and social factors on the practice of medicine. *International Journal of Health Services* 7, no. 1: 37–62.

Waitzkin, Howard. 1979. A Marxian interpretation of the growth and development of coronary technology. *American Journal of Public Health* 69, no. 12: 1,260–68.

Weiss, Kay. 1983. Vaginal cancer: An iatrogenic disease. In *Women and health: The politics of sex in medicine,* ed. Elizabeth Fee, 59–76. New York: Baywood Publishing.

Wertz, Richard W., and Dorothy C. Wertz. 1979. *Lying in: A history of childbirth in America.* New York: Free Press.

Wright, Barbara Drygulski. 1987. Women, work, and the university-affiliated technology park. In *Women, work, and technology: Transformations,* ed. Barbara D. Wright, 352–70. Ann Arbor: University of Michigan Press.

The Role of Technology in the Co-optation of the Women's Health Movement: The Cases of Osteoporosis and Breast Cancer Screening

Mariamne H. Whatley and Nancy Worcester

The women's health movement has been one of the most visible and best received aspects of the women's movement. Since the late 1960s, groups of feminists throughout the United States and the world have critiqued curative medical systems that are based on the values of the male medical establishment. Attention was drawn to the sexism, racism, classism, and homophobia of the health care system. The pivotal role of women in health care decisions for the family was identified. Health activists worked for health care services accessible to *all* women and for information that would enable women to understand their bodies and health issues so that they could be involved in health care decisions. Self-help groups, women-controlled health centers, campaigns such as that against sterilization abuse of women of color, women's health courses, national organizations, including the National Women's Health Network, and books such as *Our Bodies, Ourselves* are representative of the work of the women's health movement.

A recognition of the need for fundamental changes in both health care provision and women's role in society has been central to the analysis and work of the women's health movement. When possible, the medical establishment has ignored the women's health movement. When the demand for change could not be ignored, the medical response has been to co-opt the movement (Ruzek 1980). In the 1970s, for example, hospitals defused the call for women-controlled childbirth by promising to offer a combination of the latest technology with a warm, nurturing, home-like environment. Such birthing centers co-opted the movement against medicalized childbirth by providing surface changes that did little to alter who controlled birthing "options."

Now a decade later, with a limited population of pregnant women to draw on, medical facilities are concentrating on marketing services to healthy women with money. In the 1980s, as in the 1970s, instead of making real changes that could make health services more appropriate to the needs of all women, the medical establishment is again co-opting the women's health movement. This chapter will explore the role of technology in this co-optation by examining two specific cases.

199

The new marketing drive is based on the economic premises originally identified by the women's movement: that women use health care facilities more than men and that women often choose health care facilities and providers for the entire family. Using language and style that mimic that of the women's health movement, a new range of medical services is being promoted. For example, new women's health centers have translated the feminist call for demystification of medical technology and the right of all women to be actively involved in decisions about our own bodies into provision of consumer information. Advertisements focus on the availability of libraries, seminars, hot lines, and resource people, all in a comfortable environment. While the provision of free resources to women should be applauded, it must be remembered that hospitals will not be making any money from these services. Clearly, these much-needed resources are being used as a way to attract women to medicine's money-making services.

This paper specifically examines the role of technology in this recent marketing of services to healthy women. The examples of bone mass measurement and mammography demonstrate how expensive tests are being marketed in campaigns directly contradictory to the goals of the women's health movement. First, we look at how marketing both creates and exploits the prevention-conscious mentality and intentionally plays on women's fears. Next, we discuss criteria by which bone mass measurements and mammography can be evaluated. Then, considering the complexities and controversies surrounding these particular techniques, we explore the range of information that should be available to women when they are choosing whether to have bone mass measurement or mammography.

Prevention Consciousness

Contemporary United States society, especially the middle-class, is highly health conscious. Television advertisements in which bran cereals are pushed to prevent cancer, low-cholesterol foods to reduce heart attack risk, and exercise machines to promote "wellness," reveal the dominance of the prevention ideology in health awareness. The focus on prevention is part of an overall trend among consumers away from the sick-care model of the medical industry. This medically controlled model devotes less than 10 percent of health expenditure to environmental and occupational issues, disease detection and control, medical education and research; instead, resources are directed toward drugs, surgery, hospitals, and high-technology equipment. This sick-care model may do a miraculous job of patching up accident victims or putting a new heart into someone who has eaten an all-American diet, but it does practically nothing to keep us well. For many, the resistance to this medical model may be political, based, for example, on the analysis generated by the women's health movement; prevention becomes a way of wresting control away from doctors and returning it to consumers.

Ironically, though the emphasis on prevention originated as a way to become less dependent on the medical establishment, it is now being used as a marketing technique to attract people back in. Women are the major customers of prevention services. In her seminars on marketing women's health, Sally Rynne[1] notes that 18 percent of women's medical visits are preventive, that women are the major subscribers to the prevention/wellness type of magazines, and that the audiences at health promotion programs are predominantly women. Not surprisingly, the new women's health centers present themselves as having a prevention focus, providing specific information on the role of exercise, diet, stress management, and the judicious use of medical technology in health promotion.

The last item on that list is out of place for two reasons. Unlike the other services, medical testing is the only potential money-maker for the centers. Second, these tests clearly are not *preventive* because they are detecting a disease that is already present. Even though early detection may improve prognosis, it does not prevent the disease. For consumers, having a procedure labeled as "preventive" makes it highly attractive. Marketing of medical services and technologies can capitalize on this by deliberately blurring the distinction between early detection and prevention.

Selling the Fear Factor

In order to maximize the market value of "prevention," the condition to be avoided must be sufficiently serious. Individuals either must view the disease in question as highly prevalent or believe themselves to have a high level of personal susceptibility. Fear can become an important selling point for either true preventive measures or early detection tests.

As diseases become "popular," there is a time of intense interest, during which we are inundated with media coverage of the newest plague, whether it is genital herpes, toxic shock syndrome, premenstrual syndrome, or chlamydia. Accurate and complete information is needed about all these issues; increased awareness is essential for all individuals who want to have some control over their health. However, sensational media coverage often does little besides create fear, as the AIDS panic clearly demonstrates. Those who benefit from this popular coverage are those who offer prevention or treatments, whether they are effective or not.

If the disease is not exciting enough to make a good cover story, advertising campaigns can be conducted. For example, when the pharmaceutical company Ayerst hired a public relations firm to conduct an educational campaign on osteoporosis, a survey found that 77 percent of women had not heard of this condition (Dejanikus 1985). Now, women have not only heard of it, but they are also frightened of the seeming inevitability of postmenopausal hip fractures or of becoming like the elderly woman with the severely bent spine in calcium advertisements.

Because of media coverage, advertising campaigns, and public health education, health centers do not have to work to create awareness and fear of the diseases of interest. To gain clients, these centers only need to capitalize on that awareness and fear to sell the use of technologies for early detection. Sometimes the selling of the "fear factor" may be a deliberate strategy; in other cases it may be an accidental offshoot of another marketing approach. For example, women do not need to be told that breast cancer is a highly prevalent, very serious, and often fatal disease. Those who play on women's fears of this disease can draw them into educational seminars, breast self-exam lessons, and finally to mammography screening. As in this example, technology is often presented as the ultimate answer to women's fears, but closer examination of the assumptions behind these claims is needed.

Assessing Screening Technologies

In order to evaluate the potential usefulness of mammography or any other screening program, a number of factors must be considered. In the excitement generated by a new technology, it is sometimes forgotten that "the mere existence of unrecognized cases of illness is, by itself, insufficient reason to screen" (Berwick 1985, 1,373). The true value of a screening program is in the identification of cases that would not have been detected otherwise, or would have been detected at a time when treatment would be less effective or more expensive (Berwick 1985). Inherent in this statement is the assumption that effective treatment exists (unless it is screening aimed only at preventing spread of the disease); if the early detection does not in any way alter the course of the disease, then the value of the screening for the individual is lost. Unfortunately, enthusiastic evaluations of screening programs may attribute all cases detected to the screening, without distinguishing cases that might have been identified in other ways. Another problem is that proponents of a program might assume identification a worthy end in itself, without questioning whether early detection necessarily means a better prognosis.

An evaluation of a screening program must also measure the effectiveness of the test being used; ideally, tests in a screening program will be both sensitive and specific. *Sensitivity* is the percent of disease cases identified by the test. A high degree of sensitivity means that few cases slip through undetected; false negatives, accompanied by a potentially dangerous false sense of security, are minimized. *Specificity* is the percent of unaffected people correctly labeled. High specificity means great accuracy, and few false positives. The incorrect identification of disease could lead to unnecessary, potentially expensive and dangerous treatments and tests, as well as possible psychological harm from inappropriate labeling.

In summary, a good screening program will:

1. provide early identification of a condition;
2. be highly accurate, both sensitive and specific; and
3. lead to an improved prognosis.

In discussing bone mass measurements and mammography, we will use these criteria as part of the evaluation of these technologies.

Osteoporosis Screening

Osteoporosis is an excellent illustration of the problematic relationship between the medical system and the women who use it. In previous years the response to this prevalent and potentially serious condition has been characterized by a lack of medical attention to women's health needs. In the United States annually, more than 1.6 million fractures in women over age fifty are due to osteoporosis (Kaplan 1985). However, until recently very little information was available and most women had never even heard of osteoporosis.

The lack of research on osteoporosis could be viewed as an indication of the lesser importance ascribed to women's health issues. If around age fifty, men became at risk for a disabling disease, more effort might go into searching for answers; in fact, that is the case with the "men's disease"—cardiovascular disease. Osteoporosis has been labeled as a women's disease because, although age-related loss of bone mass occurs in both men and women, women are more likely to experience problems at an earlier age. The fact that white women are more at risk than Black women may account for the fact that this condition has finally received the attention it has.

In addition, since curative medicine has little role to play, whereas prevention is an important factor, osteoporosis does not fit the medical model in the United States. At least five years ago, for example, information indicated that limited physical activity and low dietary calcium increase risk, so logical preventive measures were available. However, this information was generally not presented by health care practitioners who were more likely to prescribe estrogen if they dealt with the problem at all.

This situation has changed dramatically in the last three years. Osteoporosis can no longer serve as an example of the neglect of older women's health issues. It might seem that feminist health activists should be applauding the response of the medical establishment. Research on osteoporosis is suddenly well funded and information is so readily available that few women could fail to be aware of this issue. Any woman approaching menopause is likely to receive information from her health care practitioner on the dangers of osteoporosis. So why are we complaining? Aren't feminists ever satisfied?

The Selling of Osteoporosis

To begin to answer that question, we can first examine the sources and content of the information. Beginning in 1982, an education campaign was sponsored by Ayerst Laboratories to create public awareness of osteoporosis as a major women's health issue. This campaign used radio, television, and magazines, including articles in *Vogue, McCall's,* and *Reader's Digest* (Dejanikus 1985). As the manufacturers of Premarin, a popular form of estrogen replacement therapy (ERT), Ayerst certainly benefited from awareness of this issue. Women who sought advice from physicians about prevention might easily end up with a prescription for ERT.

Calcium manufacturers have similarly benefited from the media attention they helped to focus on studies linking calcium deficiency to osteoporosis. In 1980, retail sales of calcium supplements totaled $18 million; with increased public awareness, these sales were expected to total $166 million in 1986 (Giges 1986). A calcium-fortified sugar-free drink mix was recently test-marketed and the addition of calcium to Tab has nearly tripled the sales of this diet cola in some markets (Giges 1986). Cholesterol consciousness may have reduced the sales of dairy foods, but the dairy industry has launched a campaign to counterbalance these losses with the theme, "Dairy foods: calcium the way nature intended" (Giges 1986). The recent cautionary note that calcium might not be effective in prevention (Kolata 1986) has not changed calcium promotion.

Two major factors may contribute to the success of osteoporosis-related advertising: the prevention consciousness in our society and the fear of aging. Many advertisements play on both of these, such as the spot for a calcium supplement that shows a healthy thirty-year-old woman transformed to a stooped sixty-five-year-old in thirty seconds (Giges 1986). While such an image capitalizes on the fear of losing youthful beauty, it draws on even deeper fears of disability leading to loss of independence. The information on hip fractures is equally frightening. For example, a popular guide to preventing osteoporosis states: "The consequences of hip fractures can be devastating. Fewer than one-half of all women who suffer a hip fracture regain normal function. Fifteen percent die shortly after their injury, and nearly 30 percent die within a year" (Notelovitz and Ware 1982, 37). The fear for women is that, even if they survive a hip fracture, they may face long years of dependence and immobility.

In contrast to the past, health care practitioners are now very aware of osteoporosis. Many of the new women's health centers offer osteoporosis counseling and the topic appears regularly in the educational programs they sponsor. In addition to providing information and counseling, these centers can now offer noninvasive bone mass measurements, billed as "screening" for osteoporosis. A projected five hundred clinics will offer this service in 1986, having grown in numbers from only twenty-five in 1984 (Cummings and Black 1986). Some advertisements for the clinics suggest that most women from forty-five to seventy should be screened for osteoporosis (Ott 1986). A belief in the benefits of early detection coupled with the fear of disability with aging make this screening very attractive for a woman who can afford the procedure.

Measuring Bone Mass

Finding a noninvasive way to predict a woman's risk for fracture may seem a benefit of medical science with which few could find fault. Certainly, the prevalence and potential consequences of osteoporosis are serious enough to justify screening. However, an evaluation of the use of bone mass measurements as a screening procedure, according to the criteria discussed earlier, reveals a very different picture. According to the criteria, it is important to determine whether the procedure provides early identification, how accurate the procedure is, and whether prognosis will be affected.

To deal with the first criterion, whether a procedure provides early identification of a condition, it is important to recognize that several techniques are currently being used to detect osteoporosis. These techniques vary in availability, cost, and reliability. The most widely available technique for osteoporosis screening, single-photon absorptiometry (SPA), is the least expensive. However, SPA measures the wrist bone, which is a different type of bone from that found in the hip and spine, where the most serious fractures are likely to occur. Extrapolation from wrist measurements is of little value, no matter how accurate those measurements are, and cannot be substituted for direct vertebrae measurements (Ott 1986; Riggs and Melton 1986). Direct measurement of the vertebral bone, possible with dual-photon absorptiometry (DPA) or computerized tomography (CT), requires a high degree of technical expertise to obtain accurate results and is quite expensive, costing up to several hundred dollars for each test.

A screening procedure that is expected to provide early detection should certainly be able to identify full-blown cases of the disease. Bone density screening would be expected, therefore, to be able to differentiate between those who do and do not have osteoporosis-related hip fractures (Ott 1986). However, these measurements are of little use in the elderly at-risk population because, as Ott (1986, 875) states:

> If the highest bone mass seen in patients with fractures is designated as the "fracture threshold," then nearly all women over 70 will by definition have osteoporosis.

Many factors besides bone mass (such as proneness to falling and the inability to protect oneself from injury during a fall) affect the chance of fractures (Cummings and Black 1986).

Given that this screening cannot identify those at risk for hip fractures, can it at least detect those who will experience a high degree of bone loss? Knowing someone's bone mass at age forty-five does not help one to predict how fast she may lose bone mass; a woman with a low bone mass may end up losing at a very slow rate and a woman with a much higher mass may end up losing rapidly (Ott 1986). Even if the rate of bone loss over a certain time span can be accurately measured, the rate will not be constant and predictable. It is known that women lose bone most rapidly in the five to six years immediately following menopause. After that, a woman's rate of bone loss slows down, again becoming similar to that of men. To monitor bone loss, expensive multiple measurements would need to be made and even then the predictive value in terms of fracture is highly uncertain (Cummings and Black 1986). Early measurements are being encouraged as a baseline by which to compare future measurements for assessing bone loss. But repeated measurements are useful only if a high degree of reproducibility is assured.

This leads to the second criterion—accuracy. Lack of reproducibility overshadows any evaluation of specificity and sensitivity. Cummings and Black (1986) point out that the reports of greatest reproducibility come from research centers, often using bone specimens, under highly controlled research conditions. Applying these techniques in clinical settings on real people is much more difficult. Any changes in equipment, technicians, software, radiation levels, or positioning of the person can alter results. For example, using computerized tomography (CT), a slight change in the area of the vertebrae measured can make up to a 30 percent difference in results (Ott 1986). The problem of not being able to provide good reproducibility in a given setting is exaggerated by the fact that the U.S. population is fairly mobile. Many women who have a baseline reading done at age forty-five will end up in different locations for future measurements.

The third major criterion for evaluation is whether the screening results would actually change the prognosis by altering the course of treatment or prevention. Knowledge of bone mass should have no impact on a woman's decision to take calcium or do weight-bearing exercise, as these are currently recommended as important preventive measures for *all* women. Therefore, information about current bone mass or rate of loss would play a role only in a woman's decision about the use of estrogen replacement therapy (ERT). However, other factors may play a much more important part in the ERT decision. For example, a woman may base her decision on increased cancer risk, contraindications, or the use of ERT for other problems, such as hot flashes or vaginal atrophy. Unless a woman's decision about ERT depends predominantly on information obtained by bone measurements, this information is of little value (Cummings and Black 1986).

This fact highlights a major risk of the screening. The new technology could easily lead to more medical intervention in the form of increased prescribing of ERT. Thus, the risks and benefits of ERT should be seen as central to the debate on the value of bone mass measurement. Hormone replacement therapy (HRT), containing both estrogen and progesterone, is increasingly marketed as safer than ERT. The addition of progesterone appears to counter the increased risk of endometrial cancer associated with ERT. However, more research is needed to determine the effectiveness of HRT in preventing osteoporosis. Even *if* screening could accurately predict osteoporosis, it is not clear how effective HRT would be in preventing bone loss.

Summary

Currently, bone mass measurements have limited clinical value, though they may have important research potential. No matter how refined the technology becomes, certain problems remain. The existence of non-invasive methods for measuring bone mass, combined with the high prevalence and serious consequences of osteoporosis, does not add up to a justification for recommending osteoporosis screenings. Nor can hip fracture be predicted using these technologies, though there may be slightly higher predictability for vertebral fractures. The only outcome of this screening may be increased ERT prescription.

By capitalizing on the fear of a disabling condition, clinical centers have been selling women an expensive technology of dubious clinical or preventive value. As one editorial on the subject appropriately concluded: "At this time, the use of these tests for screening perimenopausal women is premature, albeit profitable" (Ott 1986, 876).

Mammography: Breast Cancer Screening

It is relatively easy to conclude that any mass screening for osteoporosis is inappropriate at this stage, but assessing the value of mass breast cancer screening is far more complicated. The major questions, however, remain the same: will mammography provide early accurate detection and will early detection affect prognosis?

Breast cancer statistics have become common household knowledge: one of eleven North American women will experience breast cancer, every fifteen minutes a woman in the United States dies of breast cancer, and one-half of the women found to have breast cancer this year will not be alive after ten years (Sloane 1985). Mortality rates for breast cancer have remained static for over eighty years, while the incidence of breast cancer is increasing (Wertheimer et al. 1986). Over 75 percent of people questioned in a National Institutes of Health survey identified cancer as women's greatest health concern, with more than 50 percent specifically naming breast cancer (Wertheimer et al. 1986). Taking advantage of a climate of intense cancer-phobia, mammography can be marketed as the glimmer of hope that something can be done to reduce mortality.

With far too little research on *preventing* cancer, the focus is on detecting breast cancer before there is node metastasis. This goal is particularly challenging since breast cancer represents more than twenty pathological categories (Skrabanek 1985) and is "notoriously unsuited to generalizations" (Moore 1985). Moore (1985, 788) states:

> All clinicians know that 10–20% of breast cancers are incurable despite earliest possible diagnosis and that 10–20% will never kill the patient because they never metastasise.

It is for the group in between these two extremes that early detection might have some value.

Presently over 90 percent of breast cancers are discovered by women themselves through breast self-exam. The average size of tumor detected by self-exam is 2.5 cm. Approximately 50 percent of these cancers have lymph node involvement by the time they are discovered (Wertheimer et al. 1986). It is not possible to detect tumors smaller than 1.0 cm by palpation, but by the time that tumors reach this size, many will have metastasised (Skrabanek 1985). (To confuse the issue, although there is a relationship between tumor size and lymph node involvement, approximately one-third of tumors more than 6.0 cm do not have node involvement [Off Our Backs 1986]. In fact, women with very large tumors [greater than 6.0 cm] have better survival rates than women with smaller tumors [Skrabanek 1985].) Whereas breast self-exam cannot detect small tumors, doctors do not offer much better results. In one study in which physicians knew they were being tested, they managed to find only 44 percent of lumps hidden in silicone breasts, where they are easier to locate than in real women (Fletcher et al. 1985). Mammography is offered as the answer where physical exam seems to fall short.

Benefits of Mammography

Enthusiasm for mammography screening and well advertised guidelines are based primarily on two major studies. The Health Insurance Plan of New York (HIP) Study in the early 1960s randomized more than 60,000 women into two groups. Half of the women were offered annual physical examinations and mammography screenings for four years. The screened population was compared with the unscreened group in ten- to fourteen-year follow-ups. Mortality reduction of 25 to 35 percent was demonstrated for women in the screened population (Shapiro, cited in Kopans 1986). In the Breast Cancer Detection Demonstration Project (BCDDP) in the early 1970s, 280,000 women were offered physical examinations and mammography screening in twenty-seven centers across the United States. Of the 3,550 cancers detected, 42 percent were nonpalpable and detected only by mammography (Baker, cited in Kopans 1986). These results were supported by a recent Swedish study showing a reduction of 31 percent in mortality and of 25 percent in the proportion of Stage II (more advanced) tumors in a population receiving mammography, compared to a nonscreened control group (Tabar, cited in Kopans 1986).

In addition to claims of mortality reduction, mammography is heralded as offering information that can make therapeutic decisions more appropriate to a woman's needs and in some cases allow for more conservative treatment. Roebuck (1986) suggests that detecting tumors at an early, small stage would permit more conservative treatment, easier local control of cancer, and even a reduction in the need for radiography. On the other hand, Kopans (1986) believes that preoperative mammography would help identify those women with multifocal macroscopic disease in which conservative treatment has a higher risk of failure; in that case mammography could lead to more radical treatment.

The American Cancer Society and the American College of Radiology (ACS/ACR) recommend a baseline mammogram for all women between the ages of thirty-five and forty, followed by annual or biennial mammograms until the age of fifty and annual mammograms after fifty. In contrast, the National Cancer Institute (NCI) does not recommend mammography for women under 50 unless they have a personal or family history of breast cancer. Marketing, of course, uses only the ACS/ACR guidelines.

It is estimated that presently only 5 percent of women over fifty have annual mammograms and probably only one-third of eligible women have ever had a baseline mammogram (Hall 1986a). A recent poll showed that only 11 percent of physicians follow ACS guidelines for mammography (Wertheimer et al. 1986). With the mass marketing of mammography, the uptake could increase dramatically. Therefore, it is important to look at the potential impact of increased mammography screening on other services.

Impact of Mass Marketing of Mammography

Too few radiologists. Even the most avid proponents of mammography recognize that a high degree of training *and* experience is required both to conduct and to interpret mammographic examinations. The literature is full of reminders that even with "considerable attention to technique with experienced and careful interpretation," there is a significant false-negative rate (Newsome and McLelland 1986b) (see below) and that "rigorous attention by the technologist carrying out the study to positioning the breast" is necessary to diminish the problem of "blind areas" (Kopans 1986). Wertheimer and coauthors (1986, 1314) caution that if ACS guidelines were more closely followed, "there would not be enough radiologists, even working full time on mammography, to analyze the mammograms." Qualitatively, Hall (1986a, 54) gives an even stronger warning:

> The large number of screening mammograms currently being performed, with multiples of this number projected for the future, necessitates that many of these examinations be interpreted or acted on by radiologists and surgeons who have little or no training in this area. Although breast-imaging centers are now commonplace at neighborhood malls and mammography has become a bread and butter examination in most radiologic offices, the "considerable clinical experience" [required for mammographic interpetation] is usually lacking.

Too many biopsies? It is predicted that surgery will be affected by mass screening almost as much as radiology. The Beth Israel Hospital in Boston was performing seven breast biopsies per week in 1985 compared with one biopsy per week four years prior (Hall 1986a). In addition to a projected increase in numbers of biopsies, the surgeons' involvement has become more complicated. A team approach to cancer detection/treatment is now more appropriate than having the patient passed serially from one specialist to the next. Radiologists and surgeons must increasingly work together because nonpalpable lesions require that the radiologist accurately guide the surgeon to the area of concern (Kopans 1986). Fisher (1986) stresses that biopsies should be performed by breast surgeon specialists so that the same person could carry out follow-up surgery if that proves to be necessary. He explains that a second surgeon is at a disadvantage not knowing exactly the size of a lump removed and whether it was removed in its entirety. Thus, mammography centers must be a part of units specializing in breast cancer treatment.

An increased number of benign biopsies are an obvious consequence of a mass mammography screening program. There is no way to estimate the psychological cost or how this perpetuates the fear of cancer, but it is easy to see how the situation arises. Mammography detects nonpalpable lesions. Although chances of carcinoma may be one in fifty or one in one hundred, "malignancy cannot be excluded," so a surgeon is faced with performing a biopsy or risking a law suit. (A Massachusetts surgeon who did not perform a biopsy for a later diagnosed breast cancer recently lost a multimillion dollar law suit [Hall 1986a].)

Roebuck (1986) emphasizes that unnecessary biopsies could be minimized if breast cancer screening programs adopted a secondary intensive investigation policy, using such techniques as magnification, ultrasound, or cytological aspiration. Hall (1986a) recommends more mammography as a solution to too many mammography-inspired biopsies. He encourages close mammographic follow-up examinations for the breast abnormalities in which the chances of carcinoma are low (less than one in ten or one in twenty). But the issue of mammography and biopsy is not an easy one. In contrast to the above arguments, *Our Bodies, Ourselves* (Boston Women's Health Book Collective 1984, 495) sees biopsy of palpable lumps as a way to avoid unnecessary mammography: "If a lump is suspicious enough to warrant a mammogram, then in most cases it is suspicious enough to warrant a biopsy. . . . If the biopsy reveals the lump to be benign (as most are) unnecessary exposure to radiation will have been avoided."

Treatment dilemmas. Additionally, a breast cancer screening program is valuable only if appropriate follow-up treatment is available. Mass screening programs will drastically increase the demand for breast cancer treatment. We need to question whether it is appropriate to push more women into a medical system that already cannot take care of their needs. As a part of the 1986 Breast Cancer Campaign,[2] the National Women's Health Network has stated: ". . . many American women who are already victims of breast cancer *can't get the effective treatment they need.*" For example, in 1984, more than 5 percent of mastectomies performed were the Halstead version—an extreme, debilitating operation discredited a decade ago by both physicians and health activists. In addition, even though European studies have indicated that a dose of chemotherapy *before* breast surgery can be very effective, it is nearly impossible for a woman to have preoperative chemotherapy in this country. Instead, intensive chemotherapy after surgery is standard treatment for women whose breast cancer has spread to the lymph nodes. Clinical studies show that postoperative chemotherapy offers no real benefit for most women over fifty, the largest group of women with breast cancer.

Though psychological counseling should be an integral part of breast cancer treatments, mass mammography screening may create additional problems. Women who have breast cancer detected by mammography adapt less well to their condition. Because they could not "feel it" the first time, they live in fear that they will not be able to tell if there is a recurrence (Skrabanek 1985).

Mammography Controversies

As advertising money is being poured into the selling of mammography, the limitations, problems, and questions about mammography need to be articulated. Consumers need to be aware that the value of mammography is still being debated. Below we raise some of the issues, including accuracy, frequency, safety, and potential for prolonging life.

Accuracy. Mammography is not particularly accurate, in terms of sensitivity or specificity. In the classic HIP study, 55 percent of cancers were not detected by screening (Thomas et al. 1983). Newsome and McLelland (1986b) estimate that the "average" false-negative rate is approximately 20 percent, but conclude:

> . . . false-negative rates ranging from a low of 5% to a high, in a select group of studies, of 69% make mammography an unreliable method to ascertain the nature of a palpable mass. (Newsome and McLelland 1986a, 528)

It has been observed that the mean delay in treatment due to false-negative mammograms was forty-three weeks (Haagensen and Asch cited in Skrabanek 1985). So although the technique is marketed for its value in early detection, false negatives could stand in the way of women with palpable masses receiving early treatment.

False-positive mammogram results are "all those cases in which a suspicious lesion is not confirmed by biopsy as malignant. This is true in about 80–90% of biopsies" (Skrabanek 1985, 317). More than 3.5 percent of women mammographically diagnosed as having malignancies in the Breast Cancer Detection Demonstration Project (BCDDP) turned out not to have cancer (Sloane 1985). At least thirty-seven of these women had already had unnecessary mastectomies, though it is still not known whether these women have been told (National Women's Health Network 1983). The psychological costs of false-positive results and unncecessary mastectomies are high prices for individuals to pay in hopes that mammography may reduce mortality rates.

Frequency and baseline recommendations. The conflicting recommendations of the ACS/ACR and the NCI reflect some of the major controversies surrounding mammography screening (see above). Even those bodies promoting mammography do not agree on the age when screening should start or how often screening should be done.

The more conservative recommendation by the NCI, that women under fifty not be screened unless they have a personal or family history of breast cancer, is based on "the unknown effect of even a small amount of radiation exposure to young women and the lack of clinical trial evidence that breast cancer mortality could be decreased through periodic screening of younger women" (Baker et al. 1985). Younger breasts are more sensitive to radiation damage and the firm, dense tissue does not provide enough contrast for an accurate mammogram. Both false negatives and false positives are more common in women under fifty. Breast cancer in younger women seems to be faster, more aggressive; survival rates are lower than for older women with tumors of comparable size and similar node involvement (Off Our Backs 1986). Therefore, for mammography to work as an early detection tool, it would need to be used frequently, an approach most inappropriate in this age group. Despite the lack of evidence that mammography reduces mortality in younger women, the average age for a first mammogram is decreasing steadily and the number of young women receiving mammograms is rising constantly (Boston Women's Health Book Collective 1984). Young women are being urged to have baseline mammography in their thirties, yet we know each individual's breasts will change dramatically as a part of the aging process. Is baseline mammography valuable as a baseline or merely as a way to hook women into the screening process? Women considering baseline mammography need to confirm that their mammography can serve this purpose. No clinic sampled in the National Women's Health Network Breast Cancer Campaign (1986) was keeping X-rays for more than five years, so an early mammogram is unlikely to have value as a baseline for future comparisons.

Once a woman is a part of the screening process it is easy to encourage frequent mammograms because no one knows the optimum intervals to reduce mortality. In the BCDDP, 20 to 26 percent of cancers appeared between annual screenings. In one HIP study, 77 percent of cancers surfaced between screenings. These interval cancers (cancers appearing between annual screenings) seem to be more aggressive with worse prognosis than cancers detected by mammography (Skrabanek 1985). This could lead one to question whether mammography screening is useful for detecting such fast-growing cancers. Haagensen has suggested that screening would have to be done every four months in order to detect early stages of all breast cancers (Haagensen, cited in Skrabanek 1985). One hates to think of how advertising could use that suggestion.

ACS/ACR recommendations are for annual mammography examinations after the age of fifty. Although this appears to be a relatively noncontroversial recommendation, the ramifications need to be considered. Napoli (1983, 7) questions, "How does a study [HIP study] that only gave three annual mammographic exams provide a basis for the current ACS recommendations that women over 50 should have an annual mammography . . . presumably for the rest of their lives?" Has anyone questioned the value of annual screenings for a sixty-year-old or a seventy-year-old?

Safety. The safety of mammography has been debated since 1977 when the media seized on a medical article: "Mammography: A Contrary View" (Bailor, cited in Baker et al. 1985) in which mammography was viewed as a *cause* as much as a *detector* of cancer. Literature today assures us that with modern equipment, emitting only 0.1 to 0.8 rad for a two-view examination, "radiation risk per se should no longer be a factor in consumer and provider acceptance of mammography" (Wertheimer et al. 1986). Today's doses are significantly lower than the rads in the HIP study. However, there is no room for complacency regarding breast screening. Except for the developing fetus, the female breast is the most radiosensitive of all human tissues. Yet, there are no federal laws regulating the use of mammograph equipment (Kushner 1984, 388). In a 1982 survey, only 67 percent of Illinois hospitals offering mammography complied with ACS guidelines of less than one rad to the midbreast (Baker et al. 1985). With competition and profitability as key issues in health care provision, we cannot trust that X-ray equipment will get the maintenance it requires. As women are increasingly being exposed to mammography at a younger age and at more frequent intervals its safety must continue to be debated and monitored.

Does mammography save lives? Given the mass marketing of mammography and the publicity focused on the relative safety of new techniques, it is not surprising that most consumers are unaware of the debates surrounding mammography's life-saving potential. Clearly the HIP study, the BCDDP, and the Swedish study can be interpreted as offering a glimmer of hope that length of survival can be improved by early detection. But even such qualified enthusiasm needs to be balanced by looking at controversies surrounding the studies (i.e., many tumors "detected by mammography only" should have been detected by clinical examination; an unexplained finding was that the lowest mortality rate was found in a subgroup of women in the mammography group who refused screening [Skrabanek 1985]). It is important to recognize that intense, short-term studies pick up different information (such as a backlog of cancers "waiting to be detected") from that detected by long-term screening in a wider cross section of the population. It will take thirty- to forty-year follow-up studies to actually show that early detected cancer is "cured" rather than simply "discovered earlier."

> It is agreed that mammography is the only practical test that can detect breast cancer before it is palpable. Early detection does not guarantee cure, though it leads to longer morbidity and longer survival times due to the lead-time bias. This is often confused with better prognosis and lower mortality. [It has been] calculated that the "improvement" in 5-year survival rates since 1950, amounting to about 10% for 97% of cancers, can be explained by the fact that cancers are diagnosed an average of six months earlier. (Skrabanek 1985, 318)

Autopsy studies may help put early detection and cancer phobia into perspective by reminding us that many women have cancer without knowing it and without it killing them. In one study, as many as 6 percent of women dying of other causes were found to have breast cancer in situ and 20 percent had dysplasia. Another autopsy study found that 25 percent of women older than twenty years had invasive breast carcinoma or premalignant lesions (Kramer and Nielsen, cited in Skrabanek 1985).

Technological innovations can make useful skills appear old-fashioned and outmoded, but mammography must not be viewed as a replacement for breast self-examination. Even if mammography proves valuable in reducing mortality, we must remember that many women will not have access to such an expensive technique and that both mammography and breast self-examination can provide unique information. Breast tissue can hide a mass so that it does not show up radiographically, but it may be felt physically. In the BCDDP, 9 percent of cancers were mammographically negative but detected by physical examination (Hall 1986b). Kopans (1986) estimates that up to 20 percent of cancers undetected by mammography appear as palpable masses between annual screenings. Canadian and British studies are presently underway to assess the separate benefits of mammography and physical examination screening (Morrison 1986 and Holliday et al. 1983). It will cost a health district at least 6.5 times as much to offer annual mammography screening as compared to a breast self-examination program, so many communities will not have the luxury of evaluating mammography (Holliday et al. 1983).

Summary

There are no simple answers to the questions posed at the beginning of this examination of mammography. In some cases mammography may provide accurate early detection and this detection may improve prognosis. However, many complications and controversies remain, even while we recognize that mammography is a potentially useful tool. In our enthusiasm for its possibilities, we should not forget its limitations and dangers. As a society we must recognize that mammography screening is valuable only as a part of *good* cancer care and treatment services available to *all* women. Enthusiasm for the promise of early detection must never hide the real issue. Research must be directed toward ways of *preventing* cancer, not *detecting* it.

Conclusion

As competition among health care facilities escalates, women's health centers have developed as a way of attracting an economically comfortable, health conscious, and healthy population. Intense marketing campaigns, using newspaper and television advertisements, direct mailings, and free lecture series, promise "total" health care for women of all ages. Some of this advertising seems to echo the goals of the women's health movement, offering caring women practitioners, longer scheduled appointments, free educational programs, resource centers, and information necessary to make informed decisions, all in a comfortable environment. None of these aspects of health care is profitable in themselves, but they do serve to attract women to these centers.

The availability of a technology such as bone mass measurement or mammography can serve both as a selling point for a clinic and as a profitable service in itself. Unfortunately, these technologies are marketed not with an honest assessment of their value, but by manipulating fear of a specific disease and by playing on the tendency to confuse detection with prevention. At this point, there is very little value in offering bone mass measurement for osteoporosis screening, though the research potential of these techniques is excellent. While mammography shows great promise for early detection of breast cancer, many controversies and problems still surround its use.

Co-optation, 1980s-style, presents new challenges for the women's health movement. Now that women's health has been "discovered" as an area offering tremendous market potential, it is more important than ever that feminist activists evaluate and critique these services. Appropriation of the rhetoric of the women's health movement by the new women's health centers must not replace movement voices calling for fundamental changes in health care provision. For years activists have been saying that issues such as premenstrual tension and osteoporosis need to be taken more seriously. Now these problems are being taken seriously, but they are being used to medicalize whole new areas of women's lives. The women's health movement must continue warning that wider interest in these areas can be used against women, that drugs must not be seen as the solution to "problems," and that technological fixes cannot substitute for real prevention.

Much of the marketing of women's health care goes against all that health activists have fought for. We must not lose sight of the fact that huge expenditures are going into technology that, even if useful, will be available to only a select segment of the population. Making health care truly accessible and appropriate to *all* women is still the primary goal of the movement.

N O T E S

1. This information was obtained from notes on a seminar on marketing women's health centers conducted by Sally Rynne, a leading consultant in this area.
2. The National Women's Health Network Breast Cancer Campaign can be contacted at 1325 G Street NW, Lower Level B, Washington, D.C. 20005.

An excerpt from this chapter was first published in *Women's Health: Readings on Social, Economic, and Political Issues,* edited by Nancy Worcester and Mariamne H. Whatley, © 1988 Kendall/Hunt Publishing Company. Reprinted by permission of Kendall/Hunt Publishing Company.

R E F E R E N C E S

Baker, Larry H., Tom D. Y. Chin, and Kay V. Wagner. 1985. Progress in screening for early breast cancer. *Journal of Surgical Oncology* 30, no. 2: 96–102.
Berwick, Donald M. 1985. Scoliosis screening: A pause in the chase. *American Journal of Public Health* 75, no. 12: 1,373–74.
Boston Women's Health Book Collective. 1984. *The new our bodies, ourselves.* New York: Simon and Schuster.
Cummings, Steven R., and Dennis Black. 1986. Should perimenopausal women be screened for osteoporosis? *Annals of Internal Medicine* 104, no. 6: 817–23.
Dejanikus, Tacie. 1985. Major drug manufacturer funds osteoporosis education campaign. *Network News* (National Women's Health Network) 10, no. 3 (May/June): 1, 3.
Fisher, Bernard. 1986. 15 questions to ask before breast biopsy. *Healthfacts* 11, no. 88 (September): 4.
Fletcher, Suzanne W., Michael S. O'Malley, and Leslie A. Bunce. 1985. Phy-

sicians' ability to detect lumps in silicone breast models. *Journal of the American Medical Association* 253, no. 15: 2,224–28.

Giges, Nancy. 1986. Calcium market shrugs off study. *Advertising Age* 57 (August 11): 49, 56.

Hall, Ferris M. 1986a. Screening mammography: Potential problems on the horizon. *New England Journal of Medicine* 314, no. 1: 53–55.

─────. 1986b. Mammography (Letter). *Journal of the American Medical Association* 255, no. 22: 3,118.

Holliday, Howard W., Eric J. Roebuck, Peter J. Doyle, Roger W. Blamey, Christopher W. Elston, Jocelyn Chamberlain, and Susan Moss. 1983. Initial results from a programme of breast self-examination. *Clinical Oncology* 9, no. 1: 11–16.

Kaplan, Frederick S. 1985. Osteoporosis. *Women and Health* 10, no. 2/3: 95–114.

Kolata, Gina. 1986. How important is dietary calcium in preventing osteoporosis? *Science* 233, no. 4763: 519–20.

Kopans, Daniel B. 1986. Breast cancer detection. *Western Journal of Medicine* 144, no. 1: 73–75.

Kushner, Rose. 1984. *Alternatives: New developments in the war on breast cancer.* New York: Warner Books.

Moore, Condict. 1985. Breast cancer screening and treatment. *Lancet* 8458 (October 5): 788.

Morrison, Brenda. 1986. The periodic health examination: 3. Breast cancer. *Canadian Medical Association Journal* 134, no. 7: 727–29.

Napoli, Maryann. 1983. Breast cancer: An update. *Network News* (National Women's Health Network) 8, no. 4 (July/August): 2–7.

National Women's Health Network. 1983. Women misdiagnosed with breast cancer. *Network News* (National Women's Health Network) 8, no. 1 (January/February): 5.

Newsome, James F., and Robert McLelland. 1986a. A word of caution concerning mammography. *Journal of the American Medical Association* 255, no. 4: 528.

─────. 1986b. Mammography (Letter). *Journal of the American Medical Association* 255, no. 22: 3,119.

Notelovitz, Morris, and Marsha Ware. 1982. *Stand tall! The informed women's guide to preventing osteoporosis.* Gainesville, Fla.: Triad.

Off Our Backs. 1986. Breast cancer: Checking the fourth quadrant. *Off Our Backs* 16, no. 2 (February): 8.

Ott, Susan. 1986. Should women get screening bone mass measurements? *Annals of Internal Medicine* 104, no. 6: 874–76.

Riggs, B. Lawrence, and L. Joseph Melton. 1986. Involutional osteoporosis. *New England Journal of Medicine* 314, no. 26: 1,676–84.

Roebuck, E. J. 1986. Mammography and screening for breast cancer. *British Medical Journal* 292, no. 6515: 223–26.

Ruzek, Sheryl Bert. 1980. Medical response to women's health activists: conflict, accommodation and cooptation. In *Research in the sociology of health* care. *Volume 1: Professional control of health services and challenges to such control,* ed. J. A. Roth, 335–54. Greenwich, Conn.: JAI Press.

Skrabanek, Petr. 1985. False premises and false promises of breast cancer screening. *Lancet* 8450 (August 10): 316–19.

Sloane, Ethel. 1985. *Biology of women.* 2d edition. New York: John Wiley and Sons.

Thomas, Barbara A., John L. Price, and Patrick S. Boulter. 1983. The Guild-ford breast screening project. *Clinical Oncology* 9, no. 2: 121–29.

Wertheimer, Michael D., Mary E. Costanza, Thomas F. Dodson, Carl D'Orsi, Harris Pastides, and Jane G. Zapka. 1986. Increasing the effort toward breast cancer detection. *Journal of the American Medical Association* 255, no. 10: 1,311–15.

Ethical Decision Making in Medical Genetics: Women as Patients and Practitioners in Eighteen Nations

Dorothy C. Wertz and John C. Fletcher

New developments in human genetics have potential impacts both on women's health and on the future of society. For example, technologies that facilitate selecting the sex of the child have the potential for creating future societies with unbalanced sex ratios; genetic screening in the workplace for susceptibility to occupationally related diseases could change the character of the workforce; widespread use of prenatal diagnosis could lead to a resurgence of eugenic concerns. A proposed plan to map the entire human genome could lead to new social definitions of normality and abnormality. Of one thing we can be certain: as genetic technologies become more complex, the ethical dilemmas faced by geneticists, policymakers, and the public at large will become more complicated. Many of the new technologies will necessarily have greater impact on women than on men because they will be carried out within women's bodies. At the same time, women, who constitute one-third of the practitioners of medical genetics around the world, may have an opportunity to have an impact on policies and practices in human genetics.

In most countries, there are no formal professional standards of ethics with regard to use of new technologies in genetics. Individual geneticists have set forth their ethical views (Berg 1983, Crawfurd 1983, Schroeder-Kurth 1984, Anders 1984, Czeizel 1988), but there has been no systematic study of the actual approaches of medical geneticists to ethical problems. Medical geneticists' views will clearly carry weight as clinicians, public health departments, and patients seek to resolve ethical problems. Fletcher, Berg, and Tranøy (1985) proposed that medical geneticists around the world would benefit from collective reflection on their preferred approaches to the most difficult moral choices. In response, we studied the approaches of medical geneticists from different cultures when they were presented with ethical dilemmas concerning fourteen clinical problems and five screening situations that required a moral choice (Wertz and Fletcher 1989). In this chapter, we discuss the ten clinical cases that focus most directly on women as patients.

We expected some variation among nations, arising from cultural differences, availability of technological resources, and structure of the health care system (national health insurance versus fee-for-service). We also anticipated that the diffusion of new technologies would tend to increase consensus.

Women and Moral Reasoning

In addition to studying approaches cross-culturally, we were interested in comparing the responses of women and men geneticists. Women constituted 35 percent of our respondents. Researchers on moral reasoning (Kohlberg 1981, Gilligan 1982) have suggested that women arrive at their moral decisions by a different process of reasoning than do men. Gilligan (1982) argues that women reach conclusions about moral dilemmas on the basis of networks of responsibility rather than individual rights. She points to the different frames of reference and verbal structures that women and men in her study used when presented with both hypothetical and actual decisions.

Theories of moral reasoning have not yet been examined among a large group of persons who have undergone professional training. According to the sociological literature, medical training aims to erase personal differences in approaches to clinical situations (Light 1979, Fox 1963, Bosk 1979). Students learn an esoteric language that helps them to control physician-patient interactions. Such training may obliterate any previous differences in language or moral reasoning associated with gender. By comparing responses of women and men geneticists, we were able to test some of the prevailing theories on a within-nation as well as a cross-cultural basis.

Methodology

In order to find out what types of cases medical geneticists found most difficult to resolve ethically, one author (Fletcher) undertook fieldwork in 1984 at twenty-five genetic centers in twelve nations (Denmark, the Federal Republic of Germany, France, Greece, Hungary, Italy, the Netherlands, Norway, Sweden, Switzerland, the United Kingdom, and the United States). Geneticists at the twelve centers described five types of ethical problems that occurred most frequently in their practices. These were (1) full disclosure of psychologically sensitive information, such as XY genotype (male chromosomes) in a person raised as a woman; (2) directive versus nondirective counseling (e.g., about fetuses with "borderline" disorders such as XYY, a sex chromosome abnormality in males that may be associated with learning disabilities or antisocial behavior); (3) presenting new or controversial reproductive options, such as in vitro fertilization (IVF) or surrogate motherhood; (4) indications for prenatal diagnosis, such as sex selection; and (5) patient confidentiality versus the duty to warn third parties of harm (e.g., to warn relatives that they may carry a genetic disorder). On the basis of this fieldwork, we developed fourteen case vignettes representing these problems. Ten of these, described in detail in the appendix to this chapter, focus on women as patients or parents. They represent the first four types of ethical problems described above. The remaining cases did not focus on the woman as patient and are not reported here. It should be noted that some difficult ethical situations of importance to women are not ordinarily dealt with by medical geneticists (e.g., selecting the sex of the child before conception by sperm separation; fetal surgery; keeping brain-dead mothers alive; allowing defective newborns to die).

The questions described in the appendix were part of an international questionnaire survey of medical geneticists in eighteen nations. Our rationale for choosing countries was: (*a*) presence of ten or more practicing medical geneticists; (*b*) geographical and cultural distribution; (*c*) a medical geneticist willing to distribute and collect the questionnaires. Some geographical areas, notably Africa, are not represented because of small numbers of geneticists.

Questions were both closed and open-ended. Respondents were asked what they would choose to do from a list of possible responses to each of the ten moral problems. They then were asked to explain, in their own words, why they had chosen the particular course of action. They were asked which of the ten cases had given them the most ethical conflict and which the least conflict.

Questionnaires were pilot-tested twice, first on eleven and then on ten medical geneticists from the United States, Canada, and Spain. They were revised after each trial. The questionnaires took approximately two hours to complete. We asked respondents to set them aside for a day after completing the first half, so that they might approach the second half freshly. Questionnaires were answered anonymously.

Our criteria for selecting geneticists were: holding an M.D., Ph.D., or equivalent degree; and engaging in the delivery or administration of genetic services (testing, counseling, prenatal diagnosis, laboratory work). Although in some countries (notably the United States) counseling is sometimes done by specially trained persons who do not hold an M.D. or a Ph.D., we decided to omit these persons to have more consistency of training across the entire sample.

In each country, including the United States, our contact person tried to include all qualified medical geneticists in the survey. Lists were compiled from certifying boards, genetics centers, and the National Foundation–March of Dimes *International Directory of Genetic Services*. Of the 1,053 medical geneticists asked to participate, 677 (64 percent) returned completed questionnaires by the close of the study in February, 1987 (table 1). Eighty-seven percent of these answered all parts of the questionnaires, including stating in their own words why they had chosen particular courses of action. Eighty-one percent held M.D.s, 16 percent Ph.D.s, and 3 percent held other degrees. They had a median of fourteen years in the practice of genetics; 82 percent were members of their national genetics society; and 77 percent were board certified in countries where certification in genetics was possible (Canada, Hungary, the UK and the United States). Respondents spent an average of forty-five hours a week in genetics. Sixty-five percent were male, and 82 percent were married, with a median of 1.5 children.

TABLE 1.   Participating Nations

Country	Geneticists Asked to Participate (no.)	Respondents (no.)	Response Rate (percentage)	Women (percentage)
Australia	14	12	86	33
Brazil	51	32	63	44
Canada	73	47	64	42
Denmark	28	15	58	13
Federal Republic of Germany	55	47	85	48
France	35	17	49	40
German Democratic Republic	25	21	80	58
Greece	11	7	64	57
Hungary	18	15	83	7[a]
India	40	27	67	46
Israel	17	15	88[b]	60[b]
Italy	26	11	42[a]	36
Japan	74	51	69	18
Norway	10[a]	6	60	20
Sweden	26	21	81	29
Switzerland	10[a]	5[a]	50	40
United Kingdom	50	33	66	41
United States	490[b]	295[b]	60	33
Total	1,053	677	64	35

[a]lowest in column
[b]highest in column

Religious backgrounds were 40 percent Protestant, 18 percent Catholic, 17 percent Jewish, 12 percent none, 5 percent Buddhist, 4 percent Hindu, and 4 percent other. As a whole, they were nonpracticing, attending a median of one religious observance a year. Forty-nine percent characterized themselves as politically liberal, 15 percent as conservative, and 36 percent as both equally. In the United States, a comparison between 274 respondents and 208 nonrespondents listed in the 1986 combined *Membership Directory* of the Genetics Society of America, American Society of Human Genetics, and American Board of Medical Genetics revealed no statistically significant differences between respondents and nonrespondents in type of degree, gender, geographical area, or subspecialty. Qualitative responses, including the respondents' anticipation of the consequences of their choices, were coded, using a system developed by the authors.

Women as Patients: Results of the Ten Cases

Ten clinical cases were specifically related to women as marital partners, patients, or fetuses. These cases will be referred to by the numbers listed in the appendix to this chapter. The ten cases reflect four main types of ethical problems: disclosure of psychologically sensitive information (cases 1 to 4); directive/nondirective counseling (cases 5 and 6); presenting reproductive options (cases 7 and 8); and indications for prenatal diagnosis (cases 9 and 10). Case 1, false paternity, is frequently used in courses on medical ethics, as presenting a conflict between the husband's right to know his test results and the injunction to do no harm. Of all the cases in our questionnaire, it produced the strongest consensus, with 96 percent of the total in favor of protecting the mother's confidentiality. Consensus was so strong (≥90 percent in all nations), that this case is not shown in table 2. Eighty-two percent would tell the mother privately, without the husband present, and let her decide what to tell him; 13 percent would lie (tell the couple that the disorder is not genetic or that they are both genetically responsible for the child's disorder), and 2 percent would ascribe the child's disorder to a new mutation, a one-in-a-million occurrence. In their reasoning, most geneticists cited "preserving the family unit."

Case 2 (table 2), disclosure to parents of which one carries the gene that has caused Down Syndrome in their child, also involves the marital relationship. Frequently parents blame each other, or the parent who is the carrier feels guilty. In countries where the status of women is especially low, a woman who is shown to be the carrier could suffer greatly. Sometimes disclosure could lead to divorce. On the other

hand, nondisclosure means that relatives of the carrier, who may themselves be carriers, will be denied access to valuable information, and
the couple themselves may be denied some reproductive options, such
as artificial insemination by donor sperm. Only in Japan and Switzerland was there greater than 75 percent agreement on this case. Of the
total 677 respondents, 54 percent would tell the couple which one was
the carrier, regardless of whether they asked or wanted to know, 45
percent would tell them only if they asked, and 1 percent would not
tell them anything at all.

In case 3 (table 2), disclosure of colleague disagreements about

TABLE 2. Percentage Who Would Disclose Psychologically Sensitive Information, by Country

Country	Which Parent Caused Down Syndrome (case 2)	Colleague Disagreement about Ambiguous Test Results (case 3)	XY Genotype in a Woman (case 4)
Australia	67	50	58
Brazil	63	72	9[b]
Canada	60	66	68
Denmark	67	47	40
Federal Republic of Germany	38	78[a]	52
France	69	47	13[b]
German Democratic Republic	65	71	19[b]
Greece	72	43	14[b]
Hungary	27	60	20[b]
India	44	56	52
Israel	71	57	27
Italy	64	46	27
Japan	6[b]	61	40
Norway	67	33	17[b]
Sweden	29	48	52
Switzerland	100[a]	20[b]	0[b]
United Kingdom	41	52	37
United States	62	75[a]	64
Total	54	66	51
Number of countries with ≥75% for disclosure	1	2	0
Number of countries with ≥75% against disclosure	1	1	7

[a] ≥ 75% for disclosure

[b] ≥ 75% against disclosure

Note: Case 1, false paternity, is not shown. It produced a 96% consensus in favor of protecting the mother's confidentiality.

ambiguous results in prenatal diagnosis to a woman patient seen alone, only in the Federal Republic of Germany and the United States would more than 75 percent disclose the fact that their colleagues disagreed. Of the total respondents, 98 percent would tell her that the results were ambiguous; 66 percent would also tell her that their colleagues disagreed about the interpretation.

Case 4 (table 2) concerns disclosure to a woman who is concerned about her infertility and who, upon testing, turns out to have a male (XY) genotype, even though she has been raised as a female. In the past this condition has been labeled testicular feminization syndrome; androgen insensitivity is now the preferred term. Such women are able to marry and adopt children, and they perform the female gender-stereotypical roles into which they have been socialized. They run some excess risk of cancer if the undescended testicles are not surgically removed, but a rationale for the surgery can be developed without revealing the XY genotype. Telling the woman that she is XY could threaten her entire self-image and social being; not telling her violates her right to know the truth and may increase the likelihood that she does not have the preventive surgery. Further, not telling increases the likelihood that she will continue to seek treatment for infertility. In other words, there is a high risk of doing harm, whatever course of action one chooses. In seven countries (Brazil, France, the German Democratic Republic, Greece, Hungary, Norway, and Switzerland), more than 75 percent would not disclose. In the United States and Canada, 68 percent and 64 percent respectively would disclose. Overall, 51 percent would disclose the truth; 49 percent would not. This case was among the three that respondents reported gave them the greatest ethical conflict. In Greece and Japan it was the case that gave the greatest ethical conflict among the entire fourteen clinical cases on the questionnaire.

Case 5 (table 3) involves nondirective counseling about fetuses with Turner syndrome (XO) or XYY. Both are disorders with low burden. Girls with XO may be essentially normal, except for short stature and infertility. Sometimes there is mild mental retardation. Boys with XYY may be normal or may have learning disabilities and behavior problems that may become associated with social deviance. We chose to include sex-linked disorders in order to see whether geneticists were more likely to give fetuses of one sex the benefit of the doubt and to counsel parents to carry the fetus to term. Although at least 75 percent in each of fifteen countries agreed that counseling should be nondirective for XYY and at least 75 percent in each of thirteen countries agreed that counseling should be nondirective for XO, 14 percent would provide optimistically weighted information or advice about XYY as opposed to 7 percent for XO. This suggests that male fetuses may be more likely to be given the benefit of the doubt.

Case 6 (table 3) involves counseling in a case in which the results of prenatal diagnosis, including both ultrasound and amniocentesis, give conflicting indications about the possibility of a small neural tube defect in the fetus. Repeated tests have failed to resolve the conflict. Given the impossibility of scientific certainty about the normality of the fetus and the likelihood that a defect, if present, would not cause severe impairment, should the geneticist give advice about aborting the fetus or carrying it to term, disclose the uncertainties in the test results but refuse to give any advice, or not disclose the test results at all? There was strong ($\geq$ 93 percent) consensus in all countries that the

TABLE 3.   Nondirective Counseling: Percentage Who Would Present Full Information without Giving Advice, by Country

Country	Fetus with Low-Burden Disorder (case 5)		Conflicting Diagnostic Findings for Neural Tube Defect (case 6)
	XO	XYY	
Australia	92[a]	92[a]	100[a]
Brazil	85[a]	84[a]	84[a]
Canada	98[a]	91[a]	94[a]
Denmark	100[a]	93[a]	79[a]
Federal Republic of Germany	74	76[a]	73
France	82[a]	35	56
German Democratic Republic	52	43	48
Greece	100[a]	86[a]	100[a]
Hungary	60	33	47
India	54	77[a]	63
Israel	93[a]	80[a]	100[a]
Italy	100[a]	82[a]	91[a]
Japan	77[a]	78[a]	77[a]
Norway	67	83[a]	67
Sweden	95[a]	90[a]	86[a]
Switzerland	80[a]	80[a]	100[a]
United Kingdom	97[a]	91[a]	84[a]
United States	92[a]	88[a]	95[a]
Total	87[a]	83[a]	87[a]
Number of countries with $\geq$ 75% in favor of nondirectiveness	13	15	12

[a] $\geq$ 75% for nondirectiveness

scientific uncertainties should be disclosed (not shown in table 3). There was strong ($\geq$ 75 percent) consensus in all countries except France, the German Democratic Republic, Hungary, India, Norway, and the Federal Republic of Germany that the counselor should be nondirective (table 3). Overall, 87 percent would be nondirective, 11 percent would give advice, and 2 percent would not disclose the test results.

TABLE 4. Presenting Reproductive Options: Percentage Who Would Present Option, without Giving Advice, in Cases in which One Parent Carries Tuberous Sclerosis, a Dominant Disorder not Diagnosable Prenatally (cases 7 and 8)

Country	Sterilization		Artificial Insemination Donor	Donor Egg IVF	Surrogate Mother
	Vasectomy	Tubal Ligation			
Australia	75[a]	91[a]	100[a]	92[a]	46
Brazil	72	69	50	59	34
Canada	91[a]	89[a]	98[a]	59	37
Denmark	60	67	80[a]	80[a]	47
Federal Republic of Germany	76[a]	72	72	33	16[b]
France	47	53	81[a]	44	0[b]
German Democratic Republic	0[b]	30	55	25[b]	5[b]
Greece	17[b]	50	67	80[a]	25[b]
Hungary	39	77[a]	47	46	31
India	45	45	54	43	48
Israel	57	67	100[a]	80[a]	39
Italy	55	64	80[a]	64	27
Japan	23[b]	19[b]	26	21[b]	10[b]
Norway	50	50	83[a]	33	33
Sweden	84[a]	84[a]	90[a]	55	30
Switzerland	60	60	100[a]	80[a]	20[b]
United Kingdom	90[a]	90[a]	94[a]	63	27
United States	84[a]	84[a]	96[a]	83[a]	67
Total	74	73	83[a]	66	46
Number of countries with $\geq$ 75% in favor of presenting this option	6	6	11	6	0
Number of countries with $\geq$ 75% against presenting this option	3	1	0	2	6

[a] $\geq$ 75% in favor of presenting
[b] $\geq$ 75% against presenting

Cases 7 and 8 (table 4) involve presenting reproductive options to male and female carriers, respectively, of tuberous sclerosis. Tuberous sclerosis was chosen because it is an example of a disorder in which an intellectually normal carrier can produce a child with extreme retardation. The disorder is dominant, meaning that the children have a 50 percent chance of being affected. It cannot be diagnosed prenatally. This means that parents who wish to avoid having children with the disorder must consider reproductive options such as adoption, sterilization, or, depending on the sex of the carrier, artificial insemination by donor, surrogate motherhood, or in vitro fertilization (IVF) with a donor egg. Respondents were asked which options they would discuss, and whether they would discuss them nondirectively or give advice about using or not using them. We chose to present the case twice, once for male carriers, and once for female carriers, in order to see whether they were counseled differently. A comparison between responses indicated that, with regard to the options open to both sexes (taking their chances of having a normal child, contraception, and adoption), counseling was essentially similar (not shown in table 4). Counselors were no more likely to be directive with women than with men.

There was strong consensus in favor of discussing vasectomy, without giving advice, in six nations (Australia, Canada, the Federal Republic of Germany, Sweden, the United Kingdom, and the United States), and strong consensus against discussing it in three nations (the German Democratic Republic, Greece, and Japan). There was strong consensus in favor of discussing tubal ligation, without giving advice, in six nations (Australia, Canada, Hungary, Sweden, the United Kingdom, and the United States) and strong consensus against discussing it in one, Japan.

Some options were not comparable, however, in terms of social acceptance or technological difficulty. Thus it is hardly surprising to find more acceptance ($\geq$ 75 percent in favor in eleven nations) of artificial insemination by donor than of insemination of a surrogate mother with the husband's sperm or IVF with a donor egg. It is interesting that, of the latter two options, geneticists preferred the technically more complicated, IVF with a donor egg, which has a very low success rate. There was a strong consensus in favor of IVF in six nations (Australia, Denmark, Greece, Israel, Switzerland, and the United States) and strong consensus against in two (the German Democratic Republic and Japan). There was strong consensus against surrogacy in six nations (the Federal Republic of Germany, France, the German Democratic Republic, Greece, Japan, and Switzerland). Only in the United States would a majority (67 percent) present surrogacy as an option without being asked. In giving reasons for their responses, geneticists seemed to believe that surrogacy was in fact the most complicated option, in that it could have adverse psychological, social, and legal results for all concerned. IVF with a donor egg, in spite of enormous technical difficulties and few documented successes, was seen as producing a better outcome, free of legal and emotional problems for all concerned. It was also seen by some as psychologically healthier. As one respondent put it, "the child is so much more one's own."

Case 9 (table 5) deals with providing prenatal diagnosis to an anxious young woman (age twenty-five) who has no family history of genetic disorders or personal history of exposure to toxic substances. There are no medical or genetic indications for its use in this case.

TABLE 5. Indications for Prenatal Diagnosis: Percentage Who Would Perform Prenatal Diagnosis or Refer to Someone Who Would Perform

Country	Maternal Anxiety Only (case 9)	Sex Selection, in Absence of X-Linked Disease (case 10)
Australia	67	17[b]
Brazil	44	30
Canada	70	47
Denmark	87[a]	13[b]
Federal Republic of Germany	80[a]	4[b]
France	57	13[b]
German Democratic Republic	5[b]	10[b]
Greece	43	29
Hungary	20[b]	60
India	56	52
Israel	80[a]	33
Italy	82[a]	18[b]
Japan	18[b]	6[b]
Norway	50	17[b]
Sweden	91[a]	38
Switzerland	100[a]	0[b]
United Kingdom	89[a]	24[b]
United States	89[a]	62
Total	73	42
Number of countries with ≥ 75% in favor of performing	8	0
Number of countries with ≥ 75% against performing	3	10

[a] ≥ 75% in favor of performing
[b] ≥ 75% against performing

Nevertheless, she appears very anxious about the fetus and persists in her demands for prenatal diagnosis even after being told that in her case the potential medical risks for the fetus, in terms of miscarriage, may outweigh the likelihood of diagnosing an abnormality. Answers to this question portend the future of prenatal diagnosis. Will it become a procedure to be performed on demand, for anxious mothers who can pay for it and who want to be sure that they have perfect children? If so, this could be seen as a victory for the autonomy of women patients. On the other hand, unless resources are virtually unlimited, it would necessarily deprive women who could benefit from the service but who cannot pay for it. Responses to this question by country reflect the level of technology diffusion. The greater the resources that geneticists perceive as available and the greater their experience with the procedure (and greater experience goes hand-in-hand with perceived safety), the more likely they are to approve its use on demand. Few seemed to be aware that in so doing they might be depriving other women of the service. There was strong consensus ($\geq$ 75 percent) for performing in eight nations (Denmark, the Federal Republic of Germany, Israel, Italy, Sweden, Switzerland, the United Kingdom, and the United States) and strong consensus against in three nations (the German Democratic Republic, Hungary, and Japan).

Case 10 (table 5), use of prenatal diagnosis for sex selection, is the most controversial in the entire survey. It gave respondents the greatest ethical conflict in the largest number of countries. Paradoxically, it also gave many respondents the *least* ethical conflict, because many felt that this was "nonnegotiable." We constructed the question so as to have the prospective parents desire a son, because sons are strongly preferred in some of our survey countries and we could find no evidence of societal preference for daughters in any of the participating nations. Recognizing that parents will go to extremes in order to coerce physicians to cooperate with their wishes in such cases, we constructed a case in which a couple had four daughters and threatened to have an abortion if the geneticist refused to perform prenatal diagnosis, rather than take the 50 percent risk of having another daughter. The geneticist is thus put in the situation of presumably becoming party to an abortion if s/he refuses, and of a 50 percent probability of abortion if s/he accedes to their demand. Although this situation may appear extreme to an outsider, it reflects the mind-set of some patients who desire this service. There was a strong consensus ($\geq$ 75 percent) against prenatal diagnosis for sex selection in ten nations: Australia, Denmark, the Federal Republic of Germany, France, the German Democratic Republic, Italy, Japan, Norway, Switzerland, and the United Kingdom. Only in the United States, Hungary, and India would a majority either perform prenatal diagnosis or refer to someone who would. They would apparently do so for different reasons, however. In the United States, 68 percent of those who would perform prenatal diagnosis or refer would do so out of respect for parental autonomy; in Hungary, all fifteen of those offering prenatal diagnosis would do so in order to prevent the otherwise certain abortion of a normal fetus. In India, 61 percent cited social considerations, such as the plight of unwanted girls, the position of women in society, or limiting the population. In another five countries substantial minorities would either perform prenatal diagnosis or refer: Canada (47 percent), Sweden (38 percent), Israel (33 percent), Brazil (30 percent), and Greece (29 percent).

In their reasoning, 30 percent of all respondents said that they opposed the abortion of a normal fetus or that the interests of the fetus should be weighed equally with those of living persons. Those who would actually perform prenatal diagnosis were more likely ($p < .0005$) to set down the consequences of their actions, whereas those who would refuse or refer did not give their rationale. Stated consequences related to the fetus or parents and not to society. Of the 605 persons who gave reasons for their action in this case, only 4.7 percent mentioned the position of women in society, 0.5 percent mentioned maintaining a balanced sex ratio, 0.6 percent limiting the population, and 4.9 percent setting a precedent that would harm the moral order.

The responses we obtained in the United States and Canada contrast markedly with earlier studies finding only 1 percent in a sample of 448 (Sorenson 1976) and 21 percent in a sample of 149 geneticists (Fraser and Pressor 1977) willing to perform prenatal diagnosis for sex selection. As chorionic villus sampling, which makes fetal sexing possible in the first trimester of pregnancy, becomes readily available, medical geneticists may become even more willing to comply with this still controversial request.

The societal impact and the possibility of an unbalanced sex ratio were not considerations for most. This may be shortsighted. Although most families in the United States and Canada desire a balance between boys and girls, there is often a preference that the firstborn be a boy (Warren 1987). If parents are able to act on this preference, the process of socialization into gender roles and the power balance between genders could be profoundly affected.

Women as Practitioners

We are concerned with women as practitioners as well as patients. Many geneticists are pediatricians, and a sizable percent of these are women. Of the 677 respondents, 65 percent were male, 35 percent female. Percentages by country are listed in table 1. Women were more likely than men to have a Ph.D. and less likely to have an M.D. Women had fewer years in the practice of genetics but more hours per week in genetics. Women in the sample were younger, less likely to be married, and had fewer children than men. They did not differ significantly in regard to specialty within genetics, board certification, professional memberships, number of patients per week, hours per week spent in special activities (e.g., laboratory work), religious background, number of religious observances attended per year, or political inclination.

The qualitative portions of the questionnaires enabled us to compare the reasons given by women and men and the "richness" of these responses, for example, the total number of reasons given for an action, whether the consequences of an action were considered, whose interests were considered most important, and the perception or nonperception of conflicts between the interests of different persons or between moral principles. The first two reasons given by a respondent were each assigned one of ninety-three codes, grouped under six major headings: (1) Autonomy of the person; (2) Nonmaleficence; (3) Beneficence; (4) Justice; (5) Strict (monetary) utilitarianism; and (6) All nonmoral answers.

These headings are based on widely accepted moral principles commonly discussed in medical ethics (Beauchamp and Childress 1979). Examples of answers falling under the heading of *Autonomy* are the patient's right to decide, right to know, or right not to know. Other examples are preserving patient confidentiality and the geneticist's obligation to tell the truth. Examples of reasons falling under the heading *Nonmaleficence* are: doing no harm; preventing harm to patient, fetus, child, future children; truth-telling as a source of harm; prevention of guilt or anxiety; preserving the family unit; and not setting a precedent that will harm the moral order (the "slippery slope" argument).

Beneficence means a positive inclination to do good, as opposed to the mere avoidance of harm. Statements relating to the common good, public health, improvement of life for future generations, of working conditions, or of social equality all fall under the heading *Beneficence*. So also do the "caring" relationships described by Gilligan as so influential in women's moral thinking. Examples of these are statements of responsibility to family or society, helping to remove guilt or anxiety, providing counseling, telling the truth in such a manner as to maximize good, and helping patients prepare for the future, including preparation for a child with a birth defect or for the stresses of abortion.

Justice involves balancing the rights of individuals against the welfare of society. Statements such as "they deserve this (medical) service," or "don't waste resources" fall under the heading of justice, as do statements about equal access, the right of all to affordable medical care, or "the interests of the fetus ought to be considered equally with those of living persons."

Strict monetary utilitarianism is based exclusively on monetary arguments about efficiency, economic costs versus economic benefits, or protection of the economic interests of institutional third parties. Fewer than 1 percent of respondents gave such arguments.

Nonmoral answers were those not referring to any moral principle, for example, "I disapprove of this," or "my institution forbids this."

According to Kohlberg's research on men, the "highest" stage of male moral reasoning would involve a combination of justice and autonomy (respect for persons). If current theories of gender and moral reasoning apply to persons with professional training across cultures, we might expect that men would refer more frequently to reasons involving justice or autonomy, and women would refer more frequently to reasons involving beneficence.

In addition to coding the first two reasons given for choices of action, we coded four additional aspects of respondents' moral reasoning. These were: (1) total number of reasons given; (2) whether the possible consequences of an action were stated; (3) whose welfare was considered most important when making the decision; and (4) whether a conflict of interest or of principles was perceived when making the decision.

Gender Differences in Responses

We compared gender differences in three regards: respondents' decisions on the ten cases; the moral principles (autonomy, nonmaleficence, beneficence, justice, etc.) underlying their reasoning; and the four additional aspects of moral reasoning described above (number of reasons, consequences, welfare, and perception of conflict). Because men and women differed on a number of characteristics, whenever a significant association ($p < .10$) was found between gender and a response, we controlled for the additional characteristics on which men and women differed.[1] The only results reported below are gender differences that remained after including these controls.

There were significant gender differences in choice of action for five of the ten cases (cases 3, 5, 6, 8, and 9), in moral values for two cases (cases 6 and 9), and in three of the four additional aspects of reasoning (consequences, welfare, or perception of conflict) for three cases (cases 1, 3, and 8). These differences are described in table 6. There were no differences in the numbers of reasons given. Interestingly, there were no cross-cultural gender differences in responses or reasoning with regard to two cases where we most expected them: use of prenatal diagnosis for the purpose of selecting the sex of the child, and disclosure to a woman with XY genotype. In the United States, however, women were twice as likely as men to say they would perform prenatal diagnosis for sex selection, on the basis of respect for patient autonomy.

The gender differences in table 6 fall into three types: (1) cases involving marital relationships; (2) directive/nondirective counseling; (3) a case testing professional response to a woman patient's autonomy (prenatal diagnosis for an anxious woman). The two cases in the study that most directly involved the marriage were case 1, false paternity, and case 3, disclosure of which parent carries a translocation. In case 1, false paternity, there were no differences in choice of action; almost all respondents chose to preserve the mother's confidentiality. Women, however, were more likely than men to mention conflicts between spouses; 75 percent of women and 57 percent of men mentioned marital conflicts. In case 3, women were more likely than men to disclose which parent carried the translocation without first asking the parents whether they wished to know; 63 percent of women and 46 percent of men would disclose the information, even if parents did not ask for it. Twenty-two percent of women and 13 percent of men would also disclose the information to relatives at risk for carrying the translocation. The welfare of the extended family, including relatives at risk and their potential offspring, was the primary consideration for 45 percent of women and 29 percent of men in this case; 57 percent of women and 41 percent of men mentioned the consequences of their actions.

In regard to counseling, men of all nationalities were more likely than women to consider it "appropriate" to give directive advice in counseling (such as telling patients what they ought to do or telling patients what the geneticist would do if in their situation) when asked to state their views on a checklist of approaches to counseling (not included in tables). Men were also more likely than women to give directive advice or purposely slanted information in case 5, fetuses with borderline disorders XO and XYY, and case 6, advice about aborting or carrying to term when prenatal diagnosis produces conflicting results. In both cases 5 and 6, the majority of both men and women (83 to 95 percent) would counsel nondirectively. Approximately twice as many men as women, however, would give directive advice. There

TABLE 6.   Gender Differences in Responses, in percentage (*n* = 677)[a]

Case Description		Women	Men
Cases Involving the Marriage			
Case 1: False paternity	Mention marital conflict	75%	57%
Case 3: Disclose which parent carries a translocation causing Down Syndrome in the child	Would disclose even if not asked	63	46
	Would also tell relatives at risk	22	13
	See welfare of extended family as most important	45	29
	Mention consequences	57	41
Cases Involving Nondirective Counseling			
Case 5: Nondirective counseling about fetuses with low-burden disorders			
XO (female fetus)	Would give advice	6	14
XYY (male fetus)	Would give advice	10	17
Case 6: Nondirective counseling about conflicting diagnostic findings for neural tube defect	Would give advice	5	13
	Dominant value:		
	Autonomy	91	82
Case 8: Surrogate motherhood as option for female carrier	Would discuss without being asked to do so	35	52
	Mention consequences	34	20
Case Involving Women's Autonomy			
Case 9: Prenatal diagnosis for an anxious woman, in the absence of medical indication	Would perform	76	61
	Dominant values:		
	Autonomy	39	31
	Justice	11	22

[a]All gender differences in this table remain significant after controlling for type of degree, years in genetics, hours per week in genetics, age, marital status, number of children, religiosity.

were gender differences in dominant values underlying the responses to case 6. Women were more likely than men to refer to patient autonomy.

In case 8, counseling of female carriers of tuberous sclerosis, women were less likely than men to describe surrogate motherhood as a possibility, unless the patient asked about it. Among geneticists, fewer women (35 percent) than men (52 percent) would nondirectively discuss surrogacy as a reproductive option without being asked. More women (40 percent) than men (24 percent) would discuss surrogacy if the patient specifically asked about it; but the total percentage who would discuss it at all is similar. Additionally, 34 percent of women and 20 percent of men mentioned the possible consequences of surrogacy. Most of the consequences described were negative, both for the marriage and for the surrogate. There were no gender differences in responses about IVF with donor egg as a reproductive option.

Of the ten cases, the one most directly exemplifying patient autonomy is case 9, prenatal diagnosis for an anxious woman. In case 9, women were more likely than men to perform prenatal diagnosis for maternal anxiety, without medical or age indications; 76 percent of women and 61 percent of men would perform prenatal diagnosis. An additional 6 percent of women and 10 percent of men would refer the patient elsewhere. Women's reasons for performing prenatal diagnosis were more likely than men's to indicate respect for the patient's autonomy ("she has a right to the service," or "she has a right to decide"). Men's reasons were more likely than women's to reflect the value of justice ("don't waste resources," "equal access to services"). Although women's emphasis on the autonomy of the woman patient appeared cross-nationally, it was most marked within the United States.

Table 6 suggests a pattern of gender differences that at least partially accords with Gilligan's hypothesis that women base their moral reasoning on a network of responsibilities. Women showed greater concern than men for the marriage and the welfare of the extended family. On the other hand, women also showed more concern than men for the rights of patients to make their own decisions after nondirective counseling and the rights of patients to request and receive prenatal diagnostic services, even if the geneticist personally disagrees. Prochoice arguments in the United States and other western nations have been framed around autonomy-based issues. The western social/political context of reproductive discussions is therefore somewhat at odds with the Gilligan predictions that women will frame their decisions in terms of responsibilities rather than individual rights.

Conclusion

We originally anticipated finding agreement across cultures in regard to disclosure of laboratory results and sensitive information. We further anticipated that there would be greater consensus both within and among the four nations where genetic technology originated and has undergone the greatest diffusion (the United Kingdom, the United States, Canada, and Denmark) than within or among nations where there is less diffusion of technology. Neither hypothesis was supported by the data. Although there was indeed a worldwide consensus in favor of not concealing laboratory results, there was less consensus than we expected in regard to full disclosure of colleague disagreements or nondirective counseling. Nations with greater technological diffusion displayed no greater consensus than others.

Some general patterns emerged, however. The two nations where the health system is under greatest government control (the German Democratic Republic and Hungary) also gave the most directive counseling. The United States, Canada, and United Kingdom, on the other hand, leaned most strongly toward nondirective counseling. The United States stood alone in willingness to present surrogate motherhood as an option and almost alone in willingness to provide prenatal diagnosis for sex selection. Geneticists in the United States referred more frequently than respondents elsewhere to unlimited patient autonomy (unlimited right to decide, right to referral, right to know or not to know). In their emphasis on autonomy, they usually overlooked concerns of justice (equal access to services, wise use of scarce resources) or the common good (maintaining a balanced sex ratio or setting a precedent that would harm the moral order). In some cases, women geneticists in the United States went further than men in valuing autonomy.

When asked to rank ten issues in order of priority, geneticists placed genetic screening in the workplace, long-range eugenic concerns, and sex selection at the bottom of the list. These are precisely the issues that are of greatest concern to the public. Future actions on these issues could change the entire structure of society by unbalancing the sex ratio or limiting access to work. If a proposed project to map the human genome within the next ten years is undertaken, the eugenic concerns now given low priority by geneticists could also come quickly to the forefront.

Societal problems tend to sneak up on medicine and catch physicians unaware. The outlook on ethical problems among medical geneticists reflects a general confidence about resolving moral conflicts at the individual-familial level and a lack of will to make a contribution at the societal-political level, especially in terms of questions that involve society's interests. One explanation for this situation is that many geneticists avoid any appearance of eugenic considerations and shy away from societal issues. The emergence of even more powerful scientific and diagnostic tools, such as DNA probes, will not allow medical geneticists any place to hide from the social implications of medical genetics. In our view, medical geneticists need to consolidate their best insights of the past so that they can be prepared to contribute to the development of improved and informed ethical guidance for the complex problems of the future. Women geneticists in particular need to be concerned about the potential effects of new technologies on women. They need to consider raising their consciousness as women as well as professionals.

NOTE

1. Because of the type of data (nominal level of measurement) in our analysis, we used a stepwise logistic regression model for our controls.

REFERENCES

Anders, G. J. P. A. 1984. Counseil génétique et diagnostic prénatal (Genetic counseling and prenatal diagnosis). In *La medicine face aux nouveaux pouvoirs* (Medicine faces new possibilities). Comptes rendus du 5eme Congres de la Federation Européenne des Associations Médicales Catholiques, 15–22.
Beauchamp, Thomas L., and James F. Childress. 1979. *Principles of biomedical ethics.* New York: Oxford University Press.
Berg, Kåre. 1983. Ethical problems arising from research progress in medical genetics. In *Research ethics,* ed. Kåre Berg and Knut Erik Tranøy, 261–75. New York: Alan R. Liss.
Bosk, Charles L. 1979. *Forgive and remember: Managing medical failure.* Chicago: University of Chicago Press.
Czeizel, Andrew. 1988. *The right to be born healthy: The ethical problems of human genetics in Hungary.* New York: Alan R. Liss.
Crawfurd, Martin d'A. 1983. Ethical and legal aspects of early prenatal diagnosis. *British Medical Bulletin* 39, no. 4: 310–14.
Fletcher, John C., Kåre Berg, and Knut Erik Tranøy. 1985. Ethical aspects of medical genetics. *Clinical Genetics* 27:199–205.
Fox, Renée C. 1957. Training for uncertainty. In *The student physician,* ed. Robert K. Merton, G. Reader, and P. Kendall. Cambridge: Harvard University Press.
Fraser, F. C. 1974. Genetic counseling. *American Journal of Human Genetics* 26:636–59.
Fraser, F. C., and C. Pressor. 1977. Attitudes of counselors in relation to prenatal sex determination for choice of sex. In: *Genetic counseling,* ed. H. A. Lubs and F. DelaCruz, 109–20. New York: Raven.

Gilligan, Carol. 1982. *In a different voice: Psychological theory and women's development*. Cambridge: Harvard University Press.

Kohlberg, Lawrence. 1981. *The philosophy of moral development*. San Francisco: Harper and Row.

Light, Donald. 1979. Uncertainty and control in professional training. *Journal of Health and Social Behavior* 20, no. 14: 310–22.

Schroeder-Kurth, Traute M. 1984. Die Bedeutung von Methoden, Risikoabwagung und Indikationsstellung fuer die praenatale Diagnostik (The importance of methods, risk calculation and setting of indications for prenatal diagnosis). In *Genetik und Moral,* ed. R. Thiele. Mainz: Gruenewald Verlag.

Sorenson, James Roger. 1976. From social movement to clinical medicine: The role of law and the medical profession in regulating applied human genetics. In *Genetics and the Law,* ed. Aubrey Milunsky and George J. Annas, Vol. 1. New York: Plenum.

Sorenson, James Roger, Judith P. Swazey, and Norman A. Scotch. 1981. *Reproductive pasts, reproductive futures: Genetic counselling and its effectiveness*. New York: Alan R. Liss.

Warren, Mary Anne. 1987. *Gendercide: The implications of sex selection*. Totowa, N.J.: Rowman and Allenheld.

Wertz, Dorothy C., and John C. Fletcher. 1989. *Ethics and human genetics: A cross-cultural perspective*. Heidelberg: Springer-Verlag.

Appendix: Selected Cases for Ethical Resolution

Label	Clinical Situation

Full Disclosure of Psychologically Sensitive Information (table 2)

Label	Clinical Situation
Case 1. False paternity	You are evaluating a child with an autosomal recessive disorder for which carrier testing is possible and accurate. In the process of testing relatives for genetic counseling, you discover that the mother and half the siblings are carriers, whereas the husband is not. The husband believes that he is the child's biological father.
Case 2. Parental translocation	You identify a parent of a Down Syndrome child as having a balanced translocation. Would you tell the couple which one is the carrier?
Case 3. Colleagues disagree about ambiguous test results	Laboratory analysis of amniotic fluid cells suggests that the fetus may be a trisomy 13 mosaic. There is disagreement among the medical geneticists responsible for the analysis as to whether or not the laboratory results are artifacts of culture, in other words, false positives. Given the present state of knowledge, there is no way of resolving this disagreement scientifically within the legal time limit for termination of pregnancy, because the results of repeat tests will not be available until after 24 weeks gestational age. You were not responsible for the laboratory work in this case and have not taken one side or the other. You are, however, the medical geneticist responsible for dealing directly with the prospective mother.

(Continued on next page)

Label	Clinical Situation
Case 4. XY female	A woman undergoes diagnosis for in-fertility. Tests reveal that she is chro-mosomally male (XY). Would you tell her that she is XY, or give her other reasons for her infertility?

Nondirective Counseling (table 3)

Case 5. Fetuses with low-burden disorders: XO (Turner syndrome) and XYY	Prenatal diagnosis has revealed an ab-normal fetus. The prospective parents came to see you in genetics clinic. Do you advise them to carry the preg-nancy to term, to have an abortion, or give optimistically or pessimistically slanted information, or do you pro-vide information and let them decide?
Case 6. Conflicting diagnostic findings for neural tube defect	Maternal serum alpha-fetoprotein has been elevated in your patient on two occasions, but level II ultrasound dis-closes no abnormality, despite careful examination of the fetal head, spine, abdomen, and kidneys. The fetal karyotype is normal. Amniotic alpha-fetoprotein is elevated and acetylcho-linesterase is borderline. These re-sults raise the possibility of a small neural tube defect. What do you tell the prospective mother?

Reproductive Options (table 4)

Case 7. For male carriers: vasec-tomy and artificial insemina-tion donor	Evaluation of a child produces find-ings consistent with a tuberous scle-rosis. Upon examining the parents, you find evidence that one carries the tuberous sclerosis gene, even though intelligence seems normal. After a discussion of the risk of having an-other child with tuberous sclerosis
Case 8. For female carriers: tubal ligation, IVF with donor egg, surrogate mother	

(Continued on next page)

Label	Clinical Situation
	who might be severely affected, the couple asks you whether recurrence of the disorder can be prevented. The options are taking their chances, contraception, sterilization, adoption, artificial insemination by a donor, IVF with a donated egg, and insemination of a surrogate mother with the husband's sperm.
Case 9. Maternal anxiety only	A 25-year-old woman with no family history of genetic disorders and no personal history of exposure to toxic substances requests prenatal diagnosis. There are no genetic or medical indications for its use. Nevertheless, she appears very anxious about the normality of the fetus, and persists in her demands for prenatal diagnosis even after being informed that in her case the potential medical risks for the fetus, in terms of miscarriage, may outweigh the likelihood of diagnosing an abnormality.
Case 10. Sex selection, in absence of X-linked disease	A couple requests prenatal diagnosis for purposes of selecting the sex of the child. They already have four girls and are desperate for a boy. They say that if the fetus is a girl, they will abort it and will keep trying until they conceive a boy. They also tell you that if you refuse to do prenatal diagnosis for sex selection, they will abort the fetus rather than run the risk of having another girl.

The Meaning of Risk, Choice, and Responsibility for a DES Daughter

Susan E. Bell

Diethylstilbestrol (DES), a synthetic estrogen, was first produced in 1938. Quite quickly it was prescribed for a wide variety of medical conditions associated with estrogen dysfunction, most notably menopausal symptoms and pregnancy complications (Bell 1986, 1987, 1989). From 1940 to 1971 it was commonly prescribed to women for complications of pregnancy. At first, DES was recommended for pregnant women who had diabetes or other diseases, or a history of repeated miscarriages; ultimately, however, it was recommended for pregnant women with no apparent problems (Apfel and Fisher 1984). The Food and Drug Administration (FDA) no longer approves DES for use during pregnancy; however, it still allows prescription of DES for treatment of menopausal problems, suppression of lactation, and advanced cases of breast cancer.

The FDA withdrew its approval of DES usage in pregnancy in response to studies linking it to a rare form of vaginal cancer in DES daughters (women prenatally exposed to DES). Research also indicates that DES daughters are more vulnerable than nonexposed women to other reproductive tract problems, including miscarriages, infertility, and cervical cancer. There is a slightly increased frequency of genital abnormalities in DES sons as well, including undescended testes, epididymal cysts, low sperm count, and decreased sperm mobility. DES mothers have an increased risk of breast cancer (Apfel and Fisher 1984). Today, members of the medical profession disagree about the dimension of risk associated with prenatal exposure and the appropriate way to treat DES-related problems. Hence, DES mothers, daughters, and sons are faced with living with long-term risk and medical uncertainty.

In this chapter, I consider how one DES daughter has understood and responded to risk and medical uncertainty as well as how she became politically active about the DES issue. I show that her political activity emerged over time in response to her sexual and reproductive experiences and her understanding of her physicians' explanations of the role of DES in these experiences. Before examining this woman's experience, I briefly review some of the research about the physical

and psychological effects of prenatal DES exposure and describe some
of the political activities taken by DES daughters in general.

Physical and Psychological Effects of DES
on DES Daughters

Some of the risks faced by DES daughters are known. For example,
up to 90 percent of DES daughters have adenosis, a condition in which
cells that are normally found in the cervix are found on the walls and
surfaces of the vagina. At this time no one knows how serious adenosis
is or what will come from the condition as time passes. Furthermore,
just over 500 women (two-thirds of them with documented DES exposure) have been diagnosed with vaginal clear-cell adenocarcinoma
(vaginal cancer). The risk of DES daughters developing clear-cell adenocarcinoma is estimated to be about 1/1000 through their mid-30s.
This is a surprisingly high rate considering that up until 1966 this kind
of cancer had almost never been reported in young women. Cancer
has been found in DES daughters between the ages of seven and thirty-
four; the median age at diagnosis is nineteen (Melnick et al. 1987).
Finally, in comparison to nonexposed women, DES daughters are more
likely to have difficulty conceiving and, once pregnant, to have a miscarriage, premature birth, stillbirth, or tubal pregnancy (Apfel and
Fisher 1984; Linn et al. 1988; Senekjian et al. 1988).

Regarding other risks for DES daughters, there is less certainty.
A recent review of the medical literature found a range of expert opinions about the long-term consequences of DES exposure. Some spec-
ulate that "what is currently known [is] 'the tip of the iceberg' " (Herbst
and Bern 1981, 1) and that DES daughters will be at higher risk of
cervical, breast, and uterine cancer as they reach midlife (Apfel and
Fisher 1984, 55). Others disagree that the risks for DES daughters will
extend beyond adenosis, infertility, and vaginal clear-cell adenocarcinoma. The lack of consensus within medicine means that DES daughters live with uncertainty about the dimensions of risk associated with
their prenatal exposure to this drug.

Another type of uncertainty involves medical protocols for screening and treating DES-related problems. These protocols have changed
since 1971, when DES-exposure was first linked to clear-cell adenocarcinoma. One example of this involves treatment of adenosis. Today,
experts recommend leaving it alone and observing it. In the early
1970s, however, they proposed a number of different approaches: partial removal of the vagina; cauterization of the vagina and cervix; cry-
osurgery (freezing); periodic removal of adenosis patches by punch

biopsies (Apfel and Fisher 1984, 94–96). DES daughters must find ways to respond to and cope with changing medical knowledge and the consequences of this changing knowledge for their interactions with the health care system. Ironically, DES daughters must return to medicine—the very source of their problems—for information and treatment.

The increased likelihood of suffering from reproductive tract problems, combined with the climate of uncertainty, may contribute to greater psychological distress for DES daughters. A number of studies indicate that these women may feel anxiety, grief, anger, or fear after learning that they have been exposed to the drug (Apfel and Fisher 1984; Schwartz and Stewart 1977). In addition, they have increased rates of major depression (Meyer-Bahlburg et al. 1985a) and "appear to be at risk for disorders of sexual desire, diminished sexual enjoyment, and (associated?) difficulties with sexual partners" (Meyer-Bahlburg et al. 1985b).

Women's Health Activism and DES

Adverse experiences with DES have stimulated women to become politically active. In 1978, women's health activists founded DES Action, a national organization, to provide information and support for people exposed to DES. As part of the women's health movement, DES Action is connected to a political effort to restructure health care: "to alter the quality, quantity, content, and control of obstetrical and gynecological services on the societal level, institutional level, and in face-to-face interaction with professionals" (Ruzek 1979, 143).

Members of DES Action argue that DES was not tested sufficiently before it was released for sale, nor did DES mothers give informed consent before they took it during pregnancy. Furthermore, the drug industry and medical profession supported its use in pregnancy even after controlled studies published in the 1950s showed that DES was ineffective in preventing miscarriage; they were also slow to take responsibility for locating, screening, and caring for people exposed to DES after the publication of a report in 1971 linking prenatal exposure to DES with vaginal clear-cell adenocarcinoma (see DES Action Voice, vols. 1–5 and issues 22–35).

According to DES Action, DES daughters were originally exposed to DES in part because of the organization of medical care, the unequal access to power and information available to physicians and patients, and the attitude of some medical professionals. These same conditions exist today and contribute to the difficulties experienced by individual DES daughters. Therefore, DES Action directs its efforts to changing the medical system. It collects and distributes information, testifies at public hearings, and attempts to change laws and regulations regarding medical services for the DES-exposed.

Developing a Perspective on DES

In this chapter I interpret an interview with one DES daughter to explore how she has understood and responded to the consequences of her DES exposure at different stages in her life and to show how her identity as a politically active woman has emerged during this process.[1] The interview is one of a series of interviews that I conducted with DES daughters to study the social and emotional effects of living with risk and medical uncertainty associated with prenatal DES exposure.

To demonstrate the making of a political woman, I interpret three stories that emerged during the course of an interview with a woman I shall call "Sarah."[2] I chose to examine this interview because it illustrates the dynamic and continuing relationship between medical technology and health experiences. In this case, as with many other DES daughters, the relationship became injurious; Sarah eventually responded by becoming politically active (for another example, see Bichler 1981). Through the three stories, Sarah ties together significant events and important relationships in her life. She makes sense of what has happened to her (Williams 1984). Sarah's stories show how she has come to understand and accept her status as a DES daughter, after first denying it, and the reasons for this change. They also show how she has come to accept herself as different from women not exposed to DES, as having something in common with DES daughters, and how she became a politically active DES daughter.

Elsewhere (Bell 1988) I introduce story analysis as an approach to understanding interview material and then analyze Sarah's stories. I demonstrate the link between story structure, content, and sequence. Here, I summarize the results of that analysis.

I use the concept of "voices" to identify the transformation in Sarah's understanding of her experiences and her emerging political self. Following Mishler (1984), I identify two voices in Sarah's stories: the voice of medicine and the voice of the lifeworld. Each voice represents "a specific normative order, a particular assumption about the relationship between appearance, reality, and language" (Mishler 1984, 63). Each represents one way of knowing about health, illness, and disease. The voice of medicine seeks to understand and explain events within the framework of the biomedical model (Mishler 1981). According to this voice, health and disease are universal to the human species. Each disease has a specific etiology and can be diagnosed in individuals on the basis of objective signs and symptoms. Individual life experiences that do not relate specifically to the disease are superfluous to the voice of medicine. It frames problems in the language of medical experts and increases their mystification, thereby decreasing the ability of lay people to understand these problems. The effect of this voice is to "strip away" the social context of health and disease as well as to ignore patients' experience and self-understanding of their own problems (see Mishler 1984, 120).

The voice of the lifeworld represents the understanding of health and disease within a social context (Mishler 1986, 143). According to this voice, events become connected and meaningful depending on a person's "biographical situation and position in the social world" (Mishler 1984, 104). The self is the center of the lifeworld. Mishler argues that even though the voice of medicine is the usual explanatory framework, health, illness, and disease can become truly meaningful to people only after they have been contextualized. Thus, the two voices constantly struggle: both in medical interviews, when doctors and patients attempt to understand each other; and outside of the medical world, when people try to make sense of their problems.

As we shall see, in the first two stories that Sarah tells, the voice of medicine predominates. In the third story, she speaks in the voice of the lifeworld. This shift in voice reflects and helps Sarah to explain her politicization.

Analysis

Sarah is a middle-class white woman in her early 30s. She is married, has a two-year-old son, and is employed part-time in a professional capacity in the service sector. Her husband is employed by one of the Fortune 500 companies. They live in a suburb of a large city in the northeastern United States. When we first met, Sarah offered to talk with me about her experiences; I called her a few weeks later and went to her home to interview her. The interview lasted about one and a half hours and was tape-recorded. The interview covered a period of about twelve years in Sarah's life, beginning with the time she first found out she was a DES daughter.

Story 1: it sort of f'flitted in and out

Beginning in the first story, Sarah conveys the importance of understanding the meaning of DES exposure for her by repeating key words and phrases about knowing, learning, understanding, remembering, and thinking. For the most part, she uses negatives to describe her understanding of DES at this time of her life; DES had little meaning for her. She explains that because she "*didn't* have anything, that [she] understood was wrong with [her]" she "sort of, *denied*, almost everything about it" (emphasis added).[3]

> when I was around, 19,
> I was in college
> and I went, to a, gynecologist to get birth control
> he was, he knew that I was a DES daughter because I had
> adenosis (p) um,
> so he, told y'know he told me (p)
> I think shortly after that,
> [my mother] told me,
> um and I either said "I know already" or,
> and I was so concerned at the time about getting birth
> control,
> that I think it sort of didn't, um,
> it never really, became the major part of my life
> it sort of f'flitted in and out (p)

To describe her gynecologist's logic, Sarah uses the voice of medicine. He knew she was a DES daughter because she had adenosis. He saw the cells, identified them, and interpreted them by referring to an abstract body of knowledge. Adenosis is a common condition in DES daughters; it is uncommon in nonexposed women and therefore it is an indication of DES exposure. Her mother, too, told Sarah of her exposure to DES; this assertion is supported by her experience of taking DES when she was pregnant with Sarah. Her mother spoke in the voice of the lifeworld. She remembered taking DES because she remembered being pregnant with Sarah.

Sarah dismissed both voices: her gynecologist's and her mother's. She explains her lack of attention to the voices and her lack of concern about DES by placing these responses in the context of her life at that time: she was a nineteen-year-old college student, interested in becoming sexually active, using birth control, and growing up. In comparison to these concerns, the possibility that her reproductive and sexual organs might be damaged was unimportant. The idea merely "f'flitted in and out."

Story 2: um(p) and that's when I(p) um began to
accept the fact(p)

Sarah became actively concerned about DES ten years later after she had a miscarriage. During her first pregnancy she went into labor at five and one-half months and delivered a baby who lived only eight hours. At this point, Sarah was no longer an adolescent, exploring her sexuality. She was a married woman who had just lost a baby. In this context, she began to take her exposure to DES seriously. In order to protect future pregnancies, she would need to understand how her reproductive organs were different from those of women not exposed to DES, and how these differences could lead her body to function improperly.

Sarah begins the second story about 15 minutes later in the interview, reintroducing the theme of knowing with the phrase "t'the forefront of my mind":

> I then had some problems around, pregnancy,
> that sort of brought the whole issue of DES (p) t'much
> more t'the forefront of my mind
> and has made me much more, actively concerned about it,
> but, ah I, my first pregnancy, um, I had problems, due to
> DES
> I got pregnant
> and in the, middle of the night one night
> my, membranes broke,
> and (p) y'know [my husband] r'rushed me to the hospital
> and I delivered a baby girl,
> who lived about eight hours
> but she died
> and even then, when the, resident the (p) doctor who was
> taking care of me
> um said, in the aftermath that maybe she thought it was due
> to DES,
> um, I didn't believe her (p)

In the aftermath of losing the baby, Sarah couldn't understand why it had happened. She didn't believe her physician's explanation because, as she says: "y'didn't I still didn't understand the mechanism of how all this happens . . . and I hadn't educated myself as to . . . what was actually going on." Her doctor (this time a woman) could not make a convincing case for the link between DES and the miscarriage: "she was sort of going through a whole list of things that she thought it might be . . . and that was sort of one out of." Sarah's physician could not yet adequately account for Sarah's miscarriage in the voice of medicine; she did not yet know the specific etiology of this event.

Right after Sarah lost the baby, her mother also linked DES and the miscarriage, using the voice of the lifeworld, but Sarah rejected this account too:

> I can remember when my mother said "Maybe this is due to the
> DES"
> I said, "Now don't be ridiculous,"
> um because I did
> I mean she was feeling awful
> She was really d-
> I mean we were all distraught
> but y'know, to have her think that she had something to do
> with my losing the baby
> was more than I could tolerate,

In the aftermath, neither her doctor nor her mother could convince Sarah that her miscarriage was due to DES because she could not understand, believe, or tolerate it so soon after she lost the baby. Neither voice could penetrate Sarah's anguish; neither made sense to her.

A few weeks later, she accepted the connection. Sarah attributes her new understanding to the power of the voice of medicine. The doctor used the scientific method. She had gathered more data, sorted through them, and ordered them into a coherent whole. Sarah says:

> um she re- she had really done a lot of research
> and sort of, presented me with a whole, scheme of how this
> could have happened
> and why she thought it was related to the DES
> then it was clear that it probably was,
> um (p) and that's when I (p) um began to accept the fact (p)
> y'know once it made sense,

Sarah understood and accepted the explanation because it was presented in the logic and language of science:

> um, that I had an incompetent cervix[4]
> and that, the incident of that is (some ?) the incidence of
> that is so much more higher in, DES daughters
> um, because all the facts of the, miscarriage, fit with
> incompetent cervix

The connection between DES and the miscarriage was Sarah's "incompetent cervix." The physician linked them for Sarah using the voice of medicine: DES causes women to have incompetent cervices and women who have them are more likely than other women to have miscarriages. Sarah had an incompetent cervix; therefore she had had a miscarriage. Sarah's response to this proposition was acceptance because "it made sense."

However, a closer reading of the story indicates that Sarah's transformation from not knowing to knowing and accepting the serious consequences of exposure to DES hinged on her ability both to understand rationally what had happened, and why, and to experience a pregnancy and miscarriage. Sarah's use of the word *sense* eloquently ties the two voices together, for *sense* has two meanings. It refers to something that can be grasped, comprehended, and known, as well as to the ability to receive mental impressions through the actions of a body's sense organs (sight, taste, smell, pain, etc.) or through changes in the condition of the body (*Webster's Third New International Dictionary*). Logic and reason were not sufficiently powerful to induce a change in Sarah's attitude, nor was experience alone. Sarah could accept her identity as a DES daughter because she had had "some problems around pregnancy" (a miscarriage), and because subsequently her doctor presented her with a logical explanation of this. Not until Sarah lost a baby, a loss for which she had been entirely unprepared, could she accept the possibility of risks associated with DES, regardless of how these risks were explained to her.

With her acceptance, Sarah began to take her identity as a DES daughter seriously. She accepted responsibility for her miscarriage. This is evident in her use of the voice of medicine to explain her circumstances ("I had an incompetent cervix"). Even though the term "incompetent cervix" is a standard medical term, the adjective "incompetent" has "negative and judgmental connotations" (Fox 1983, 462).[5] It blames the victim for the problem.

As long as Sarah framed her understanding in the language and logic of medicine, she could neither locate the cause of her miscarriage outside herself nor begin to draw a connection between her condition and that of other DES daughters. She remained isolated—blaming her body for the miscarriage and identifying it as incompetent. Instead of recognizing her similarity to DES daughters, she recognized her difference from other (normal and competent) women.

Story 3: I no longer can be, blithe about it, and
say "not me"

In the third story, Sarah shows how, over time, she has been able to incorporate the doctors' findings into her lifeworld. She integrates them by giving them meaning grounded in her experience and by drawing causal connections beyond the technical explanations provided by her physicians. She accounts for her miscarriage as follows: Medicine had prescribed DES to her mother. Thus medicine was responsible for Sarah's exposure to DES. Furthermore, medicine had caused her miscarriage by exposing her to DES and then failing to warn her of reproductive risks associated with this exposure.

Sarah's active concern about DES led her to contact DES Action:

> (p) heard an ad on tv or the radio (p)
> and I think I it if they had the tape number
> and I called up
> and asked for information
> and they sent me their little packet
> and I, joined
> and then a while later
> they sent me a card,
> um that they were having a coffee one of the the one of
> those like the one that you went to,
> um and I couldn't go to that
> um, but then I sort of felt like I had made an obligation to
> meet these people
> and, so I went ahead and met them you know
> and liked them
> and thought I it was someing [sic] something that I wanted
> to be more involved in
> (p) and have stayed that way

Her request for information was consistent with a central goal of DES Action: to let DES daughters know about the need for medical screening and follow-up care, to refer them to physicians familiar with DES-related problems, and to provide them with reviews of medical and scientific studies about DES. In turn, Sarah accepted DES Action's request that she join the organization. She thereby acknowledged that she had something in common with other DES daughters. They, like she, faced the risk of reproductive difficulties and cancer because of the physiological effects of DES.

At first, however, Sarah was not ready to acknowledge that her concerns were similar to those of DES Action. Although she was invited to become active, to go to a meeting, and to share her experiences with others, she felt she couldn't. She was not yet ready to talk about what had happened to her. Until she could talk about her experiences, she could not understand "the politics of the DES experience" (*Coalition News,* August 1978, 3), or become an active member of DES

Action. Sarah was not yet ready to join others protesting the abuses of medicine.

Nonetheless, Sarah felt an "obligation to meet these people" and so she did, found she liked them, and became more involved. She joined the women's health movement. For Sarah, this meant understanding and accepting the iatrogenic role of medicine in her life. By becoming an active member of an organization in the women's health movement, Sarah joined others to educate patients and doctors, to transform power relations between them, and to change the medical system more generally.

In the third story, Sarah criticizes the actions, logic, and power of medicine. In other words, she criticizes the voice of medicine. First, she criticizes her doctors' actions during her pregnancy and begins to shift the blame for her miscarriage:

> , well, the more I had ti- the more removed I got
> from what had happened to me
> and the longer it, the more that time went by then, the
> angrier I got about, some of the things that happened to me,
> um, and the, I really felt like (p)
> the fact that I that' that I shouldn't have lost that first
> baby
> and that something different should have been done (p)

She is now able to use her anger and her intuition ("I really felt") to reinterpret the cause of her miscarriage.

There is some ambiguity in this section of the third story. The phrase, "I shouldn't have lost that first baby," could refer to Sarah's own sense of responsibility for the loss. She had been "blithe," had "actively put [DES] out of [her] mind" and had not "educated" herself. Yet, in the larger context of the story, her admonition could also refer both to the first error, when DES was prescribed to her mother, and to the second, when her doctor should have known that she was at a greater risk of having a miscarriage and protected her. Medicine should have been more aware of the consequences of DES exposure, then and now: "something different should have been done."

Next, Sarah criticizes the logic of medicine:

> you know and and the the little things along the way
> like not being, like being advised, to take the pill (p)
> that it most likely wouldn't hurt me (p)
> you know it's not clear whether it wouldn' or it wouldn't
> but prudence would say, use some other method of birth

control (p)

There has been considerable controversy within medicine over the most appropriate method of contraception for DES daughters. There are, as yet, "no data [to] indicate that any contraceptive method carries a risk of ill effects among DES-exposed women greater than the risk in the unexposed population" (Noller, Townsend, and Kaufman 1981, 95). According to the logic of science, it is appropriate to prescribe birth control pills to DES daughters. Sarah's physician had correctly applied a body of knowledge to Sarah's individual case when he had prescribed birth control pills to her. Nevertheless, the DES Task Force recommends that use of birth control pills "must be viewed in a prudent fashion, and the decision to use them made only after careful consideration of alternate methods, patient preference, and medical judgment" (U.S. Department of Health, Education and Welfare 1978, 16). After educating herself, Sarah had learned that her physician's advice, "to take the pill . . . that it most likely wouldn't hurt [her]," while not wrong, omitted a step. He had been imprudent; he had not, apparently, explored the use of other methods of birth control. He had not given her all the information so that she could reasonably decide for herself.

Sarah's use of the word *prudence* implies that she has become familiar with the literature on DES (Dutton 1984) and signals a shift in voice. She uses the voice of the lifeworld (*prudence*) and criticizes her physician for adhering to the voice of medicine (if there is no statistical evidence that birth control pills are harmful, it is safe to prescribe them). Sarah is critical of her physician's advice and the way he came to his recommendation (see Apfel and Fisher 1984).

Finally, Sarah criticizes the power of medicine. According to her, medicine does not inform or educate women about risks associated with DES. In fact, it encourages them to be "blithe" about the risks and thus to be passive and dependent.[6] "DES women are patronized, to some extent, . . . by their medical care." They "shouldn't be." In this respect the voice of medicine mystifies problems, decreases women's ability to understand them, and thereby strengthens its power over women.

Sarah's alternatives to these three problems involve, first, education. She would "help, obstetricians, be more aware," so that they wouldn't, out of ignorance, prescribe dangerous medications or fail to use precautions for DES women.[7] She would inform other women of specific problems associated with DES exposure, because "there are women out there who don't know . . . that this is a problem." She

would educate herself, because she is "more interested in being educated about [DES]." Despite the lack of scientific evidence about problems for DES daughters later in life, she is worried:

> oh w'well I'I'm fairly convinced at this point
> that we'll have problems, a'at each, age period
> you know if not a m'm', middle age then through menopause
> then some, something else some problems will occur along the
> way (p)

In sum, women and their doctors should be educated about medical
knowledge and the limits of this knowledge, so that they can act reasonably and prudently, now and in the future.

Beyond education, however, changing the power relationships between doctors and patients is another alternative both in the present
and future. Through collective action, Sarah wants to "help DES
daughters be more assertive and get better medical care (p) right away,"
and to help herself stay "on top of what the next step might be." As
a member of DES Action, Sarah advocates change in physicians' and
patients' ways of thinking, acting, and relating to each other.

Sarah ends the third story by looking ahead to the future, by acknowledging the uncertainty and risk that lie ahead. Unlike some physicians who do not take into account the possibility of long-term
consequences (Herbst and Bern 1981), Sarah can no longer "blithely"
think "that since [she] was past the age where most people get [DES-
related] cancer that there was nothing more (p) for [her] to think about."

For Sarah, being a DES daughter has come to mean accepting risk
and uncertainty for the rest of her life. The uncertainty is not hers
alone; she recognizes that it is shared by other "DES women" and the
medical profession. The third story, thus, moves beyond the view of
doctors as sole experts and embraces a new vision: to seek and to
share the wisdom of the lifeworld alongside the expertise and uncertainty of medicine. To accomplish this both depends upon and neces-
sitates becoming political. For only in and through the women's health
movement can the structural changes implied by Sarah's view be put
into practice.

Beyond Sarah's Experiences

I have focused on the experiences of one DES daughter because her
experiences have implications for our understanding of the relationship
between women and medical technologies more generally. In our cur-

rent medical care system, technologies play a dominant role. However, the long-term consequences of these technologies are uncertain (Bell 1989). As Dutton (1987, 54) observes, "no amount of advance testing" can reveal all possible effects of medical technologies, because some are too rare and others may be delayed or cumulative. This pattern of uncertainty means that patients and doctors must make decisions about immediate treatments in light of the possibility of exposing themselves (and their offspring) to unknown future risks. The relationship between women and technologies is dynamic, even for specific technologies, such as DES, and in individual cases, such as Sarah's.

Aside from uncertainty about long-term consequences, there is uncertainty regarding responses to these consequences, once they appear. Changing protocols for the diagnosis and treatment of iatrogenic diseases and disorders, such as DES-related adenosis, illustrate the limits of medical knowledge. These protocols also demonstrate the extent to which both doctors and patients make choices that are limited and constrained by particular social and historical contexts.

As we have learned through the example of DES, specifically through Sarah's experiences, the voice of medicine cannot adequately respond to these uncertainties. This voice depends on physicians' ability to generalize and to diagnose and treat problems without reference to individual experiences. The uncertainty inherent in medical technologies requires that risks and benefits be evaluated on an individual basis, through the voice of the lifeworld. Thus, patients' biographies and positions in the social world are crucial factors in decision making.

Taken together, Sarah's stories show how the voice of medicine and the voice of the lifeworld can be balanced. While patients may come to a variety of resolutions, Sarah's stories show how an integrated understanding can lead to empowerment and political action. Feminist oriented self-help groups, such as DES Action, can lessen dependence on medical expertise, foster a sense of control, and create a collective way of responding to uncertainty.

NOTES

This chapter summarizes the argument developed fully in "Becoming a Political Woman: The Reconstruction and Interpretation of Experience Through Stories," which appears in Alexandra Dundas Todd and Sue Fisher, eds., *Gender and Discourse: The Power of Talk* (Ablex, 1988). Research for this chapter was made possible by a postdoctoral fellowship from the National Institute of Mental Health (5 T32 MH 1426-08) and a grant from the faculty research fund,

Bowdoin College. Thanks are due to Kim Yanoshik for her editorial comments and suggestions.

1. For a comprehensive discussion of story analysis, see Bell, 1988.
2. My use of the word "stories" is not meant to imply that this account is fictional, nor that I disbelieve the respondent. Instead, I use this word to emphasize the structural features of these sections of the interview. For more on the aspect of the account, see Bell, 1988.
3. The transcripts preserve many features of the participants' manner of speaking but are not fully equivalent to speech (see Mishler 1984). False starts, hesitations, and repetitions are retained in the text. Silences shorter than one second are indicated by a comma, ",". Longer silences are marked by "(p)". Nonlexical utterances, the interviewer's talk, and the length of silences are omitted here. Copies of the complete transcripts of the three stories are available from the author upon request.
4. An *incompetent cervix* is a medical term that *Dorland's Illustrated Medical Dictionary* defines as a cervix that "is abnormally prone to dilate in the second trimester of pregnancy, resulting in premature expulsion of the fetus (middle trimester abortion)."
5. I am indebted to Catherine Kohler Riessman for this reference.
6. See Danziger, 1986, for a discussion of different types of doctor-patient encounters during pregnancy.
7. By being aware during the second pregnancy, her obstetrician prevented the loss of the second baby. This physician had taken a number of precautions because of Sarah's DES exposure and her "incompetent cervix." In addition, Sarah had educated herself and found a physician who was an expert in caring for DES daughters during their pregnancies.

REFERENCES

Apfel, Roberta J., and Susan M. Fisher. 1984. *To do no harm: DES and the dilemmas of modern medicine.* New Haven: Yale University Press.
Bell, Susan E. 1986. A new model of medical technology development: A case study of DES. In *Research in the sociology of health care.* Volume 4, ed. J. Roth and S. Ruzek, 1–32. Greenwich, Conn.: JAI.
———. 1987. Changing ideas: The medicalization of menopause. *Social Science and Medicine* 24:535–42.
———. 1988. Becoming a political woman: The reconstruction and interpretation of experience through stories. In *Gender and discourse: The power of talk,* ed. A. D. Todd and S. Fisher, 97–123. Norwood, N.J.: Ablex.
———. 1989. Technology in medicine: Development, diffusion, and health policy. In *Handbook of medical sociology.* Fourth edition, ed. H. E. Freeman and S. Levine, 185–204. New York: Prentice-Hall.
Bichler, Joyce. 1981. *DES daughter.* New York: Avon.
Coalition for the Medical Rights of Women. 1978. *Coalition News,* August.

_____. *The rock will wear away*. 1980. San Francisco: Coalition for the Medical Rights of Women.

Danziger, Sandra Klein. 1986. The uses of expertise in doctor-patient encounters during pregnancy. In *The sociology of health and illness*, ed. P. Conrad and R. Kern, New York: St. Martin's.

DES Action Voice. 1979–88. San Francisco: DES Action National.

Dutton, Diana. 1984. The impact of public participation in biomedical policy: Evidence from four case studies. In *Citizen participation in science policy*, ed. J. C. Petersen, 147–81. Amherst: University of Massachusetts.

_____. 1987. Medical risks, disclosure, and liability: Slouching toward informed consent. *Science, Technology, and Human Values* 12:148–59.

Fox, Howard A. 1983. The incompetent cervix: Words that can hurt. *American Journal of Obstetrics and Gynecology* 147:462–63.

Herbst, Arthur L., and Howard A. Bern, eds. 1981. *Developmental effects of diethylstilbestrol (DES) in pregnancy*. New York: Thieme-Stratton.

Linn, Shai, Ellice Lieberman, Stephen C. Schoenbaum, Richard R. Monson, Phillip C. Stubblefield, and Kenneth J. Ryan. 1988. Adverse outcomes of pregnancy in women exposed to diethylstilbestrol in utero. *Journal of Reproductive Medicine* 33:3–7.

Melnick, Sandra, Philip Cole, Diane Anderson, and Arthur H. Herbst. 1987. Rates and risks of diethylstilbestrol-related clear-cell adenocarcinoma of the vagina and cervix: An update. *New England Journal of Medicine* 316:514–16.

Meyer-Bahlburg, Heino F. L., and Anke A. Ehrhardt. 1985. A prenatal-hormone hypothesis for depression in adults with a history of fetal DES exposure. In *Hormones and depression*, ed. U. Halbreich and D. M. Rose, New York: Raven Press.

Meyer-Bahlburg, Heino F. L., Anke A. Ehrhardt, Jean Endicott, Norma P. Veridiano, E. Douglas Whitehead, and Felix H. Vann. 1985. Depression in adults with a history of prenatal DES exposure. *Psychopharmacology Bulletin* 21:686–89.

Meyer-Bahlburg, Heino F. L., Anke A. Ehrhardt, Judith F. Feldman, Laura R. Rosen, Norma P. Veridiano, and Ilse Zimmerman. 1985. Sexual activity level and sexual functioning in women prenatally exposed to diethylstilbestrol. *Psychosomatic Medicine* 47:497–511.

Mishler, Elliot G. 1981. Viewpoint: Critical perspectives on the biomedical model. In *Social contexts of health, illness, and patient care*, ed. E. G. Mishler, L. R. AmaraSingham, S. T. Hauser, R. Liem, S. D. Osherson, N. E. Waxler, 1–23. New York: Cambridge University Press.

_____. 1984. *The discourse of medicine: Dialectics of medical interviews*. Norwood, N.J.: Ablex.

_____. 1986. *Research interviewing: Context and narrative*. Cambridge: Harvard University Press.

Noller, Kenneth L., Duane Townsend, and Raymond H. Kaufman. 1981. Genital findings, colposcopic evaluation, and current management of the diethylstilbestrol-exposed female. In *Developmental effects of diethylstilbestrol (DES) in pregnancy*, 81–102. *See* Herbst and Bern 1981.

Ruzek, Sheryl Burt. 1979. *The women's health movement.* New York: Praeger.

Schwartz, Ruth W., and Nancy B. Stewart. 1977. Psychological effects of DES exposure. *Journal of the American Medical Association* 237:252–54.

Senekjian, Elizabeth K., Ronald K. Potkul, Keith Frey, and Arthur L. Herbst. 1988. Infertility among daughters either exposed or not exposed to diethylstilbestrol. *American Journal of Obstetrics and Gynecology* 158:493–98.

U. S. Department of Health, Education and Welfare. 1978. *DES task force summary report.* DHEW Publication No. (NIH) 79-1688.

Vessey, M. P., D. V. I. Fairweather, Beatrice Norman-Smith, and J. Buckley. 1983. A randomized double-blind controlled trial of the value of stilboestrol therapy in pregnancy: Long-term follow-up of mothers and their offspring. *British Journal of Obstetrics and Gynecology* 90:1,007–17.

Williams, Gareth. 1984. The genesis of chronic illness: Narrative re-construction. *Sociology of Health and Illness* 6:175–200.

Hospitals and Hospices: Feminist Decisions about Care for the Dying

Alice Lind

> Women and humane values can no longer be devalued, trivialized, marginalized and/or privatized. A feminist synthesis which affirms "feminine" strengths and what positive "masculine" values that do exist must challenge and transcend the masculinist social order. Then and only then can the power of love in the sense of caring about ourselves and others begin and continue to exceed the love of power over others. (Heide 1985, 146).

Caring has not been traditionally recognized as a principle for making health care decisions. Instead we in the health care professions have relied on the notions of justice, avoiding harm, and autonomy when we respond to moral dilemmas. Underlying the notion of autonomy, or self-determination, has been the concept of respect for persons. But respect and caring are very different. Respect allows us to stand apart from our clients, observing the differences between us. Caring requires that we observe the similarities, in our attempt to "apprehend the reality of the other" (Noddings in Grimshaw 1986, 216).

The importance of maintaining caring relationships has traditionally been ignored in today's medical system in favor of "the relative overvaluing of procedures and techniques" (Heide 1985, 35). The loss of caring in health care has resulted in decisions about people that are not rooted in humane values. Nowhere has this been more apparent than in the care provided for dying persons.

A basically paternalistic assumption guides the practice of most health care providers in acute care settings, which is that the health care provider has the authority to control and direct the type of activity that will take place. If a client presents a hospital's emergency department with a life-threatening condition, it is assumed that person must desire all the modern medicine available to sustain his or her life. If a patient in a coronary care unit develops a life-threatening arrythmia, shock will be applied to restore the heart's normal rhythm. When an ambulance is called for a person whose breathing has stopped, the emergency medical technician will insert a breathing tube and begin artificial resuscitation.

This assumption, however, is not necessarily shared by the clients who request services from the health care system. People who enter hospitals may simply be looking for an end to their chest pain, an easing of their shortness of breath, or respite for the family members who have been providing around-the-clock care. But with medical technology's rapid advances, and increased regulation on the appropriate use of medical facilities, hospitals are intent on cure rather than comfort.

Ethical decisions about how and where to die take place in this setting, in spite of the divergent assumptions held by health care practitioners and their clients. The President's Commission for the Study of Ethical Problems in Medicine identified the "technological approach to medical care" as "perhaps the single most significant factor" in changing the nature of decision making (President's Commission 1982, 33).

The hospice movement arose out of a need for more humane care for dying persons. Prior to the 1950s, more deaths occurred at home than in hospitals. There typically came a time in a person's illness when the physician had no further curative treatment to offer, and at that point, he would counsel the family to keep the patient comfortable and when appropriate to call the priest. In the previous century, families could obtain narcotics without a prescription, and female family members were accustomed to providing care for dying patients at home. Institutional care was necessary only when a patient had no family support or was impoverished (President's Commission 1983, 17).

As medical advances took place in this century, it became more and more difficult for a physician to recognize the end and cease treatment on a dying patient. Care became increasingly institutionalized, until in the 1980s, only 13 percent of patients die at home (Greer 1985, 7). In many cases, patients die in hospitals contrary to their own wishes. Certainly some patients want every possible therapy in an attempt to cure illness or sustain life, but others do not. Furthermore, some patients are never consulted about their wishes for treatment. The failure to include patients in these decisions can result in tragically unwanted therapy, and solitary deaths in foreign environments. For the predominantly female caregivers, such conflicts produce moral dilemmas at an astounding rate.

The hospice movement arose out of a need to regain control over a normal life event from physicians and institutions. Its philosophy, promulgated by the pioneering Cicely Saunders, was that death could be a comfortable, dignified experience. Hospice care stressed the palliation of symptoms as well as the inclusion of the family in the plan of care.

Hospice was developed to serve as an alternative to modern technological medicine, yet current practitioners of hospice care find some uses of technology philosophically acceptable. What values distinguish hospice from traditional medicine, and how is technology used in these settings? The answer lies in the principle of caring in decision making. This chapter explores my nursing experiences in both worlds, and discusses the moral constructs that guide my practice.

Many people assume that work in an intensive care unit (ICU) is stressful, and that work with dying patients is depressing. Because I have sought out such work, I am often asked why I chose those particular fields. I will offer an account of my personal reflections about my work, rather than an objective recitation of quality of life statistics, or a review of the current literature.

As a senior nursing student, I worked as a nurses' aide in a large city hospital and spent most of my time in the intensive care units. My favorite unit quickly became the one with the most critical patients, those who had had open heart surgery or some major trauma. I liked the busyness of it, the importance of the work the nurses did and the authority they conveyed. When I graduated, I was offered a job in that unit.

Many nursing educators and administrators are aware of the "reality shock" that happens when the idealistic nursing student joins the very real work setting of a hospital. Having studied philosophy along with the nursing curriculum, I was probably even more idealistic than most. In a paper for a course in Phenomenology and Existentialism, I wrote about the nurse's role as therapist in determining "the meaning of the illness for the patient and family." The initial assessment of a patient, I said, should include social, spiritual, intellectual, and emotional factors. The values I held as a nursing student imbued this paper with optimism; the goal of wholeness and independence for both the patient and the nurse was a central theme. As I started working, I quickly learned which of my ideals would be valued and which were extraneous.

For example, in my first few months of work, I cared for a patient who was unconscious and dying. I had been taught that unconscious patients may be aware of their surroundings and what is said in their presence; I also felt it was important not to let people die completely alone. Since we only allowed visitors into the intensive care unit three times a day for fifteen minutes, I provided extra contact time by sitting in my patient's room, holding her hand, and talking to her. The other nurses thought my actions peculiar; the nurse's aide asked me what in the world I was doing; the charge nurse decided that because I was not busy, I should take care of another patient as well. They were much more comfortable if I sat at the nurses' station, watching patients from a distance. After several months, I began distancing myself from patients as they did: by physically removing myself, joking about the patients, or talking over them as we performed tasks.

The physical layout of the unit was a disorienting one. Three of the rooms were enclosed in glass, making the patient feel like a fish in a bowl. The other six beds were separated only by curtains, which were controlled by the nurses. Most often, they were pulled far enough to protect patients from viewing each other, but were open at the foot of the bed so that the nurses could watch, hawklike, from the desk.

When a patient died in that unit, the curtains were pulled securely around the other beds while the nurses placed the body on a stretcher, covered it with a frame and a drape, and pushed it discretely out of the unit. We showed little feeling about the patients who died, and if the relatives required much time consoling, we called the chaplain.

The ethical dilemma that arose most frequently during my first year of nursing was in defining death. Until 1979, Texas, where I was in practice, did not have a "brain death statute." In other words, even if patients had irreversible and complete loss of brain function, they would not be declared dead if their respiratory and cardiac functions were being maintained mechanically (Robertson 1983, 116). It was frequently left up to the families, then, to decide when or if to "pull the plug." It was a very difficult decision, as data were not available to determine when a patient was beyond hope of improvement, and frequent stories of supposedly "brain-dead" patients waking up from their comas suggested hope.

Technology began to lose its rosy glow as I saw more patients being kept alive on machines when it was apparent to me that they were dying. One motorcycle accident victim came into the hospital, was resuscitated in the emergency room, and entered the ICU on a ventilator. He had no evidence of brain activity beyond the minimum required to keep his heart beating. After taking care of him in the unit for several weeks, we realized he would never regain consciousness: brain tissue leaked onto his dressings. Yet his family was unable to make the decision to remove the breathing machine that supported his life, and the doctors were afraid of the legal consequences. The situation angered me; I felt powerless to act. By today's standards, the patient was dead, and yet we could not allow him to die. Nurses began taking small risks. One nurse tried turning down the percentage of oxygen the patient received from the ventilator; another would suction or clean out the breathing tube without giving deep breaths of oxygen between suctioning. Although these actions seemed risky, they did not seem to contribute to the patient's death. He finally died when a fever overcame his minimal functions.

Daring acts of guerrilla nursing that attempted to shorten a patient's suffering were damaging in several ways. To proceed in this manner meant one could maintain the illusion of control without openly acknowledging one's power or powerlessness in the situation. And ultimately one found that technology gave a very illusory power at best. The real power we could have attained was the power to change the process of decision making: listening for the obstacles to a decision that needed making and supporting the family when they asked the physician for the information they needed. Instead we gave up that power by acting as if the decision was fixed, and that we were only instruments of someone or something higher in the chain of command.

The feminist author Starhawk distinguishes two uses of power as "power-over" and "power-from-within." Power-over is the power based on rules and authority: the "popular conception of justice." Power-over allows one to make decisions for others, even to the extent of causing pain and suffering. There is no room to consider the consequences of one's actions, only the laws that govern them. Power-from-within, the feminist source of power, is based on integrity. Integrity implies caring, an honoring of the other so that no action is considered apart from its consequences (Starhawk 1982, 34–35).

Acting within that caring, we could have recognized the community of support that existed within the nursing team. It was not up to someone in a position of authority to grant us more power; it was up to us to recognize the shared power of the patient, his family, his physician, and every nurse in the unit. Together, we could have come to a humane decision much sooner.

Since my first year of working in intensive care, many improvements have been made in the way care is provided. For instance, most units now have open visiting hours, a greater degree of privacy, and more consideration for the factors that lead to disorientation. However, technology is still so much a given that it is almost impossible to respect individual control and autonomy. It is taken for granted that every patient will be connected to a machine that monitors the heart continuously, thus giving him or her a tether of six feet. Intravenous (IV) lines for administering fluid are started and restarted without asking permission or explaining their purpose. When patients pull lines and tubes out, their hands are restrained by cloth ties, and if they get restless and try to climb over the siderails, a vest with long straps secures them to the bed. At times, technology is used as a threat. One physician encouraged a patient to cough by showing him a tube twice the diameter of his nares; "The nurses will have to put this down your nose if you don't start coughing."

Just as technology is used to control patients, it is used to control their families. When a nurse in an ICU tells a family member they cannot visit because of a procedure, it has a mysterious weight. Families are afraid to touch their loved ones, and not every nurse encourages them to do so. We like the awe we inspire by manipulating the tubes and wires and numbers; it is another distancing maneuver, putting us closer to physicians and farther from patients and families.

High-technology medicine has attained a prestige that is far out of proportion to its capacity to improve human life. Technology has been used to justify the hegemony of physicians and to reinforce the hierarchical structure in medicine (Grimshaw 1986). As Barbara Ehrenreich and Deirdre English (1973) relate in the classic essay "Witches, Midwives, and Nurses," when the "regular" physicians took over the healing practice from women, the functions of caring and curing were "split irrevocably." Doctors took over the function of curing and assigned caring, with a lower economic value, to nurses. Medicine then became a masculine profession, with the ideal doctor having traits of "intellect and action, abstract theory and hard-headed pragmatism" (Ehrenreich and English 1973, 40).

Nursing tried to emulate medicine, by incorporating these masculine values of scientific, linear thinking, by encouraging a professional model of practice that separated nurse from patient, and by buying into a hierarchy with the male doctor–decision maker at the top and the patient at the bottom. The mystification of knowledge that results from the use of technology at the bedside is very seductive to many nurses, as it was to me when I was a nursing student. I recall being very surprised to meet a nurse who was returning to work on a general medical floor after several years in a coronary care unit: it seemed like a step down, a relinquishing of power.

The ability to use technology is greatly rewarded in ICU. Those nurses who are trained to use the most complex equipment are entitled to a few fringe benefits—higher pay when they are called in to work with the machines, more hours allocated for education, and so forth. The ability to use the various machines is a criterion used in job applications. The nurse who is honored and respected by peers is more often the one who is skilled with machinery than the one who takes the extra time to comfort a patient or counsel a family member.

The modern intensive care unit is imbued with masculine values, despite the fact that the majority of the nurses who direct patient care are women. In a setting in which split-second thinking can save or lose a life, the value of nurturing must take second priority. Rules about the behavior of professionals and their patients gain new importance, and the authority of the physician is seldom questioned. As Starhawk emphasizes, suffering can result from such a system.

Marie, a friend and former co-worker, had been a hospice nurse for several years when she decided to return to the hospital to refresh her knowledge in the use of technology. In the first month of orientation to the emergency room, an elderly woman was admitted in very critical condition. As Marie began her initial assessment, she noticed the physician approaching with life-saving equipment. Marie drew him aside and informed him that the patient did not want to be resuscitated.

"How do you know?" he asked.

"I asked her if she wants us to pound on her chest when her heart stops, and she said no."

"Good grief! You can't ask her that!" the physician replied. "This is an emergency room!"

The values inherent in the operation of an intensive care unit become most obvious in the act of attempting to resuscitate a patient whose heartbeat and breathing have stopped. In the act of resuscitation, clinicians must adopt a "depersonalizing attitude" toward the patient in order to carry out the violent actions required. This task is made easier by the "corpse-like appearance of the patient" (Nolan 1987, 10). Unfortunately ICU nurses are forced to "depersonalize" patients hundreds of times over the course of several years of work; this attitude can then extend to the other patients they care for, who are in fact all potential "corpses."

Both nurses and patients face the idea of resuscitation with mixed emotions: dread and hope. "Attempts at resuscitation . . . carry risks of the most fearful aspects of death: pain, isolation, violence, and loss of control." But at the same time, resuscitation implies control over death, and can be confused with the ability to cure the underlying illness. "Patients desperately wish for modern technology to extend clinicians' power over death and illness, and the symbolic features of resuscitation do little to dispel such hopes" (Nolan 1987, 10).

No wonder it is so difficult to discuss withholding resuscitation with a dying patient. Thus, nurses who work in ICU are faced every day with the prospect of resuscitating dying patients who may not have been consulted about their wishes. The crucial problem is that technology is applied to dying people in an amoral way: it is used without regard for the values of the client.

I left one ICU job for another when I decided that, morally, I could not work in a setting in which I would not choose to be a patient.

After several years, it seemed I could never act in complete accord with my moral beliefs and work in the structured environment of an intensive care unit. I started volunteering for a hospice agency. I felt it expiated my guilt in some way, and provided a sense of balance. After two years of volunteering, my attraction for hospice work overcame my fear of a radical career change, and I became a hospice home-care nurse.

Here I encounter people with equally life-threatening disease, facing similar decisions, but in a radically different setting. Just being present in someone else's home lends itself to asking permission and yielding authority.

Clients (*patient* reflects passivity) are referred to hospice care in a number of different ways: through their physicians, a discharge planner at a hospital, a family member or friend, or self-referral. A client does not have to accept that he or she is dying in order to receive hospice care. In fact, some of our clients are still actively seeking treatment for their diseases. However, most want to stay out of the hospital as long as possible, and need some assistance to do so.

"Dying must be defined in order to be reacted to as dying" (O'Hara-Devereaux et al. 1981, 19). In other words, it is usually up to the physician to recognize that regardless of medical treatment, the client is within six months of dying. However, various obstacles may interfere with a physician's referral to hospice care: a lack of knowledge about hospice, a resistance to yielding authority for their patient's care, and sometimes even anger that patients are refusing treatment. Ironically, a recent article in the *New England Journal of Medicine* promotes hospice by reassuring physicians that they do not need to give up control when they make a referral: "When the primary physician serves as the leader of the medical hospice team, all other objectives will be better served." The article describes the physician's role as "pivotal and crucial," encompassing all the activities—symptom management, referral, support for the hospice team as well as the family—that are usually accomplished by an entire staff (Bulkin and Lukashok 1988, 377).

Our hospice team consists of nurses, home health aides, social workers, a physical therapist, a chaplain, and a team of volunteers. A registered nurse is generally the first person to meet the client. The initial assessment involves identifying problems and making referrals to the appropriate team member. Problems are confirmed and prioritized with the client and family, and frequently include physical symptoms, psychosocial issues of the client and caregivers, and spiritual concerns.

We establish goals with the client, which are based on the problems identified. Pain is a common problem for hospice clients. A team member's goal might be to reduce the pain to a minimum; the client's goal might be to stay awake during the day in order to stay as active as possible; the family member's goal might be uninterrupted sleep during the night. Together we try to develop a plan that addresses each of our goals. In hospice philosophy, the family and client are together the "unit of care": it is assumed that the family may need care and counseling while they participate in the care of the dying person (Blues and Zerwekh 1984, 101).

It is also within the hospice philosophy for the caregivers to empower their clients. Blues and Zerwekh (1984, 36–37) discuss several methods for enhancing a client's self-awareness and decision-making ability, including life review, writing journals, and meditation. Within the first week or two of visiting, we try to discuss the ultimate choice: where does the client want to be at the time of death? For some people, this is an easy subject to address, and is the reason for choosing hospice care. For others, it is very threatening. Without pushing an agenda onto clients by forcing them to come to terms with the dying process, we can still explore the fears around death, the client's past history with family members or friends who have died, and the caregiver's expectations of what will occur.

It is difficult to advocate for a client who is not clear about his or her wishes, or for one who is clear about his or her wishes but does not want to act on them. One of my first clients wanted never to return to a certain hospital, but did not have a physician who could admit him to a different one. He lived alone, so it seemed unrealistic to act as if he could remain at home as he got sicker. On every visit, I brought up the question of choosing another doctor, but he consistently claimed he didn't need one because he was not going back to the hospital. He got increasingly angry with me until he began refusing my visits. The planning for his final days was never completed. When he eventually did get sicker, he returned to the hospital he hated.

If I worked with a similar client today, I would not push him to make a plan for an outcome he feared so much. Instead, I would explore the fear with him: "What was it like being in the hospital? What was the scariest thing that happened to you there? What would make staying in a hospital easier for you? What did the doctor say that frightened you so much?" I am more sensitive now, also, to knowing when a client would rather relate stories from his past than plan for a future that seems terrifyingly brief. "There is no greater gift you can give a person than to sit down and listen to his story" (Blues and Zerwekh

1984, 30). It is the only real way we, as healthy professional caregivers, can begin to understand the experience of the dying client. This receptivity is the essence of the caring relationship that allows us to act in a moral way toward our clients.

The decisions made about the use of technology are thus made in a moral context. In contrast to the hospital setting, technology is never a given in hospice care. Because clients are now leaving hospitals "quicker and sicker," a plethora of technology is available for home use, from pumps that regulate the flow of intravenous fluid, to ventilators that assist or control breathing. But for hospice clients, technology is used only within the context of their goals.

For example, intravenous fluid is an option when a client is no longer able to eat and drink. Food carries great symbolic meaning for clients and their families; many families become very distressed when the client's appetite has vanished. When cajoling and encouraging fail to get results, some families become desperate. In general, when hospice clients quit eating, it is because they are close to death. Under these circumstances, it would be cruel to force a person to eat or drink, so the family asks about giving fluid through an intravenous line.

Since IV fluid is so commonplace in hospitals, people frequently assume it to be without risk and with great benefit. The hospice nurse needs to provide more realistic information to the client and family about the process of dying with and without IVs. We provide information about the side effects of hydration: IV fluid can cause discomfort due to additional work required of the heart, pressure from swelling that may cause pain, and the possible need for more tubes to drain the extra fluid. The dehydration that can occur as the client's oral intake decreases can eliminate some of these problems and have the effect of producing a "natural anaesthesia" as the client becomes sleepy.

Most clients choose not to have IV fluid, and the family concentrates on making the client comfortable with frequent mouth care. However, if the client's desire is to live just a few extra days or weeks, or if the symptoms associated with dehydration prove worse than those related to the intravenous fluid, the hospice staff assists the client to attain his or her goals.

Another example of technology used in home care is the patient-controlled analgesia pump. This is a small programmable pump that allows the client and family to regulate a constant flow of injectable pain medicine. The nurse who sets up the pump receives physician orders for the hourly rate of infusion, along with a range of rate increase if necessary. It is usually possible to calculate a dose large enough to keep the client comfortable while allowing enough alertness to interact with the family. The goal is to prevent the peaks and valleys of pain control that occur with oral pain medicine. In general, clients and families are so delighted with this effect that they wonder why all clients don't use this method. Of course, hospice nurses must advocate vigorously in order for the physician to relinquish control over the administration of medication.

Additional technology that we use is similarly focused on comfort and on making it easier for a client to stay at home. We frequently use special mattresses to prevent skin breakdown, or rarely, a bed that is made out of constantly circulating beads that prevents any pressure against the skin. A transcutaneous electric nerve stimulation (TENS) unit is sometimes used for pain. It generates an electric signal that may interrupt the pain sensation at a local area. If the client desires a specific technological aid, we are quite aggressive in our efforts to secure it in order to promote comfort.

Hospice nurses have had to become comfortable with a variety of technological devices. However, we never allow the machines to come between us and the human being we are taking care of. Marie, a former hospice nurse, worked with a very sick person in the intensive care unit one weekend. She took report from the night shift nurse, who walked into the patient's room with her. Marie introduced herself to the patient, reminded him that it was Saturday, and told him that she would be taking care of him all day. Marie said, "The night nurse looked very suspicious, as if she was worried I wouldn't be able to take care of a patient unless I looked at the medication pumps before I looked at the patient."

The first principle of hospice care is "Dying is a normal process" (Blues and Zerwekh 1984, 97). I feel privileged to get close to people who are dying. I feel especially privileged when I am present at the time they die. I don't know that I had ever witnessed a death while I was working in intensive care: usually my eyes were focused on the heart monitor or the breathing machines. But I have watched people die naturally in the past two years, and it is a remarkable experience. No two deaths are the same, and they do not always go as smoothly as planned. But there is a definite change that takes place when a person who has been struggling to hang on to life relaxes and lets go. It is a moving, spiritual experience, regardless of the belief systems of the caregivers.

When nurses and physicians ignore the spiritual aspect of death, they can pretend they are in control of the dying person's experience. For me, this illusion was quickly dispelled by encounters with people who could maintain control under very difficult circumstances: pain, weakness, and family stress. I have been amazed by the strong women clients I have met in hospice; several seemed to choose the time and place of their death, and were active in their family roles until they died. Our role as hospice workers was to assist them in maintaining their control, to empower them by minimizing the symptoms and teaching them what to expect, and to listen to them describe what they were experiencing.

The ability to work with people without controlling them is based on feminist morality. Josephine Donovan describes the work of Kathryn Allen Rabuzzi and Sara Ruddick on women's epistemology, which underlies the feminist moral vision. They speak of the positive ability to wait passively, and the humility that arises when we give up control (Donovan 1987, 174–75). The injudicious use of technology to remove control from a dying person is immoral from a feminist standpoint.

Feminist values also guide our relationships with each other as a team. The hierarchical structure is replaced by a spirit in which the person who provides personal care is as important as the administrator. This spirit makes our work with each other as a hospice team as complex as our work with our clients. The agency I work for recently went on a retreat to explore our philosophy, our goals, and our relationships. We spoke of the intimacy of our work with clients, the rewarding yet costly nature of the work. We talked about the value we place on trust and being present with each other. The metaphor we used for the agency as a whole was the body: we must nurture the sense of connectedness.

Some hospitals, recognizing the stress nurses work under, provide support groups for their staff. However, unless support groups are ongoing and mandatory, as they are in most hospice programs, it can add stress to try to get away from patient care to attend a meeting. And it is very rare for a hospital to offer a full-day retreat for nursing staff. With the current budget crises most hospitals face, there is limited support for attending continuing education, let alone something as esoteric as a retreat.

I feel more comfortable in my role as a hospice nurse not only because of the different kind of care I give, and not only because of the support and nurturance I receive from the women I work with, but also because of the inherent values in hospice. The use of caring as a real principle for action can be seen in hospice work, in the sense of "apprehending the reality of the other," in its rejection of suffering, and in its "consideration of the relation between means and ends" (Grimshaw 1986, 220–21).

Dying is an intimate process. We can use technology to separate ourselves from the process, or use it to allow more closeness. We can teach families to do many of the things people do in hospitals—give shots, control infusions of drugs, manage skin care—and thus put them in as intimate a relationship with the dying person as they are willing to accept.

As hospice nurses, our style of teaching reflects the value of egalitarianism and our nonauthoritative stance. My sister, a pediatrician, told me about a study on patient compliance she had seen. (The word *compliance* itself implies a hierarchy of decision making.) The study revealed that patients are more likely to trust a physician's experience with a drug or treatment than they are to believe a scientific study. This was bound to change my sister's practice; she even used personal authority to convince her own children about appropriate treatment of an injury. (Aunt Alice is a nurse, and she thinks you should put your finger under cold water.) It came as no surprise to me that patients rely on our past experience. Many families ask for a "normalization" of the dying process: "Does everybody feel this way? Have you ever seen a patient like this before? Does this work for most of your patients?" Teaching would be to no avail if we did not observe and use the client's system of learning.

As a moral theory, the ethic of care best fits a "contextual" model, which speaks to real people dealing with real issues in a particular culture. Instead of focusing on abstract principles of action, an ethic of care focuses on the characteristics of a moral person (Tronto 1987, 658).

Wilma Scott Heide, a feminist nurse described these qualities as "excellences"—eschewing the word *virtue,* which is from the Latin *vir* for man. Her biographer chooses three excellences important to Heide: interdependence, nurturance, and courage. "Courage includes a willingness to risk, resoluteness, determination, steadfastness. . . . It is simply that willingness to do, consistent with feminist values, what needs to be done" (Haney 1985, 159).

Courage is not evident in my description of the actions we took to try to shorten the suffering of a brain-dead patient in the intensive care unit. Courage requires a sense of our real power as women, that power we have as enablers, as advocates, from "being with" instead of "doing to" our clients. It takes a great deal of courage to allow people to die in the manner they choose, not to intervene when we don't agree with the choice. As one nurse stated, "I feel that we sometimes impose our own middle-class values on clients" when we try to convince them to do what we feel is right. Then we step back and ask ourselves, "Who are we making feel safe, the client or the nurse? Who are we making comfortable?" Courage means we do not act out of fear of legal consequences, but out of respect and caring for the individual.

"To put feminism in the center of the stage of morality is to bring women into the center as subject, as agent, as actor" (Haney 1985, 176). Women and nurses must act as moral agents for the health care revolution to continue. We have too long acted as if we were passive recipients of moral decisions. Recognizing ourselves as actors will promote liberation.

The revolution is accelerating as hospice nurses move back into mainstream health care. Marie took a job in the intensive care unit and startled the other professionals there into taking a look at their assumptions. I am beginning a new role in a residential setting for persons with AIDS. Not all of my new clients will be ready for palliative therapy alone; some may want aggressive technological treatment. But all of them, as much as they are able, will be empowered to choose their living and dying.

The caring philosophy of feminism provides a hopeful vision for the future of health care. The vision is here now as hospice. If we do not allow the hospice philosophy to become diluted as hospice care becomes commonplace and regulated, it can serve as a standard for all health care.

BIBLIOGRAPHY

Blues, Ann, and Joyce Zerwekh. 1984. *Hospice and palliative nursing care.* New York: Grune and Stratton.
Bulkin, Wilma, and Herbert Lukashok. 1988. Rx for dying: The case for hospice. *New England Journal of Medicine* 318, no. 6: 376–78.
Donovan, Josephine. 1987. *Feminist theory.* New York: Ungar.
Ehrenreich, Barbara, and Deirdre English. 1973. *Witches, midwives, and nurses: A history of women healers.* Old Westbury, N.Y.: Feminist Press.
Gilligan, Carol. 1982. *In a different voice.* Cambridge: Harvard University Press.
Greer, David, and Vincent Mor. 1985. How Medicare is altering the hospice movement. *Hastings Center Report,* October 15, no. 5: 5–9.
Grimshaw, Jean. 1986. *Philosophy and feminist thinking.* Minneapolis: University of Minnesota Press.
Haney, Elizabeth Humes. 1985. *A feminist legacy: The ethics of Wilma Scott Heide and Company.* Buffalo, N.Y.: Margretdaughters.
Heide, Wilma Scott. 1985. *Feminism for the health of it.* Buffalo, N.Y.: Margretdaughters.
Lenz, Elinor, and Marbara Myerhoff. 1985. *The feminization of America: How*

women's values are changing our public and private lives. Los Angeles: Jeremy Tarcher.

Nolan, Kathleen. 1987. In death's shadow: The meanings of withholding resuscitation. *Hastings Center Report* (October): 9–14.

O'Hara-Devereaux, Maray, Len Hughes Andrus, and Cynthia Scott, eds. 1981. *Eldercare: A guide to clinical geriatrics*. New York: Grune and Stratton.

President's Commission for the Study of Ethical Problems in Medicine. 1982. *Making health care decisions*. Washington, D.C.: Government Printing Office.

President's Commission for the Study of Ethical Problems in Medicine and Biomedical and Behavioral Research. 1983. *Deciding to forego life-sustaining treatment*. Washington, D.C.: Government Printing Office.

Robertson, John. 1983. *The rights of the critically ill*. Cambridge, Mass.: Ballinger Publishing Co.

Smith, Ruth L. 1985. Feminism and the moral subject. In *Women's consciousness, women's conscience*, ed. Barbara Andolsen, Christine Gudorf, and Mary Pellauer. San Francisco: Harper and Row.

Starhawk. 1982. *Dreaming the dark: Magic, sex, and politics*. Boston: Beacon Press.

Tronto, Joan. 1987. Beyond gender difference to a theory of care. *Signs* 12, no. 4: 644–63.

Part 3
Occupational and Environmental
Technologies: Research and
Resources for Change

Introduction

Myra Marx Ferree

There are few people today who are not aware that the environment in which they live and work may have consequences for their health. The widespread health risks of asbestos in schools or smoking in offices have drawn some media attention, and particularly dangerous settings such as Times Beach or Love Canal have been the focus of sustained concern. Some jobs have been long recognized as presenting special health problems, such as black lung for coal miners, asbestosis for shipfitters, and brown lung for textile workers. Other jobs, created by newer technologies, are just beginning to be scrutinized for the health consequences they may have. For example, data entry jobs that demand eight hours of keyboard use and sustained attention to a computer screen may generate wrist and eye strain of such serious extent as to produce permanent disabilities. The production of computer chips demands assembly work with a microscope in an atmosphere filled with a variety of potentially noxious chemicals. Plastic packaging exposes workers to fumes, and electronic components assembly demands solvents.

Which of these technologies have particular impacts on women's health? The answer to that question depends as much on the way gender is used to organize the workplace as it does on the specific physiological differences between women and men. The conditions under which women live and work are frequently different from those facing men. The sex-typing of jobs puts women workers into different occupations and industries, while women's lower wages mean that women supporting families may have to live in poorer, more dangerous neighborhoods (near highways, with higher carbon monoxide exposure from car exhaust systems or in center cities, with older housing and higher crime rates). Women with children are responsible for their nutrition and health care more directly than are fathers, and women with paid jobs often also have unpaid work at home placing physical and emotional demands on them. When women's health is affected by technology, these physiological and psychological effects are mediated by the special social circumstances of women's lives. Because society is organized on gender lines the practical consequences of many technologies are different for women than for men.

The example of the health consequences of computer technology may illustrate the contrast between effects that are gender-specific because of sex differences in physiology or psychology and those that reflect the gender arrangements in which the particular technologies are implemented. Only a few of the potentially negative effects computers could have on women's health will be inherently gender-specific. For example, the possible increase in miscarriages or birth defects due to prolonged VDT radiation exposure for pregnant women will be different from, though not necessarily greater than, the negative reproductive consequences such exposure may have for men. Nevertheless, many effects of technology will be different for women because of the nature of the work they do. Women make up over 80 percent of the clerical labor force, and clerical workers are disproportionately subject to eyestrain from sustained focus on a screen, tendonitis or back problems from poorly designed keyboards and chairs, and stress-related disorders incident upon repetitive tasks that demand a high level of accuracy. This in turn reflects the overall relations of control that give women little authority to structure their own work. At this level, male management's view of women workers as short-term employees who may be made to work intensively for a few years and then replaced at low cost when they "burn out" means that it will be women who spend eight hours a day at data-entry terminals, suffering boredom and backache, with little chance to stretch, talk, or change tasks.

While computers are a very obvious form of new technology with dramatic effects on the nature and structure of work, their very novelty makes it difficult to have any clear picture of what their physical and mental health hazards or benefits will turn out to be. Research has hardly begun even on the reproductive health risks, and the broader picture of gender-related hazards in the social construction of computer work has yet to be sketched out. Moreover, the prominence of computers and microchips has tended to obscure the continuing significance of other forms of technology. While not necessarily new, their consequences for women's health are still understudied and poorly understood. The gender and class biases of existing research throw even what we think we know into question.

The focus of this part is on this often-neglected aspect of technology: the gender context in which workplace and environmental practices affect health. The effect is not direct and simple, nor are the technologies themselves. Manufacturing processes, for example, involve technologies in production (e.g., assembly lines, time clocks) as well as in the products (e.g., TV sets, microchips). Some health hazards relate more to the former (Fifield et al.), others arise from the latter

(Bertin; Dew et al.), especially regarding the chemicals used, all of which will end up disposed of somewhere in the environment (Nelson). The women's health movement (Mellow) provides a perspective for examining the gender context of concern and choice in which decisions to use technologies are made. Despite the diversity of the technologies with which the authors deal, there are several themes that run through these chapters.

First, the authors highlight the significance of the political and economic relations surrounding the use of technologies, rather than depicting them as uniformly good or bad. Consequently, no individual technological development takes center stage as either a demon or a "deus ex machina" for future progress. The chapters in this section concentrate on factors that shape how technology is used and the political and social relationships that determine their effects. They point out how little we know about the health impacts of technologies, partly because consideration of these consequences has played so small a role in the decision to use them.

Second, they consider gender similarities as well as differences in the impact and consequences of technologies on the health and well-being of women and men, rather than polarizing experience along gender lines. In some previous studies men's health has been disregarded and in other cases women have been ignored, particularly when stereotypes of women and men as reproducers, nurturers, and paid workers intervened to shape research and policy. In contrast, these papers look critically at the relevance of gender for the academics' and activists' responses to technology as well as for the real health consequences for people in a variety of jobs and settings.

Third, health effects of technology are viewed as both mental and physical, separately and in interaction. Mental consequences include the positive psychological effects from access to certain forms of technology along with the debilitating stress, depression, and negative self-image that may result from being controlled or contaminated by it. These mental effects are integrated into the total picture of health outcomes. None of the chapters falls into the trap of considering health merely the absence of a diagnosed disease; all offer a more complex and comprehensive view of well-being, one more in accord with that of the women's health movement.

Finally, all the chapters emphasize the importance of social activism in creating change in law, in policy, in workplace practices, and in the economic and social structures that disproportionately place health burdens on women. Women emerge not as victims, nor as saviors, but as subjects of their own lives, struggling to protect their own health and livelihoods. The challenges are manifold, but the variety of resources for and routes to a more healthy world that women have already discovered offer a recurrent note of optimism. Collective organization in several different forms—in unions, in the women's health movement, and in environmental activism—provides a crucial source of strength for these struggles.

The first theme, evaluating the political and economic context in which technology is implemented, is central to Joan Bertin's article on how so-called fetal protection policies are used to include or exclude workers. Although employers have attempted to keep women out of certain jobs defined as high-risk to a real or potential fetus, Bertin shows that the definitions of hazard are not based on objective scientific evidence so much as on a political and economic assessment of costs. Women's own health risks—reproductive and otherwise—rarely enter these calculations. The gender bias that tends to treat only women as responsible for their children encourages everyone to overlook the fact that men also have reproductive systems and that hazardous chemicals affect sperm as well as fetuses. Thus women are offered the nonchoice of being sterilized or losing their jobs, while employers are protected from the costs of cleaning up their workplaces and chemical exposures to men continue to put the next generation at risk.

Bertin's chapter thus also brings to the fore the second theme, namely, that the sex differences in physiological risks may be small but the social and political structure of gender exposes men and women to very different consequences of any given technology. Women, not men, are assumed to be able to choose not to work and so it becomes politically acceptable to make sterilization a condition of continued employment for women only. Gender stereotypes suggest an artificial division between mothers and women who work in "men's" jobs and thus obscure the outrageousness of the "choice" offered. No one would find an employer's demand that male workers be castrated to keep their jobs to be "biologically justified" no matter what level of risk to men's reproductive system was found. While female sterilization has become a medically simpler operation than it once was, it is still more drastic and dangerous than male sterilization (vasectomy). Because childbearing still shapes social womanhood, female sterilization, like male castration, implies a removal of one of the most gender-defining aspects of a body. Despite these medical and social costs, the demand for female sterilization is treated as a "cheap" fix for hazardous conditions. Thus employers use gender expectations and stereotypes to protect themselves from workers' demands for a safer workplace and to transfer the costs to the women workers themselves.

The differential impact on women of the political and economic relations in which technology is used is also clearly evident in the chapter by Fifield, Reisine, Pfeiffer, and Affleck, which draws particular attention to the class context of the workplace. Rather than looking at any one specific technology, Fifield and her coauthors consider how the well-being of women with rheumatoid arthritis (RA) is affected by their ability to continue to work despite the disease and how technology can be used to either enhance or diminish their chances of employment. The consequences of job loss for women have been understudied because it is assumed that paid work is not psychologically important; however, these authors find that women with equally severe disease who are no longer able to work are more depressed and experience more pain than women who have been able to hold on to their jobs despite their illness.

The ability to keep working despite having RA is found to be less a function of the severity of the disease than of the stringency of the work environment. Women with a given level of disease who have more control over the timing and other conditions of their work can keep their jobs while women with less control are excluded from the labor market as disabled. Both social class and gender shape the amount of control workers have and thus the extent to which their work environment is disabling them. Workers with control can use technologies to help themselves keep working (e.g., specially adapted cars) while workers who are controlled see technology being used to exclude them (e.g., time clocks, computer-monitored keystrokes). The technologies with the greatest impact on women's experience of the disease are thus also those which structure the workplace for the "able-bodied," and Fifield et al. see workers' collective efforts to humanize the workplace as also making it a less handicapping environment for women with RA.

The potential costs of using hazardous chemicals for workers involved in manufacturing technologically sophisticated products is central to the paper by Dew, Bromet, Parkinson, Dunn, and Ryan. As in the paper by Fifield et al., health is defined broadly as both mental and physical well-being. Like Bertin, Dew et al. make clear how gender biases have shaped this field of research. These authors note that most studies of the toxic consequences of solvent exposure have been done on male workers and that industry standards reflect this. Moreover, low-level exposures to solvents and experiences of occupational stress may have some symptoms in common, such as headaches, malaise, and declines in performance on certain tasks. Because stress and solvents could combine to produce more negative outcomes than either would alone, the authors study both in interaction with each other. While the two turn out to have separate, noninteracting effects, each is shown to be a significant contributor to women's ill health, particularly in regard to certain symptoms. Thus women who have sometimes been described as having "hysterical" symptoms because of the stress they were under might in fact have been suffering the undiagnosed consequences of solvent exposure.

Solvent use in industry is increasing with the growing emphasis on plastics and electronics manufacturing, where women are disproportionately represented. We should therefore expect to see a rise in the number of cases where low-level solvent exposure could account for experiences of fatigue, headaches, and inability to concentrate. As Dew and her coauthors note, without further research on how solvents affect women, even the women workers themselves may inappropriately blame their symptoms solely on the stress in their lives.

The theme of understanding health as an integrated experience of mental and physical well-being, evident in the approach both Fifield and Dew and their coauthors take to workplace disabilities, is expanded in Lin Nelson's chapter on environmental degradation. While the physical health risks of pollution are great, so too are the psychological costs of uncertainty. The dangers posed by radiation and chemical exposure are cumulative and the advice offered by experts is often contradictory, so short-term choices are agonizingly difficult. Refusing to think about the issues at all may sometimes seem the only way to protect one's mental health, but Nelson shows that this is no real option at all.

Nelson's paper also makes clear the particular relevance of this issue for women while acknowledging that most of the hazards are shared by women and men. Clean air, clean water, clean food are not gender-specific needs, though in some societies, including our own, women may have less access to resources to meet these needs. Neither women nor men have any monopoly on the risks environmental pollution poses to the long-term survival of the species, nor are the dangers to the environment women's special responsibility to clean up. It is women's social position as mothers, not any special closeness to nature, that often puts them on the front line in fighting pollution in their neighborhoods and towns. Women's local networks are especially practical in mobilizing grassroots campaigns, and when women do not work directly for the employer who has created the hazard, they may be greater risk-takers and radicals in their resistance. Nelson shows how gender matters in the forms activism takes and in the responses to those women who are engaged in protest ("hysterical women" or "healers"), but also suggests some of the dangers of using gender-based appeals (e.g., protecting home, family, and children) to mobilize women for environmental activism. Among other things, protecting the planet from pollution is not something for which women can or should be held responsible.

Nelson also discusses the practical and psychological consequences of one physiologically sex-linked consequence of environmental pollution, namely the presence of dangerous chemicals in women's breast milk. On one level, this is merely an indicator of what enormous levels of chemical exposure men and nonlactating women also face. On another level, it is a practical problem for women who want to do the best possible thing for their infants and are deciding whether or not to nurse. On yet another level, it is a symbolic return to the idea of women as polluted and dangerous people, with consequences for women's body-image and self-esteem. A resolution of the problem will thus have to proceed on all of these interconnected levels. Nelson explores some of the ways that these links can be made politically without returning to stereotyped views of women and nature.

Gail Mellow's paper on the women's health movement picks up the theme of the significance of social activism for health that Nelson's chapter also highlights. By focusing on the diversity of structures, interests, and perspectives in the movement, Mellow encourages us to see feminism as touching all aspects of all women's health. The key feature of the movement is self-help, which Mellow shows to have expanded its meaning over time even among activists. While self-help once denoted merely self-care, it now includes researching and developing sources of information, making choices about risks as well as treatments, expanding the range of health care alternatives to choose among, and challenging the monopoly of professionals over the definition of good health care.

As Mellow also makes clear, social activism for women's health does not necessarily pit feminists against health care professionals; indeed, increasingly, feminists *are* health care professionals. Alliances between grassroots activists and sympathetic researchers and practitioners are becoming more common, and growing numbers of women who want to change the way health care is provided have entered the health care professions. The impact of feminism on medicine and public health is hard to ignore, whether in the reemergence of midwives as a viable occupation or the organizations of physicians and of nurses that press for change. The relationship of the women's health movement to the "experts" is therefore necessarily more ambivalent, because some of "them" are "us."

The structures and strategies of the movement increasingly reflect this ambivalence. While acknowledging co-optation as a legitimate concern, Mellow emphasizes the influence of activists upon the experts and highlights the potential for transforming health care occupations by changing the expectations and demands that their clients place on them. The decisions to develop, implement, regulate, or export health care technologies are increasingly placed under scrutiny by informed feminist critics inside and outside the professions. In this context, technologies can be demystified for users and professionals alike, and understood as both helpful and harmful. The study of social activism thus returns us to the first theme of this section, the social and economic relationships that give technology its force and direction.

In sum, all of the chapters in this part contribute to our understanding of the gendered context in which occupational and environmental technologies are implemented. They therefore expose the foundation of stereotypes on which decisions about technology often rest, whether this is an assumption that only women have reproductive systems, or that only men suffer from solvents, or that women are close to nature and so have a special responsibility to protect the environment. All of the chapters recognize important similarities in the effects of technology on women and men, while also identifying structures that distribute these consequences differently and that disproportionately direct our attention to their effects on one gender or the other. The chapters are attentive to the way that experts have defined or disregarded the consequences of technology in gender terms, and they emphasize the importance of collective organization by the persons affected to change these definitions and prescriptions. All of these chapters also contribute to our understanding of the health efffects of technology by their integrated focus on both body and brain. By showing physiological and psychological consequences to be interconnected at many different levels, these papers direct our concerns with the work technologies of the future to their potential impact on the whole person.

The chapters in this part thus not only inform us about social activism, they suggest some important directions for women's health efforts in the future. While feminists have not ignored the impact of technology on women's health, this concern has rarely led to studies such as these. As these chapters demonstrate, for feminists to narrow their consideration of the positive and negative impacts of today's technology to the few instances in which biology itself dictates a differential result, as in childbirth, would be to miss a wide range of important gendered consequences. These chapters make an important case for a much wider agenda for the women's health movement, and a broader and more inclusive view of the implications of technology for women's mental and physical well-being.

Women's Health and Women's Rights:
Reproductive Health Hazards in the Workplace

Joan E. Bertin

The American Cyanamid Company plant is in Willow Island, West Virginia, on a stretch of the Ohio River crowded with chemical plants. The surrounding area is economically depressed, and the population is heavily dependent on the chemical industry for employment. Five to six hundred workers have been employed at American Cyanamid. Their union scale wages lift them substantially above the standard of living of many of their neighbors. Until 1974, this plant employed no women in production work.

By 1978 approximately twenty-five women worked at the American Cyanamid plant. Early that year, they were called into meetings in small groups and were informed about a new company medical policy. The purpose of the policy was to protect the fetus from exposure to hazardous chemicals if a woman worker became pregnant. As a result of the policy, women would be excluded from most jobs in the plant. Those with the lowest seniority faced likely termination. A company official reportedly said that the policy was supported by the federal government and that the other chemical plants in the region would adopt similar policies.

The policy applied to all women between the ages of fifteen and fifty regardless of their marital status, sexual orientation, or childbearing intentions. The only ones not affected would be those who could present medical verification of sterility. Birth control, even a spouse's vasectomy, would not suffice. In response to questions, a company doctor told women that they should not get sterilized in order to secure their employment. Nonetheless, tubal ligations were described, and the women were assured that their insurance would cover the costs. No one offered any other suggestions as to how any of these women could secure their employment and their economic well-being.

Subsequently, the scope of the policy was substantially narrowed, but by then five women had already submitted to surgical sterilization in order to protect their right to jobs. A year later the department where five women had undergone sterilization to secure their employment was closed, allegedly for "business reasons" (Office of Technology Assessment 1985, 251–58; *Christman et al.* v. *American Cyanamid Co.* 1980).

289

These events occurred at a facility that had been cited for violations of federal occupational safety and health law,[1] and whose own
records revealed exposures to levels of toxic substances which federal
regulators and independent health professionals generally agree pose
a risk to adults of both sexes (Occupational Safety and Health Admin.
1978; U.S. Environmental Protection Agency 1985b).[2]

In 1979 these facts captured public attention. Since then, the question of occupational reproductive hazards and "fetal protection" policies in particular have been the subject of Congressional hearings,
scholarly commentary, several court decisions, and studies by the U.S.
Congress Office of Technology Assessment, the President's Council on
Environmental Quality, and others. Regulatory guidelines were attempted, but abandoned (45 Fed. Reg. 7,514 (1980); 46 Fed. Reg. 3,916
(1981)). Notwithstanding all this activity, the questions posed by these
policies have yet to be resolved satisfactorily, while the need for solutions persists. In January, 1987, some manufacturers of semiconductor
chips announced an intention to limit employment of women workers
in response to a study purportedly showing an increased risk of miscarriage in such employment. Unlike the earlier situations, which mostly
involved male-intensive industries in which women were viewed as a
marginal element of the workforce, this most recent example involves
an industry that is substantially populated by women. The earlier cases
invited speculation that so-called fetal protection policies forced those
women who wished to function in a "male" world literally to sacrifice
their "femaleness." The newer situation, in contrast, suggests that
women are always marginal workers and that their rights and interest
in employment must always yield to their paramount responsibility as
childbearers.

Initially, public attention focused on exclusionary policies of the
American Cyanamid version because of the cruel choice they posed
for women workers: your fertility or your job. But these policies also
raise crucial scientific and legal questions: what evidence supports the
proposition that women (or fetuses) are uniquely susceptible to the
harmful effects of toxic chemicals or are susceptible at lower levels of
exposure? Did Congress and state legislatures, when they enacted broad
prohibitions against sex discrimination and an expansive right to a safe
and healthy workplace, intend that pregnant workers were not to be
covered to the same extent as all other workers?

To date, these questions have been addressed only in part, and in
a not wholly satisfactory way. This chapter will describe the nature and
extent of the problem posed by exclusionary policies and the judicial
and other responses to them, and will then propose legislative actions

and public policy initiatives to enhance workers' rights to reproductive freedom, occupational safety, procreative health, and nondiscrimination in employment.

The Scope of the Problem

Hundreds of thousands of lucrative jobs are closed to women workers as a result of exclusionary policies. Many of the country's largest corporations have adopted such policies, and in some companies the policies affect large numbers of jobs (Becker 1986, 1226). The Lead Industries Association has publicly opposed the employment of fertile women since 1974 (Stellman 1977, 178), and almost a million jobs are at stake in that industry alone.

Many of the policies bar all women of childbearing age or capacity from certain jobs, a rule that affects women for most of their working lives. However, the average woman bears only two children, and most working women plan the timing of those births. Many blue-collar women bear children early in life, before they begin work. For example, in 1977, only 1 percent of married, blue-collar working women aged thirty or over expected to bear a child within the next year (U.S. Bureau of the Census 1978). Thus, concern for specific workplace effects on pregnancy cannot rationally be directed at the entire female workforce, and women cannot be viewed as permanently potentially pregnant or as powerless to control conception and childbirth.

The Premise of Fetal Hypersusceptibility:
Fact or Stereotype?

"Fetal protection" policies assume that the fetus is uniquely susceptible to injury from hazardous workplace exposures or that it is susceptible at lower exposure levels than those that would threaten adult workers. Some companies have adopted policies solely on the basis of this unexamined assumption, rather than on the basis of an actual examination of the biological effects of specific chemicals or conditions. A review of the scientific literature on the reproductive and other health effects of occupational exposures reveals that the assumption of heightened or unique fetal risk, while sometimes validated, frequently relies more on stereotypes than on facts, and that the adverse health effects of toxic chemicals are rarely confined to the fetus in utero.

Toxic substances can affect the normal development of the fetus at three stages of the reproductive process. Gametotoxins are substances that cause malformations of the *egg or sperm* prior to conception, thereby impairing the exposed individual's ability to produce a healthy fetus. Mutagens are chemicals that cause alterations in the chromosomal structure of the DNA molecule in the *male and female* reproductive cells, which can be manifested by abnormal fetal development and genetic defects in later generations. Teratogens are substances that operate directly on the fetus and impair normal growth after conception (Stellman 1979; Paul and Himmelstein 1988, 922–27).

The male spermatozoa may be particularly sensitive to chemical and other injury. The testes, vulnerably located in the scrotal sack outside the body, are the "sperm factories" where sperm are constantly being produced. It takes about seventy-two days for each sperm to mature through the type of cell division called meiosis, known to be one of the body processes most susceptible to chemical toxicity. Exposure of men to chemicals or physical conditions such as radiation may cause mutations in sperm (changes in the hereditary information they carry); may cause sperm deformities, slow movement, or reduction in sperm numbers; may affect hormones essential to reproduction; and may alter sexual behavior.

In 1977 male workers at an Occidental Chemical Company plant in California reported an unusually low birth rate in their families. Subsequent testing showed that fourteen of twenty-five tested men were either sterile or had extremely low sperm counts. The affected men had all worked with the pesticide dibromochloropropane (DBCP) (U.S. Dept. of Labor 1980, 305–7). Subsequently, DBCP was banned for almost all uses, based on the human data showing "low and zero sperm counts, on animal test data indicating DBCP was a carcinogen in laboratory animals, and on laboratory studies demonstrating DBCP caused heritable genetic damage" (U.S. Environmental Protection Agency 1985a).

The following year, the Occupational Safety and Health Administration (OSHA) examined the health effects of workplace exposure to lead, from which women are commonly excluded, and concluded with regard to reproductive health:

> Germ cells can be affected by lead which may cause genetic damage in the *egg or sperm* cells before conception and which can be passed on to the developing fetus. The record indicates that genetic damage from lead occurs prior to conception in *either father or mother.* The result of genetic damage could be failure to implant, miscarriage, stillbirth, or birth defects. (43 Fed. Reg. 52,959–60 (1978), emphasis added)

Similarly, the United Nations Scientific Committee on the Effects of Atomic Radiation (UNSCEAR) concluded that, in addition to risks posed by in utero radiation exposure, preconception *paternal* irradiation could result in "from 2 to 10 congenitally malformed liveborn children, per rad of paternal radiation, with about five times this number of recognizable abortions and about 10 times the number of losses at the early embryonic stage" (UNSCEAR 1977; 9). The Environmental Protection Agency's (EPA) Teratology Policy Workgroup recently conducted an internal study of nineteen pesticides regulated because of fetal effects, and five industrial chemicals. EPA concluded that "if a pesticide is extensively tested for health effects, it is likely to show additional positive effects other than teratogenicity . . . [and] teratogenicity was never the most sensitive effect, except in the case of one pesticide" (U.S. Environmental Protection Agency 1985c, 25).

Recent concern over miscarriage rates in the semiconductor industry demonstrates the problem regarding selective assessment of hazards. Among the chemicals widely used in the industry are glycol ethers, which are known to cause reproductive injury in male animals (National Institute of Occupational Safety and Health 1983). A recent compendium identified the wide variety of toxic substances used in the industry and documented numerous hazards that have been recognized for a number of years (La Dou 1986). Whether employment in this industry poses a risk of miscarriage to pregnant women is still unknown. However, the existence of other occupational health hazards is well established, and these risks are not addressed by policies excluding or limiting the employment of potential mothers.

Selective concern for female aspects of reproduction is particularly peculiar in light of the record of indifference to workplace hazards evidenced by some industries with exclusionary policies. For example, in 1973, the Manufacturing Chemists Association kept the link between vinyl chloride exposure and angiosarcoma, a fatal form of liver cancer, "confidential in order 'to minimize unwarranted speculation' " (U.S. Dept. of Labor 1980, 273). At the same time, some industries barred women from jobs involving vinyl chloride exposure (Becker 1986, 1226). Similarly the Lead Industries Association (LIA) and many of its members maintained at OSHA hearings that the permissible blood lead level for all workers should be 80 micrograms per 100 grams of blood, a level that OSHA found would result in "severe lead intoxication" (43 Fed. Reg. 54,415–16, 52954 (1978)). At the time of the OSHA hearings members of LIA were in general noncompliance with OSHA standards (43 Fed. Reg. 54,435 (1978)), and many enforced exclusionary policies against fertile women.

These and other examples reveal starkly the problem of selective vision in acknowledging workplace health hazards: hazards are often ignored or minimized, except when they involve female aspects of reproduction. Then, employers act quickly to exclude fertile or pregnant women workers on the basis of preliminary, inconclusive, and sometimes speculative information. The prevalent assumption is that any exposure is unsafe for the fetus unless and until its safety is conclusively proved. In most other contexts, chemicals are presumed safe until proven otherwise. Once the proof is in, chemicals that are particularly harmful to men (i.e., DBCP, kepone) have been banned, while women have been barred from working around chemicals suspected to cause fetal harm. In sum, these patterns reinforce the notion that the workplace must accommodate the needs of men but not women, and that society requires and benefits from the paid labor of men, but not that of women. Men, however, are wrongly presumed invulnerable to the effects of chemical exposures until conclusive and undeniable evidence of hazard has been amassed, while fetuses are always assumed vulnerable. For women, but not for men, the primary obligation is defined as the production of healthy children, and male contribution to this process is ignored.

Federal Laws Implicated by Fetal Protection Policies

The Occupational Safety and Health Act, 29 U.S.C. §651, *et seq.* (OSH Act) requires employers to maintain a workplace "free from recognized hazards that are causing or are likely to cause death or serious physical harm" (29 U.S.C. §654 (a)(1)). It also requires the secretary of labor to promulgate health and safety standards to assure, to the extent feasible, "that no employee will suffer material impairment of health or functional capacity . . ." (29 U.S.C. §655 (b)(5)).

The OSH Act contemplates that workplace protection from toxic exposures will be achieved primarily through standard-setting. OSHA is empowered to set permissible exposure limits, to require monitoring of the workplace and the individual, and to prescribe medical surveillance and medical removal protection (with wage rates retained), among other things, in fulfilling the standard-setting obligation. However, the standard-setting process has proved to be slow and laborious: in the first thirteen years of its existence, OSHA developed standards for only twenty-three chemicals. (The *Registry of Toxic Effects of Chemical Substances* compiled by the National Institute of Occupational Safety and Health [NIOSH] lists some 59,000 chemicals.) Some standards have been invalidated as a result of industry challenge, and others are still in litigation.

Workers also gain protection under the OSH Act from the Hazard Communication Standard (29 C.F.R. §1910.1200) promulgated in 1983, the so-called right-to-know act under which chemical manufacturers and importers must provide workers with information about chemical hazards, and distributors must do the same for customers (Office of Technology Assessment 1984). In addition, the Environmental Protection Agency also affects the health of workers through its responsibilities for the protection of farm workers under the Federal Insecticide, Fungicide and Rodenticide Act (FIFRA), its responsibility for the regulation of occupational exposure to ionizing radiation under the Atomic Energy Act, and its general responsibility for the control of pollutants and the transport and disposal of toxic substances. EPA has broad regulatory authority over toxic substances pursuant to the Toxic Substances Control Act (TSCA), which is not specifically designed to regulate occupational exposures but has implications in the employment context, as comprehensive regulation of a chemical will have an impact on its use in the workplace.

Title VII of the Civil Rights Act, 42 U.S.C. §2000e, *et seq.,* and many similar state laws prohibit sex discrimination in employment, including discrimination on the basis of "pregnancy, childbirth, and related medical conditions." Discrimination is defined simply as different treatment, regardless of motive. Thus, a practice or policy that openly treats women differently, even if for purportedly benign purposes, would be apparently discriminatory under Title VII.

Nothing in any of these statutes indicates any Congressional intent to offer pregnant employees less or different legal protection. The laws are comprehensive in their design, the OSH Act, for example, promising a "clean and healthful workplace" to "every working man *and woman*" (emphasis added), and Title VII comprehensively prohibiting sex discrimination and other forms of discrimination in employment. These statutes would appear to disallow exclusionary policies, not only because such policies are discriminatory on their face but also because of their inherent admission that a hazardous condition exists. Read together, these laws appear to require that employers protect the health of *all* employees in a nondiscriminatory fashion, *i.e.,* to provide whatever degree of workplace safety and health protection is necessary to safeguard fully the employment rights of all workers. The validity of this proposition has implications beyond cases involving sex discrimination: although women (or their fetuses) have been the main focus of exclusionary employment practices, Blacks have also been targeted by employer medical policies on the theory that certain genetic characteristics may predispose them to occupationally induced illness. (Severo, 1980; Office of Technology Assessment, 1983).

Three federal courts of appeals have ruled on the legality of exclusionary employment policies under Title VII, and a fourth is currently considering the issue.[3] The appellate decisions to date all agree that policies that target pregnant or fertile women are discriminatory, even if the purported justification is a benign one related to health protection. Two courts accept the notion that some defense should be available, but in both cases the burden on the defense appears to be substantial (*Hayes* v. *Shelby Mem. Hosp.* 1984; *Wright* v. *Olin Corp* 1982).[4] For example, employers would have to show that the chemical or condition poses a significant or unreasonable risk, not just a speculative or hypothetical risk; that exposure at hazardous levels is likely to occur; that the risk is confined to the fetus in utero, i.e., the male reproductive system is not similarly susceptible to injury; and that such a substantial body of expert opinion in relevant fields supports this conclusion that "an informed employer could not responsibly fail to act." Neither of these courts explicitly describes the other kinds of risks to male reproductive health that would serve to undermine the validity of a female-specific policy. Heritable injuries clearly qualify, and other injuries such as infertility, damage to sperm, and sterility might also. *Hayes* indicates that a failure of consistency in overall health protection indicates that a fetal protection policy is a pretext for discrimination.

Even an otherwise justifiable policy would be unlawful if there is an alternative that would provide protection with a less discriminatory effect. An alternative is almost always available: engineering controls, product substitution, personal protective devices like respirators, voluntary transfers, and disability leave are all possible alternatives. The courts have not yet decided to what expense an employer can be put to provide nondiscriminatory approaches to workplace hazards.

One court has held that the OSH Act's "general duty clause" does not bar all exclusionary policies. In *OCAW* v. *American Cyanamid* (1984), the Court of Appeals for the District of Columbia held that the OSH Act's requirement that employers furnish workplaces "free from recognized hazards . . . likely to cause . . . serious physical harm" was not clearly intended to prohibit the use of exclusionary policies to limit reproductive hazards, but was aimed instead at chemical or other exposures posing direct individual health threats. This decision did not address the ability of OSHA to promulgate occupational exposure standards that would preclude use of exclusionary policies or fatally undermine the rationale for such policies. OSHA's authority in this regard has been upheld in another decision of the District of Columbia Court of Appeals. The court sustained OSHA's determination that lead adversely affects both male and female aspects of reproduction and held that OSHA "has statutory authority to protect the fetuses of lead-exposed working mothers. Harm to fetuses, as OSHA contends, is a material impairment of the reproductive systems of the parents." (*United Steelworkers of America* v. *Marshall* 1980). This court went further in affirming the degree of protection potentially afforded by the statute: "fertile women can find statutory protection from . . . discrimination [resulting from exclusionary policies] in the OSH Act's own requirement that OSHA standards ensure that '*no* employee will suffer material impairment of health. . . .' " This statement reflects this court's clear understanding that, even if hypersusceptible, fertile and pregnant women are entitled to the full protection of the OSH Act, at least so long as OSHA sets comprehensive standards.

The Need for Additional Legal Protections

Existing law should offer men and women adequate protection against work-related reproductive hazards and sex discrimination, but the courts have been reluctant to enforce the laws as fully as their language permits, and there is thus a need for unequivocal legislative direction. Some possible approaches and their implications are explained below.

The most obvious and direct way to address exclusionary policies is to require employers to provide a safe workplace and to prohibit use of exclusionary policies or sterility requirements to achieve that end. Such legislation would affirm its intent to protect against injury to the reproductive or sexual system, including impairment of the ability to produce healthy children, to the same extent that it protects against all other injuries or physical or functional impairments. And it should define injury to reproductive health broadly, to cover men and women and consequences for the offspring of either.

Such legislation should also directly prohibit the use of exclusionary policies and any other employer practices that might induce workers to alter their bodies in order to qualify for employment. This would legislatively reverse the decision in *OCAW* v. *American Cyanamid Co.* (1984), discussed previously, and make clear the legislative intent that employers bear the primary responsibility for carrying out the purposes of the law by improving workplace conditions, not by excluding certain workers.

Environmental legislation, which emphasizes regulation of chemical substances themselves, could be similarly revised explicitly to encompass unequivocal protection against reproductive injury, broadly defined to include injuries to adult males and females and to future offspring of either, and to prohibit any kind of exclusionary or other policy that shifts the burden for health protection to the individual from the maker or user of the chemical.[5]

Fair employment laws could also unequivocally define exclusionary policies, or policies that have similar effects, as discriminatory and therefore unlawful employment practices, to make clear that health-related employment needs must be resolved on a nondiscriminatory basis.

The law should safeguard the right of women workers to remain fertile (if they wish to do so) without negative economic consequences, and ensure that workplace health protection is afforded to all in a nondiscriminatory fashion. Emergencies may be handled either by suspending production until the hazard can be controlled, or, if complete control is impossible, by offering employees paid disability leave or transfers with no loss of pay or benefits. The law should remove any incentive to identify workers as hypersusceptible, while at the same time recognizing the possibility of hypersusceptibility and protecting individuals by assuring that no loss of rights or employment-related benefits can flow from their biological characteristics. This approach would be consistent, for example, with the legislative proscription on discrimination on the basis of handicap or disability. Although employers might prefer to avoid the costs associated with accommodating disabled employees, Congress has recognized their right to equal employment opportunity, at least to the extent of requiring reasonable accommodation.

Thus, employers may develop and enforce medical programs that affect job placement, but they must do so in a way that does not unfairly disadvantage workers because of sex or race and in a way that reasonably accommodates workers who are disabled within the meaning of the law. An employer may adopt a policy that provides transfer opportunities for workers whose job placement threatens their physical well-being, so long as the policy is voluntary, fairly administered, and does not have a disproportionately adverse effect on a particular group of employees. For example, a worker with a back condition might require a job that does not entail heavy lifting, a worker with a skin sensitivity to a particular substance ought not to have to work with the substance, and a worker with arthritis might need a light duty assignment. In some states, it is no defense to a charge of handicap discrimination that the employer was trying to prevent future injury or otherwise to protect a disabled employee.[6]

The rationales offered for exceptions to full application of these legal principles and in support of exclusion generally fail to withstand close scrutiny. Paramount among these is the necessity to avoid liability for injury to future children of women workers. Companies that have these policies, however, are frequently unable to cite a single instance in which such a lawsuit has been brought.[7] In contrast, numerous widely reported charges have been pressed by male workers that *their* workplace exposures have resulted in injury to their children.[8] This is not surprising, given the fact that more men than women are employed in many of these industries, and that men experience much greater cumulative occupational exposures per child born than do women.[9]

Hazardous chemicals abound in the chemical, petrochemical, and other heavy industries, which have most often adopted exclusionary practices. The production process, the use of products by consumers, and the disposal of waste by-products all involve significant risks intrinsic to the nature of these businesses. The recent discovery of dioxin contamination from disposal of industrial waste underscores this point. The Agent Orange claims, the Love Canal episode, the diethylstilbesterol (DES) lawsuits, and the problems resulting from asbestos exposure, kepone contamination, and the discharge of polychlorinated biphenyls (PCBs), all reveal the multiplicity and magnitude of risks that chemical and other manufacturing entails.[10] These and other examples reveal that the hazards posed by toxic chemicals extend beyond the work environment, beyond fetal risk, and beyond women. Policies that focus exclusively on women, as if they were the only "problem," deceptively suggest that the hazards posed by toxic chemicals are confined to this subgroup of the population. The goal of real protection is undermined by the perpetuation of this profit-oriented illusion.

One court has succinctly explained why the fear of liability should not excuse blatant sex discrimination:

> In today's litigious society, the potential for litigation rests in almost every human activity. For example, every employer faces the risk that a pregnant employee will encounter a workplace activity that would not normally be hazardous to a nonpregnant employee, but which could prove injurious to a developing fetus. These hazards range from slippery floors to uncontrolled cigarette smoke, asbestos, known and unknown carcinogenic materials used in the workplace and a plethora of other hazards of modern society. The employer is, of course, free to protect itself from financially ruinous lawsuits by purchasing insurance and by maintaining the degree of care required by law. (*Hayes* v. *Shelby Mem. Hosp.* 1984, 1553 n. 15)

An employer's best protection is to prevent foreseeable injury. The employer who conscientiously monitors the workplace environment, informs employees fully, abates known hazards, and when necessary

offers voluntary transfer without loss of pay or benefits will be best
insured against an adverse judgment. The law does not require an
employer to have a crystal ball—only to be prudent and diligent. That
this standard is frequently not satisfied is all too apparent from the
history of litigation over toxic exposures generally. Perhaps the formulation of policy and legislation regarding reproductive hazards will
provide an opportunity to insist that no less should be expected from
those whose profit-making activities expose others to potential hazards. Placing this burden on employers would result in cost-shifting,
as the increased costs associated with the requirement of a safe workplace ultimately get passed on to consumers. In this way, the product
or service more accurately reflects the true cost of production.

In sum, exclusionary policies exist both because of cost considerations and because of stereotypes; because women are viewed both
as marginal workers and as more physically vulnerable, and thus more
expensive employees. The costs may be those associated with cleanup,
with voluntary temporary transfer systems, with compound substitution of nontoxic materials, with more sophisticated and wearable personal protective equipment protection, or with insurance. Male
vulnerability, often ignored, ought to be as much a reason to incur
these costs as the danger to women and fetuses. The money necessary
to abate risks might be spent in various ways, but necessarily directed
at the goal of affording full employment rights without sacrificing safety
or bodily integrity. Congress has already mandated this approach: "even
a very high cost could not justify continuation of the policy of discrimination against pregnant women which has played such a major part in
the pattern of sex discrimination in this country" (U.S. Senate 1977,
11).

NOTES

This chapter is adapted from a paper presented at a conference, Reproductive
Laws for the 1990s, held in New York on May 4, 1987. The paper, with com-
mentaries, appears in a volume called *Reproductive Laws for the 1990s*, edited
by Sherrill Cohen and Nadine Taub and published by Humana Press, Clifton,
N.J. in 1989.

1. This citation was ultimately sustained with regard to the employer's failure
   to provide adequate training on the use of respirators. The company con-
   tended that the government had failed to prove exposures above the permissible levels because it had not taken readings *inside* respirators, and
   prevailed on that argument, notwithstanding the ironic result of the two

diverse holdings. An appeal was taken and the case was ultimately settled. *Secretary of Labor* v. *American Cyanamid Co.,* OSHRC Docket No. 79-2438.

2. Regarding risks of lead exposure generally, see Federal Register 43 (1978): 52,952–53,014. Recent evidence indicates that adult males may be at particular risk for cardiovascular disease from exposure to very low levels of lead. Federal Register 50 (1985): 9,386–9,408.

3. Litigation has focused on Title VII because private individuals cannot enforce the provisions of the OSH Act, a function reserved to the Department of Labor.

4. In the other case, *Zuniga* v. *Kleberg Co. Hosp.,* the court found an alternate basis to rule for the plaintiff and thus did not rule on the question of defense.

5. In particular, the Toxics Substances Control Act, 15 U.S.C. § 2601, *et seq.* grants the Environmental Protection Agency broad regulatory authority over chemical substances or mixtures; registration of pesticides comes under EPA jurisdiction pursuant to the Federal Insecticide, Fungicide and Rodenticide Act, 7 U.S.C. § 136, *et seq.*

6. Some conditions, such as obesity, may constitute a disability for employment discrimination purposes, even without an underlying medical cause and even though not a disability for purposes of receipt of rehabilitation services.

7. This kind of evidence is notably lacking from the record in the reported cases on this issue that have gone to trial: *EEOC* v. *Olin Corp.,* 24 FEP Cases 1615 (W.D. N.C. 1980), affirmed in part, reversed in part, and remanded *sub nom. Wright* v. *Olin Corp.,* 697 F.2d 1172 (4th Cir. 1982), and *Zuniga* v. *Kleberg County Hosp.* S.D. Tex., Civ. Action No. 77-C-62, Jan. 26, 1981) reversed, 692 F.2d 920 (5th Cir. 1982). *See also* deposition of Robert M. Clyne, M.D., May 16, 1983, p. 191, in *Christman* v. *American Cyanamid Co.,* 1980.

8. Lawsuits brought by male veterans who served in Vietnam and were exposed to the herbicide "agent orange" exemplify this point. Some actions allege birth defects in subsequently born children, miscarriages, and "serious maladies in servicemen." *See,* e.g., "Five Makers of Agent Orange Charge U.S. Misused Chemical in Vietnam: Companies Replying to Suit, Say Federal Negligence is Responsible for Any Harm to Veterans and Kin," *New York Times,* January 7, 1980. Male workers at a plant in Renssalaer, New York, also allege that their exposure to the herbicide oryzalin has resulted in birth defects in their children. They filed complaints with OSHA and the Environmental Protection Agency. "Union, Citing Birth Defects, Asks Ban On a Herbicide," *New York Times,* November 9, 1979.

9. A comparison of occupational experience preceding live births in 1976 reveals that the occupational exposure per conception is at least twice as great for males as for females. The calculation is based on the assumption that the working population procreates at the same rate as the nonworking population, an assumption that is probably far more true for men than for women. Thus, this figure represents a conservative estimate of the differences between male and female occupational exposure per birth. See V. R. Hunt 1979, 23–24.

10. Similarly, the semiconductor industry faces claims by residents of Santa Clara County, where water supplies have been contaminated by underground waste storage tanks.

BIBLIOGRAPHY

Becker, Mary E. 1986. From *Muller* v. *Oregon* to fetal vulnerability policies. *University of Chicago Law Review* 53, no. 4: 1219–73.
Christman v. *American Cyanamid Co.* 1980. Civil Action No. 80-0024P (N.D. W. Va.) *Second Amended Complaint* (filed Dec. 5, 1980).
Hayes v. *Shelby Memorial Hospital*, 726 F.2d 1543 (11th Cir. 1984).
Hunt, Vilma. 1979. *Work and the health of women.* Boca Raton, Fla.: CRC Press.
La Dou, Joseph, ed. 1986. *State of the art reviews: Occupational medicine: The microelectronics industry.* Philadelphia: Hanley and Belfus.
National Institute of Occupational Safety and Health. 1983. *Glycol ethers, 2-methoxyethanol and 2-ethoxyethanol. NIOSH Current Intelligence Bulletin 39.*
Occupational Safety and Health Administration, U.S. Department of Labor. 1978. Final standard for occupational exposure to lead. *Federal Register* 43:52,952–53,014.
Office of Technology Assessment. 1985. *Reproductive health hazards in the workplace.* Washington, D.C.: Government Printing Office.
———. 1984. *Preventing illness and injury in the workplace.* Washington, D.C.: Government Printing Office.
———. 1983. *The role of genetic testing in the prevention of occupational disease.* Washington, D.C.: Government Printing Office.
Oil, Chemical & Atomic Workers International Union v. *American Cyanamid Co.*, 741 F.2d 444 (D.C. Cir. 1984).
Paul, Maureen, and Jay Himmelstein. 1988. Reproductive hazards in the workplace: what the practitioner needs to know about chemical exposures. *Obstetrics and Gynecology* 71, no 6: 921–38.
Severo, Richard. 1980. Genetic tests by industry raise questions on rights of workers. *New York Times,* February 3.
Stellman, Jeanne Mager. 1979. The effects of toxic agents on reproduction. *Occupational health and safety,* April, 36–43.
———. 1977. *Women's work, women's health: Myths and realities.* New York: Pantheon Books.
U.S. Bureau of the Census, Department of Commerce. 1978. Fertility of American women: June 1977. *Current population reports,* series P-20, no. 325.
U.S. Department of Labor. 1980. *Protecting people at work: A reader in occupational safety and health.* Washington, D.C.: Government Printing Office.

U.S. Environmental Protection Agency. 1985a, January 9. Intent to cancel registrations of pesticides containing dibromochloropropane (DBCP). *Federal Register* 50: 1,122–30.

————. 1985b, March 7. Regulation of fuel and fuel additives: Gasoline lead content. *Federal Register* 50:9386–408.

————. 1985c, May 1. *Report of the teratology policy workgroup.* Excerpted in *Inside EPA Weekly Report,* July 5, 11–13.

U.S. Scientific Committee on the Effects of Atomic Radiation. 1977. *Sources and effects of ionizing radiation.* New York: United Nations.

U.S. Senate (1977). *Report No. 95–331,* Senate Subcommittee on Labor, Human Resources Committee. Washington, D.C.: Government Printing Office.

United Steelworkers of America v. *Marshall,* 647 F.2d 1189 (D.C. Cir. 1980), *cert. denied sub nom. Lead Industries Ass'n Inc.* v. *Donovan,* 453 U.S. 913 (1981).

Wright v. *Olin Corp.,* 697 F.2d 1172 (4th Cir. 1982).

Zuniga v. *Kleberg County Hospital,* 692 F.2d 986 (5th Cir. 1982).

Workplace Disability:
Gender, Technology, and the Experience
of Rheumatoid Arthritis

*Judith Fifield, Susan Reisine, Carol A. Pfeiffer,
and Glenn Affleck*

> Getting back to work is getting back to the mainstream. RA patients need
> something to get up and look forward to. We need to be motivated to
> "keep on goin on." You give up and you feed the disease. I want to work,
> to travel, to attend social events—otherwise you give up. I can't lay here
> in this bed, become satisfied with the condition and get where I want. I
> have to be a little bit dissatisfied with the condition.

This fifty-four-year-old unemployed black woman with the chronic disease rheumatoid arthritis (RA) expressed the concerns of many of her
fellow sufferers. Many women with RA perceive benefits of being in
paid employment, of being in the "mainstream." Getting back to work
or maintaining work in the face of RA is not, however, simply a matter
of the will to work or the severity of the disease.

As this woman went on to say, holding a job often depends on the
conditions under which the work is carried out. She was perfectly able
to do clerical work, but she needed flexible hours, and at times was
unable to work up to the quotas set in the office. She needed more
autonomy over the scheduling of her work, a characteristic of the work
environment that is not evenly distributed across all jobs. She, like
many others, was constrained to seek work in an environment that is
handicapping for women with RA. While such women have a serious,
often incapacitating sickness, the degree of disability they experience
is as much a feature of their technological and social environment as
their medical condition.

This chapter will explore the technological and relational barriers
that emerged in our study of the work environments of 131 women
with RA. The first two sections will look at the theoretical and medical
issues raised by RA; the next will discuss how gender and class structure technological and social environments. The illness experience of
these women with RA will then be analyzed in terms of their structured
locations. Finally, suggestions for social interventions will be made.

Theoretical Background

Although the dominant western medical model would lead us to believe otherwise, sickness is not a matter of disease alone (Young 1982a). Rather, it is composed of two distinct processes. Sickness includes the underlying pathophysiology and alterations in bodily states that produce disease and symptoms of disease and also the separate process by which individuals perceive, evaluate, and respond to symptoms in different ways. People vary in the amount of pain they perceive, if and how they reduce activity, when and how they define themselves as sick (Mechanic 1978). People can also respond to non-disease-related alterations in bodily states such as feelings of anger or anxiety "as if" they were symptoms of disease. Psychological distress, group definitions of disease, previous experience, and socialization processes are all thought to affect symptom perception (Barsky 1979; Linn et al. 1985; Tessler and Mechanic 1978). Kleinman (1983) has described this separate process of response to or perception of symptoms as the illness experience (Kleinman 1983).

We use this approach to draw attention to the fact that sickness has both a distinctly biophysiological (disease) as well as an experiential (illness) component. We believe, however, that to understand the illness experience, it must be considered within the constraints of existing social structures that shape the everyday life of individuals. When structural factors are excluded from the analysis, explanations of differences in individual's perceptions, evaluations, and response to symptoms will tend to locate the source of difference within the individual. As a result, they quite naturally suggest interventions that stress individual adaptation rather than social structural change.

We suggest that for women with RA, structural factors located in the workplace play an important role in shaping their illness experience. Consequently, we argue that interventions must be directed toward those factors as well as toward the disease process itself. Our study suggests an understanding of disease that differs from that of the dominant western medical model. It also suggests alternative strategies for intervention in RA, and a revision of the popular notion of RA as an invariably "crippling arthritis." While our inquiry will be based in part on quantitative analysis, it will be supported as well by the words of the women speaking from within their experience of the disease.

Medical Background

Rheumatoid arthritis is a chronic, often debilitating disease that includes inflammation in the joints and limitation in joint function. Women are affected two to three times more often than men with a peak incidence between the ages of forty and sixty. The disease of RA is characteristically accompanied by an illness experience including pain, morning stiffness, fatigue, and work disability (Rodman et al. 1983, 38). It is, in fact, a leading cause of functional disabilities and work loss (Bombardier and Tugwell 1983; Krute and Burdotte 1978). Little is known about how the loss of work shapes the person's experience of RA. Does it lead to increased reports of symptoms as studies in the nondiagnosed population have found (Verbrugge 1982)?

Medical research has found that the indicators of illness associated with RA (pain, fatigue, morning stiffness, and work disability) are neither random nor related solely to the severity of disease (Fries 1983). Among the more commonly reported causes of symptom exacerbation among RA patients are stress, excessive activity, and lack of exercise (Affleck et al. 1987; Rimon 1985). One study found that certain characteristics of paid work, such as having minimal schedule freedom and little control over the pace of work, are better predictors of work disability in RA than are characteristics of the disease itself (Yelin et al. 1980a; 1980b). This suggests that a process separate from the disease is operating to distribute the illness of RA across the population of persons with RA. Identifying social factors that appear to put people at risk for exacerbation of symptoms, or that put barriers in the way of their continued employment, will make an important contribution to the ongoing management of the condition.

For instance, the implementation of workplace technology can be either enabling or disabling. It can be done in ways that grant workers discretion over their work pace, their movement within the workplace, and their work hours. Conversely, it can be implemented in ways that increase constraints and pressures on workers. We stress that it is the structuring of workers' time and energy in the work process and not technology in terms of particular tools, machines, or techniques, that forces many women with RA out of the work force.

Salaman (1981), Edwards (1979), Machung (1984), Acker and Van Houten (1974) link this structuring of the work process to the historical development of gender and class relations. They argue that it takes the form of increasing institutionalization of methods of control via rules and regulations governing workers' time. Owners and managers gain as class conflict is controlled and the profit margin is protected and some men gain as male privilege is reinforced. Most workers, however, lose as their autonomy in the workplace is eroded. While this decreases options for all workers, it is especially hard on those with diseases such as RA whose ability to hold a job may depend on flexible schedules.

By focusing on the connections between the macro-level structures of class and gender and the micro-level experience of the illness associated with rheumatoid arthritis, we hope to contribute to the development of a structural understanding of illness, seeing the "person disabled within a handicapping environment" (Altman 1986).

Structuring of Paid Work

One's paid work, by virtue of its particular location within the social relations of production determines the amount of autonomy and rewards accrued. Jobs vary in the degree to which they offer control over the product, the production process, the activities of and the material benefits of labor (Wright 1978; Kalleberg and Griffin 1980). Control can be exercised in numerous ways including machine pacing of work, the imposition of daily production quotas, and such Tayloristic practices as the fragmentation and routinization of work (Salaman 1981). Owners and managers have extensive control over the product, the production process, the activities of labor, and material benefits while workers have proportionately little.

Gender relations contribute further to the social structuring of work. The normative assignment of women to housework and child-care creates barriers to their full and competitive participation in the market (Sokoloff 1980). Barriers include inadequate day care and non-participation by other family members in household work, such that women are left with the bulk of the care of others in the home even when they work outside. Other barriers include employers' perceptions of women as less serious or less able workers than men; thus women are less apt than men to obtain positions that offer control and authority, regardless of their occupation (Wright et al. 1982; Sokoloff 1986; Wolf and Fligstein 1979). Women are paid less than men for work of comparable worth and are segregated into the lowest-paid market sectors, occupations, and jobs within firms. Women are also disproportionately exposed to machine-based control as they are crowded into typically "women's work." Machung (1984) has described the case for clericals.

> For managers, those who design, manufacture, sell and administer the new technology, automation does mean more control over labor costs, faster and more complete information and higher levels of expertise, responsibility and salary. But for clericals, automation means something completely different: more routinized jobs, more standardized work, greater pressure, and less sociability. (1984, 132)

These factors combine to disadvantage women in the competition for autonomy and the rewards of the market (Reskin and Roos 1985; Bielby and Baron 1984; Treiman and Hartmann 1981). Minority women are doubly disadvantaged as they have the added effect of race working to crowd them into the least desirable work assigned to women (Mullings 1984).

Because of these class, race, and gender factors the range of illness risks associated with paid work are not randomly distributed. Previous research has linked the lack of workplace autonomy among men with an increased risk of developing coronary heart disease (Karasek 1979). Both men and women who perceive low work autonomy experience increased headaches, hypertension, and depression (Hall and Savery 1986). Being out of the paid work force, however, is associated with more illness than is being employed (Verbrugge 1982). Among the non-employed, those with a preference for work appear to be more adversely affected in terms of illness (Verbrugge 1982).

People with RA may also be at risk for increased illness when their class location greatly limits personal control in the workplace. They may be at risk for more symptoms as a result of the stress associated with a lack of control or as a result of the inability to obtain the proper balance of rest and activity. As Yelin et al. (1980a; 1980b) found, they may also be at risk for an increased probability of exclusion from work. If the exclusion is personally distressing, it too can be a source of symptom exacerbation.[1]

Gender places additional barriers in the way of individuals with RA. Employers are less likely to invest in women workers (Corcoran and Duncan 1979; Bielby and Baron 1985). Women may be more likely than men to be excluded either because they are viewed as expendable, or because they are unable to establish control and autonomy vis-à-vis their employers. The combination of this gender-based risk and the class-based risk discussed above may explain the fact that women with disabilities (not specifically RA) experience more unemployment and underemployment than do comparable men (Vash 1982).

In light of these findings, we expect women with RA to be at risk for worse illness outcomes (e.g., more work disability and higher reports of pain and depression) to the extent that their paid work places them in a handicapping environment. This environment would be one that offered insufficient control and autonomy to accommodate the needs of RA patients. They are, in effect, placed in a relationship to the tools and procedures of their work that is disabling rather than enabling. Their work environment is incompatible with the maintenance of paid employment. Once excluded from work, women with

RA are expected to be at greater risk of increased perception of symptoms due to the economic and social psychological distress that accompanies work exclusion.

In our study we expected to find that the disabling characteristics of the work environment were important factors in exclusion and its consequences. We expected disease characteristics to play an important role, as well. It is the relative importance of these factors that we explore here.

Sample and Methods

The 131 women who participated in this study are all patients with definite or classical RA who attend either a large rheumatology clinic at a teaching hospital or a private rheumatology practice.[2] They were each contacted by their physicians about participation in the study and then interviewed by two members of the research team. Each woman was interviewed twice. One interview was conducted by telephone with a structured format regarding the details of the woman's work history, and one was conducted in the home and focused on her beliefs as to the causes of the disease, her experience of symptoms, and her process of coping with the disease. It was during the in-home interviews that the women spoke in depth about their experience of the disease, i.e., their illness. The quotations are taken from those interviews.

Evaluations of disease characteristics were obtained from the attending clinicians. Each patient's clinician was asked to fill out a physical assessment form developed by the project directors and the clinic faculty. The severity rating was based on the American Rheumatism Association's criteria of degree of joint erosion, deformity, and muscle atrophy. The drug therapy variable was also based on the physician's report of being on one of five remittive agents. These drugs are intended to produce a remission in the disease and therefore could be important in explaining work capacity.

The class location of the respondent's reported occupation at onset was measured by the Hollingshead scale and collapsed into three categories for this analysis: professional, white-collar, and blue-collar.[3] The control over production question asked respondents how much control they had over the pace of their work, what was produced, and what tools were used (responses could be "superior," "self and superior," "self and co-worker," or "self alone"). The control over work activities question asked how much discretion the person had over taking a break, leaving to go to the doctor, taking a day off, a week off, or deciding when to come in to work (response categories were "without permission," "inform supervisor," "get permission," or "couldn't do"). High control should create a relationship to work that allows for accommodation of the temporal constraints of RA, including morning stiffness and flares in symptoms. The physical nature of work was based on the respondent's report of mostly mental, partly physical, and mostly physical work.

The dependent variable "work exclusion" was measured by the respondent's report of having been employed at the onset of the disease and still being employed at the time of the interview versus having been employed at the time of onset and no longer employed at the time of the interview. Persons no longer employed were considered to be excluded from work, a category that encompasses both those technically unemployed (out of work and seeking employment) and those out of the labor force entirely.

Pain was measured by the question "How much pain have you had in the last week?" A visual analogue scale was used that allowed respondents to rate their current pain from zero to one hundred. Depression was measured on the Center for Epidemiologic Studies–Depression Scale (CES-D), an instrument that is specially constructed to avoid questions that elicit symptoms characteristic of a chronic disease. It has high internal consistency and test-retest reliability, with minimal correlations between the test and age, social class, or sex (Radloff 1977). A score of sixteen and above is generally interpreted as reflecting clinical depression. Studies have reported a mean score of 9.25 for a general population and 24.42 for an inpatient psychiatric population using the CES-D (Radloff 1977).

Results

The average respondent was a white woman of middle age with at least one year of college, a family income of $23,000, with moderately severe disease of greater than five years duration. Only 5 percent of the sample was Black or Hispanic. Surprisingly, the majority (58 percent) of this sample of women was still working. At onset, twenty-five (19 percent) women were employed in professional occupations, seventy-three (56 percent) in white-collar, and thirty-three (25 percent) in blue-collar work. While the majority of professional women (48 percent) and a substantial minority of white-collar women (28 percent) reported high control over the production process (the pace of work, what was produced, and how it was done), they were not characteristic of the sample. The majority of white-collar (45 percent) and blue-collar women (67 percent) reported little or no control over those factors. The majority of women in all three work locations (88 percent professional, 81 percent white-collar, and 97 percent blue-collar) reported low to moderate control over their work activities (including work schedule and discretion over leaving work for rest or physician visits). The majority of professional (68 percent) and white-collar women (62 percent) reported work that was part mental and part physical, while blue-collar women (52 percent) reported predominantly physical work.

It is interesting to note that being defined as professional does not necessarily imply control in all spheres of work. Professional women and many white-collar women reported high control over the production process but only low to moderate control over their time. Blue-collar women report little or no product control but moderate time control. They also do predominately physical work. As Sokoloff (1987) and others have shown, this finding may reflect the extent to which, despite certain nominal occupational attainments, women as a group remain in subordinate positions. Gender as a system of control may depress the autonomy of women as a group such that they are not accorded control in the workplace equal to comparably placed males.[4]

Our first hypothesis posited that the exclusion from work (loss of work since disease onset) experienced by these women with RA would best be explained by the extent to which their work environment disabled them. Specifically, we expected that a low degree of control over the technological process and the activities of work would better explain work loss than would characteristics of the disease. This hypothesis was tested using multiple classification analysis. The results are displayed in table 1.

Controlling for current age, income at onset, and education at onset, four variables emerged as significant predictors of work exclusion. Low control over the activities of work at onset and current disease severity were the strongest predictors of work exclusion. As expected, the control factor was more important than the severity rating. Other significant predictors were the class location of work at onset and disease of greater than five years' duration. The physical nature of the work itself was not significant as a predictor. It is moderately correlated with blue-collar work ($r = .46$, $p < .01$), which emerged as the better predictor of the two, but a weaker predictor than was autonomy over work schedule, which had the strongest relationship with a beta of $-.36$.

The relative importance of autonomy and physical work is an important finding because it contradicts popular notions of how disease disables workers. People may assume that the problems blue-collar workers face in continuing employment are primarily physical (i.e., blocked access to the facility, or inability to lift weight or operate machinery). While certain technologies (e.g., special chairs, variable-height work stations, electric beds) obviously ease the physical barriers to work, autonomy over one's activities at work is more important in determining the ability to maintain employment. Being able to come in late and to go home late if it is a particularly stiff morning, to leave one's machine or desk or patients as needed, to have discretion over sick time, vacation time, and doctor visit time, all appear to be more important than the physical technology of the work or the severity of the disease. These women are not merely "unemployed"; they have been pushed out of their work by the socially created conditions of their work process.

TABLE 1. Analysis of variance of work exclusion in women with RA: controlling for age, education, and income at onset of RA

	% Excluded	Beta	N
Severity			
Mild	26		(30)
Moderate	38		(65)
Severe	64	0.28**	(33)
Duration of RA			
< 5 years	39		(43)
> 5 years	43	0.04**	(85)
Remittive Therapy			
No	42		(24)
Yes	42	0.00	(104)
Occupation			
Professional White-Collar	39		(97)
Blue-Collar	50	0.09*	(31)
Physical Nature			
Mental	34		(34)
Mental/Physical	43		(72)
Physical	52	0.12	(22)
Production Control			
Low	37		(61)
Medium	48		(30)
High	46	0.10	(37)
Activity Control			
Low	65		(43)
Medium	34		(67)
High	15	0.36**	(18)
Grand Mean = 42% excluded			

$R^2 = .35$
*$p < .05$
**$p < .01$

These findings are illustrated by the experience of a Hispanic woman with mild disease who was unable to remain in paid work as a sewing machine operator.

> When the disease began I didn't know what it was. I was sitting at a sewing machine for forty hours a week. I was thinking of taking off some time and having it checked out but the kind of job I did have, there wasn't any coverage, no insurance or anything, so if I did leave I would lose the income. It wasn't a big-paying job. I make $150 per week, and take home $130, so I have to be careful and take in the forty hours in order to come home with something. I was turned down for disability.

Although her clinically mild disease did not meet the official eligibility requirements for disability she was nonetheless disabled by both the conditions of her work and the paucity of benefits it provided. Not only was she locked into a job that kept her in the same position for hours and hours (leading to joint stiffening in many people with RA) but she was also constrained to keep trying to work even with these difficulties as she could not afford to miss time. There was no compromise situation available to her. It was either work under the prevailing conditions or be excluded from paid work altogether.

The fifty-four-year-old unemployed clerical worker who spoke of her desire to "get back into the mainstream" also spoke about the process of her exclusion and its relation to issues of autonomy, control over time, and respect for workers. Referring to a job she was unable to keep due to office quotas, she said:

> That wasn't work at your own pace—you had to do a certain amount of work a day. I worked a full-time job for twenty years and they told me I wasn't capable of doing anything and that is what got me. . . . they didn't give me medical disability, they called it "inability to meet standards."

Note the emphasis on her as the source of her work inability rather than work standards that were too restrictive for a woman with a chronic disease.

Compare these excluded women with two white women still working at the time of interview. The first woman is a health physicist with moderately severe disease. She describes a great deal of control over the pace of her work, her relation to the tools and procedures of her work, and her work environment, but little control over her schedule. If a power plant needs to be tested on a particular day she must be there "even if she has to crawl." Regarding the issues she can control, she says:

> Out in the field, I've told my boss, I'm not going to schlep those boxes—it's not worth it to me. If you can't deal with it on my expenses, it's too bad . . . but I will do it when I can get someone. There were several months when I couldn't do certain samples 'cause I couldn't hold the bottles—so the lab paid $70 a sample to send them out to be done and they didn't say anything to me. Apparently my work was worth that to them.

While she may need to "crawl to work," this woman's situation is vastly different from those of the two workers above. She is in charge of the test and she decides that she must go. She also has discretion over the conditions of her work, and importantly, her employer treats her in ways that validate her worth as a worker. These perceptions of value and discretion stand in stark contrast to the perception of the first two workers as "damaged goods."

A second example of a woman with a great deal of control and autonomy is a forty-nine-year-old nurse-consultant with moderately severe disease. She moved from staff nursing, which was much more hands-on and was tied to a less flexible schedule, to her current job where she is able to

> plan a day in a well-thought-out fashion, get up and move around frequently, sit in a well-supporting chair, have a car with power steering, power windows, and a seat that is just right. I was also able to obtain household help.

This woman illustrates another way in which the class location of work offers control that enables rather than disables. She was able to make a lateral move within the professional ranks of nursing that carried with it more of the control over health technology that she required. On the other hand, service work, low-level clerical and health care work offer limited options for such lateral moves.

Among eight women in the study, all of whom were employed as health care workers at onset, those still working were the four professional registered nurses (RN) who now work respectively as, a consultant, a school nurse, an administrator, and a teacher. Those no longer employed were a technical nurse (LPN) and two nurses' aides who were engaged in direct patient care and were not allowed discretion over their schedule or the tools of their work. The fourth unemployed health care worker was a registered nurse who had worked very little since her marriage and unsuccessfully tried reentry after the onset of the disease.

The experience of these women strongly suggests that structured work factors are important factors along with disease factors in the process of their exclusion from paid work. However, as we found, in the multivariate analysis, work factors are more important as predictors than are disease factors.

Just how important work factors are as a cluster was tested by looking at their ability to explain the variance in work exclusion for the entire sample, after disease variables and the covariates of age, education, and income at onset had explained all that they could. The Venn diagram in figure 1 shows the relative importance of the three clusters of variables. Disease variables explain 7 percent of the total variance in work exclusion found in this study, the covariates explained another 7 percent, and work factors accounted for twice as much as either of these two clusters alone (15 percent of the total variance). There was very little overlap between the clusters, as the shared variance was only 6 percent. There were no interactions between the variables. That is, people were not boosted into a higher category of risk if they were in two risky categories simultaneously. They would have only the additive risk of those two categories, not a multiplicative risk.

These findings contradict popular notions of how disease severity and work conditions influence disability. People assume that work characteristics are exclusion risks only for those with severe disease. This analysis suggests that, on the contrary, work characteristics can be a

Figure 1. Apportioning variance explained in work exclusion. These results were obtained using multiple classification analysis. The total variance explained in work exclusion was .35.

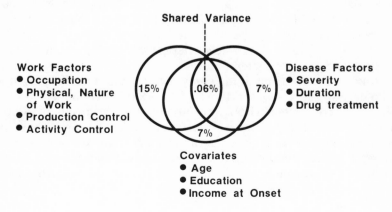

risk for exclusion at any level of severity. The worker may be at risk long before the disease progresses beyond the mild or moderate stage. Similarly, work characteristics can be of sufficiently low additive risk such that people with high disease severity can continue to work. This finding supports those who argue that the western medical model needs to be reconceptualized, as it does not acknowledge a separate, independent effect for social factors on illness outcomes.

Consequences of Exclusion

Community studies suggest that one of the consequences of exclusion from paid work is an increase in the illness experience in terms of perceived symptoms. The women in this sample reinforced this notion as they spoke of the perceived psychological and physical health benefits associated with work and the negative effects of exclusion. As pointed out earlier, the symptoms of RA increase with stress for many people. The mechanism by which stress affects symptoms is not known, but it is thought that it either alters immunity resulting in more disease, or that it causes people to focus on the symptoms they have (Rogers et al. 1982; Baker 1981). We hypothesized that the increased economic and social psychological distress that accompany the loss of work would adversely affect the illness experience of these women in terms of increased pain and depression.

In figure 2 we examine the consequences of exclusion from work on the experience of pain among these women with RA. For the sample as a whole, employed women report significantly less pain than do those excluded. They are not, however, pain free. It is important to note that the disease severity cannot explain the lower levels of pain. While on average workers are more likely to have milder disease, the difference in reported pain is found among those with both moderate and severe disease. Pain increases with disease severity for both workers and women excluded from work, but much more sharply for the latter group. These data suggest that both severity and work status have an effect on pain. They also suggest that it is possible to continue working with even severe disease and high levels of pain, but that exclusion is associated with more perception of pain. The causal connections cannot be worked out with this cross-sectional data, but the words of one working woman support the notion of pain as a consequence of exclusion.

> When I was home alone on the pity pot I would really feel bad. But when I was out to work and getting involved with the activities of the day—I'd

forget about it. I'd still have the pain, but I'd forget about it. (middle-aged nurse administrator)

The effects of work exclusion on depression, another common consequence of RA, are similar. In figure 3 we examine the depression scores of those women still working and those excluded, while controlling for disease severity. The workers have significantly lower depression scores in all categories of disease severity. Depression increases with the severity of the disease for both groups, but among employed women only those with the most severe disease score above the general population mean for depression. In contrast, even those women with mild disease who are excluded from the work force have elevated levels of depression.

An examination of the mean depression scores (fig. 3) suggests that while the excluded women score above the normal population in all categories of severity, their average score is less than would indicate clinical depression (a score of sixteen or above). A look at the full range of scores, however, finds 40 percent of the excluded above the cut-off score of sixteen for a diagnosis of clinical depression, while only 12 percent of the workers score above that point. Disabling environments that figure so heavily in work exclusion for these women also reveal themselves in the experience of pain and depression. These

Figure 2. Consequences of work exclusion for women with RA: felt pain scores by disease severity and work status.

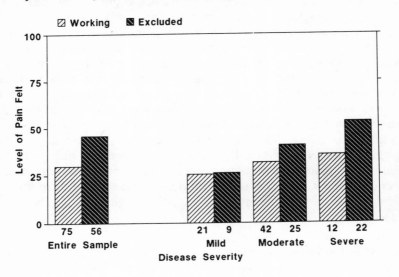

Figure 3. Consequences of work exclusion for women with RA: CES-D depression scores by disease severity and work status.

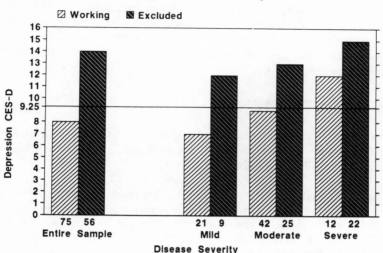

findings are further supported by those of Reisine et al. (1986). They were able to show that these same women suffered less role impairment if they were employed and less depression from the impairments they had, concluding that their work provides a buffer to the depression that so often accompanies RA.

Just as the workers above clearly understood the factors that had excluded them from their work, so they understood the connection between that exclusion and their symptom perception.

> I want to work—I'm willing to work, but what I've got won't allow me to—to do the kind of work I'm used to. It's kind of scary. I don't know which morning I'll be able to get up and get dressed and go out to work. I just can't even get a shower. The pressure—just thinking about it brings it [the symptoms] on more. (middle-aged machine operator)

> I went into a complete depression. Produce or get out! (fifty-four-year-old clerical)

Much of the earlier work on depression and RA established a connection between the two but suggested that depression was a function of the disease alone (Anderson et al. 1986). A more recent study reports that over time, the strongest predictors of change in depression in RA patients are declines in income, less education, and disease of longer duration (Hawley 1987); however, this study fails to relate low education and income loss to job exclusion. Our study goes a step further by suggesting that depression is a consequence of structured, handicapping environments. Lower levels of income and education may be surrogates measuring the effects of access to less flexible and autonomous jobs, not some characteristics of the individuals that directly affect depression.

Implications for Intervention

Interventions that go beyond those suggested by the western medical model have already been urged by some major figures in arthritis research, as the following quotation attests:

> Serologic and chemical abnormalities may provide information about pathogenesis, and physical and anatomic variables may aid in diagnosis, but it is the social, psychological, vocational and sexual consequences that make the ultimate difference between adequate and inadequate treatment, humane and uninterested care, and enablement and disablement. (Ehrlich 1983)

The findings of this study clearly point to the salience of paid work for women and their experience of RA, and underline the need for workplace interventions as a part of "humane care." While class and gender relations structure the home and the workplace in ways that are disadvantageous for women in general, they can be seen as having unique disadvantages for women with chronic disease.

As many as one-quarter of patients with RA (which affects women two to three times more often than men) and up to two-thirds of patients with other rheumatic diseases are denied disability benefits each year (Abeles 1987). A major obstacle for them is the fact that disability eligibility is based on a medical model that their conditions do not meet. The eligibility problem is compounded for women because they may be either outside the labor force altogether or employed part-time. Teachers, largely female, do not pay social security in some states. Consequently, even if they do meet the medical criteria, they are not eligible for either of the government disability programs that are tied to social security. They must draw on their pensions which often provide inadequate monthly benefits (Cook 1987). We argue that structural sources of disability must be considered when evaluation for disability takes place. We do not, however, argue that being granted disability is either desired by or desirable for many women with RA. Women benefit both psychologically and physically from being in paid employment, even with a chronic disease.

If health care providers and professionals who design intervention strategies are to provide humane care they must become more aware of the structural sources of disability and how the handicapping environment reveals itself in the illness experience. Interventions must go beyond the technology used in production (i.e., typewriter keyboards, chairs, etc.) to the technology used to control the work force (timecards, keystroke monitoring). Health care professionals should recognize that while the redesign of the physical workplace may aid some, the redesign and redefinition of the social relations that structure the work environment will potentially aid many more.

This will not, however, occur unless the problem is raised in circles that go beyond those suggested by the traditional western medical model. A first step toward the kind of social intervention that is needed is for chronically ill workers themselves to recognize the roots of their exclusion and its consequences. They must then turn to their co-workers, their unions, and other concerned groups for aid in legitimizing their concerns. Within this context, health care practitioners can be important contributors to the kind of social change that is necessary in treating the illness experience associated with RA.

NOTES

This research was supported by grants from the Arthritis Foundation and the National Institutes of Health. The authors are indebted to Myra Marx Ferree for her thoughtful comments and critical editorial advice on this manuscript. We would also like to thank Howard Tennen, Carol Goodenow, and Kathleen Grady for their contributions to this study, as well as the many women with RA who shared their experiences with us.

1. The term *exclusion* was chosen over *disabled* or *unemployed* for two reasons. First, it puts the emphasis on the structural source of the loss rather than the individual. Second, it is a broader term than *unemployed*. *Excluded* includes those officially unemployed, that is, out of work but looking, as well as those not included in unemployment statistics, as they are not looking for work. In the case of those with RA they may be unable to look, or may be discouraged as they are unable to find accommodating work.

2. The American Rheumatism Association has adopted criteria to establish uniform diagnostic procedures in all of the rheumatic diseases. In RA there are four diagnostic categories, each having certain criteria that must be met before a person can be considered as having that category of RA. The four categories are classical, definite, probable, or possible RA. The clinical

322   Healing Technology

faculty advising on this study recommended the inclusion of only the most positive diagnostic categories of classical and definite. See Rodman et al. (1983) for a more complete discussion of these criteria.
3. Hollingshead's (1958) occupational scale was used to locate respondents' work in the class structure. Respondents' own occupation was used. For the purposes of this analysis occupational groups 1 and 2 were labeled professional, groups 3 and 4 white-collar, and groups 4, 5, and 6 blue-collar.
4. This also suggests that status-ranking criteria for assigning class location, as used in this analysis, may not be the best approach, as these measures do not capture the dimensions of control thought to structure illness outcomes. The use of occupation as an indicator of class location is, itself, problematic. See Wright (1980) for a Marxist perspective on the problem. See Marsh (1986) and Garnsey (1978) for a discussion of the difficulties involved in using occupation as an indicator for women who are so often outside the work force. See Goldthorpe (1983) for an opposing view. Przeworski (1977) has proposed a scheme for the inclusion of both women and the disabled in what he calls the "excluded class."

REFERENCES

Abeles, Micah. 1987. Unpublished grant application, University of Connecticut Health Center. Citing personal communication with the former Social Security Administration chief medical officer, Dr. Herbert Blumenfeld.
Acker, Joan, and Donald R. Van Houten. 1974. Differential recruitment and control: The sex structuring of organizations. *Administrative Science Quarterly* 19, no.2: 152–63.
Affleck, Glenn, Carol Pfeiffer, Howard Tennen, and Judith Fifield. 1987. Attributional processes in rheumatoid arthritis patients. *Arthritis and Rheumatism* 30, no. 8: 927–31.
Altman, Barbara. 1986. Definitions of disability in empirical research: Is the use of administrative definition co-opting the results of disability research? Paper presented at the American Sociological Association meetings, New York, New York, August 31.
Anderson, Karen, Lawrence Bradley, Larry Young, and Lisa McDaniel. 1986. Psychological aspects of arthritis. In *Textbook of rheumatology*, ed. R. Turner and C. Wise, 178–213. New York: Elsevier Science.
Baker, G. H. B. 1981. Psychological management. *Clinics in Rheumatic Diseases* 7, no.2: 455–67.
Barsky, Arthur. 1979. Patients who amplify bodily sensations. *Annals of Internal Medicine* 91, no.1: 63–70.
Bielby, William, and James Baron. 1987. Undoing discrimination: Job integration and comparable worth. In *Ingredients for women's employment policy*, ed. C. Bose and G. Spitze, 211–29. Albany: State University of New York Press.

Bombardier, Claire, and Peter Tugwell. 1983. Measuring disability: Guidelines for rheumatology studies. *Journal of Rheumatology Supplement* 10, no.10: 68–73.

Cook, Patricia. 1987. Personal communication with member of the Connecticut Governor's Taskforce on Women and the Workplace.

Corcoran, Mary, and George Duncan. 1979. Work history, labor force attachment, and earnings differences between the races and the sexes. *Journal of Human Resources* 1, no. 14: 3–20.

Edwards, Richard. 1979. *Contested terrain: The transformation of the workplace in the twentieth century.* New York: Basic Books.

Fries, James F. 1983. Toward an understanding of patient outcome measurement. *Arthritis and Rheumatism* 26, no.6: 697–704.

Garnsey, Elizabeth. 1978. Women's work and theories of social stratification. *Sociology* 12, no.2: 223–44.

Goldthorpe, John H. 1983. Women and class analysis: In defence of the conventional view. *Sociology* 17, no.4: 465–88.

Hadler, Norman. 1985. *Arthritis and society.* London: Butterworths.

Hall, Kenneth, and Lawson K. Savery. 1986. Tight rein, more stress: Authority with strings attached puts managers under severe pressure. *Harvard Business Review* 64, no.3: 160–64.

Hawley, Donna. 1987. Anxiety and depression in rheumatoid arthritis: A four year study of 400 RA patients. Paper presented at the Arthritis Health Professionals Association national meeting, Washington, D.C.

Hollingshead, August B., and Frederick C. Redlich. 1958. *Social class and mental illness.* New York: Wiley.

Kalleberg, Arne L., and Larry J. Griffin. 1980. Class, occupation and inequality in job rewards. *American Journal of Sociology* 85, no.4: 731–68.

Karasek, Robert A. 1979. Job demands, job decision latitude and mental strain: implications for job redesign. *Administrative Science Quarterly* 24, no.2: 285–308.

Kleinman, Arthur. 1983. Editor's note. *Culture, Medicine and Psychiatry* 7, no.1: 97–99.

Krute, Aaron, and Mary Ellen Burdette. 1978. 1972 survey of disabled and non-disabled adults: chronic disease, injury and work disability. *Social Security Bulletin* 41, no. 4: 3–17.

Linn, Margaret, Richard Sandifer, and Shayna Stein. 1985. Effects of unemployment on mental and physical health. *American Journal of Public Health* 75, no.5: 502–6.

Machung, Anne. 1984. Word processing: forward for business, backward for women. In *My troubles are going to have trouble with me,* ed. Karen Brodkin Sacks and Dorothy Remy, 124–139. New Brunswick, N.J.: Rutgers University Press.

Marsh, Catherine. 1986. Social class and occupation. In *Key variables in social investigation,* ed. Robert G. Burgess, 123–52. London: Routledge and Kegan Paul.

Mechanic, David. 1978. Sex, illness, illness behavior and use of health services. *Social Science and Medicine* 12B, no.3: 207–14.

Mullings, Leith. 1984. Minority women, work and health. In *Double exposure: Women's health hazards on the job and at home*, ed. Wendy Chavkin, 121–38. New York: Monthly Review Press.

Przeworski, Adam. 1977. Proletariat into a class: The process of class formation from Karl Kautsky's *The class struggle* to recent controversies. *Politics and Society* 7, no.4: 343–401.

Radloff, Lenore. 1977. The CES-D scale: A self-report depression scale for research in the general population. *Applied Psychological Measurement.* 1, no.3: 385–401.

Reisine, Susan 1985. The impact of RA on the homemaker. Paper presented at the annual meeting of the Arthritis Health Professionals Association. Los Angeles, June 4.

Reskin, Barbara, and Patricia Roos. 1985. Status hierarchies and sex segregation. In *Ingredients for women's employment policy*, ed. Christine Bose and Glenna Spitze, 3–22. Albany: State University of New York Press.

Rimon, Ranan, and Riikka-Liisa Laakso. 1985. Life stress and RA: A 15 year follow-up study. *Psychotherapy and Psychosomatics* 43, no.1: 38–43.

Rodman, Gerald P., H. Ralph Schumacher, and Nathan J. Zvaifler. 1983. *Primer on the rheumatic diseases.* 8th ed. Atlanta: Arthritis Foundation.

Rogers, Malcolm P., Matthew H. Liang, and Allison Partridge. 1982. Psychological care of adults with rheumatoid arthritis. *Annals of internal medicine* 96, no.3: 344–48.

Salaman, Graeme. 1981. *Work organization and class structure.* New York: M. E. Sharpe.

Sokoloff, Natalie. 1980. *Between money and love: The dialectics of women's home and market work.* New York: Praeger.

———. 1987. The increase of black and white women in the professions: a contradictory process. In *Ingredients for women's employment policy*, ed. Christine Bose and Glenna Spitze, 53–73. Albany: State University of New York Press.

Tessler, Richard, and David Mechanic. 1978. Psychological distress and perceived health status. *Journal of Health and Social Behavior* 19, no.3: 254–62.

Treiman, Donald, and Heidi Hartmann. 1981. *Women, work and wages: Equal pay for jobs of equal value.* Washington, D.C.: National Academy Press.

Vash, Carolyn. 1982. Employment issues for women with disabilities. *Rehabilitation Literature* 43, no.7–8: 198–207.

Verbrugge, Lois. 1982. Work satisfaction and physical health. *Journal of Community Health* 7, no.4: 262–83.

Wolf, Wendy, and Neil Fligstein. 1979. Sex and authority in the workplace: The cause of sexual inequality. *American Sociological Review* 44, no.2: 235–52.

Wright, Erik O. 1978. *Class, crisis and the state.* London: Verso.

———. 1980. Class and occupation. *Theory and society* 9, no.1: 177–214.

Wright, Erik O., Cynthia Costello, David Hachin, and Joey Sprague. 1982. The American class structure. *American Sociological Review* 47, no.6: 709–26.

Yelin, Edward, Robert Meenan, Michael Nevitt, and Wallace Epstein. 1980. Work disability in R.A.: Effects of disease, social and work factors. *Annals of Internal Medicine* 93, no.4: 551–56.

Yelin, Edward, Michael Nevitt, and Wallace Epstein. 1980. Toward an epidemiology of work disability. *Milbank Memorial Fund Quarterly/Health and Society* 58, no.3: 386–415.

Young, Allan. 1982. The anthropologies of illness and sickness. *Annual Review of Anthropology* 11:257–85.

Effects of Solvent Exposure and Occupational Stress on the Health of Blue-Collar Women

Mary Amanda Dew, Evelyn J. Bromet, David K. Parkinson, Leslie O. Dunn, and Christopher M. Ryan

Organic solvent exposure is one of the most common toxic exposures in the workplace (Axelson, Hane, and Hogstedt 1980). Solvents are found in adhesives (e.g., glues, cements) and paints used in manufacturing new products, they are used in lubricating agents for production equipment, and they serve as major cleaning agents both for equipment and for newly finished products. Unlike worker health hazards that are unique to a specific technology and thus can be studied within the context of that technology, solvent exposure is a potential health threat to workers employed in such diverse settings as electronics, jewelry, textiles, boot and shoe, rubber, paint, and dry cleaning industries.

We already know that high levels of solvent exposure have acute, toxic effects on the central nervous system (Baker and Fine 1986; Cavanagh 1985). Case reports of exposed workers began to appear during the nineteenth century (Elofsson et al. 1980), and these reports and additional clinical studies have described the disorientation, euphoria, giddiness, convulsions, and even death that can result from high-level occupational solvent exposures (Browning 1965). More recently, a number of large-scale, epidemiologic studies have shown that, even at relatively low levels, solvent exposure may lead to health problems (e.g., Axelson, Hane, and Hogstedt 1976; Lindström 1973), and government standards for worker exposure are present in many countries. Unfortunately, there is now some indication that exposure at levels even lower than government standards may remain associated with (*a*) a variety of somatic complaints, including fatigue, headache, and irritability, (*b*) symptoms of psychological distress, and (*c*) neuropsychological deficits, particularly in the areas of manual dexterity and analyzing and synthesizing visual information (e.g., Elofsson et al. 1980).

Both the research findings and the government standards are based on studies of male workers; the consequences of such exposure for women have never been systematically studied. The paucity of research on the potential health effects of solvent exposure in women is all the

327

more striking given that over six million women in the United States—
14 percent of the female labor force—are employed in blue-collar occupations, many of which involve exposure to chemicals. It may be
tempting to suggest that solvent exposure has only recently become a
women's health issue, and therefore a research issue, as the female
work force has expanded into previously male-intensive jobs. However,
as Hunt (1979, 97) notes when remarking on the traditional lack of
concern for women's health in industry, "it is scarcely necessary to
invoke some new rising tide of women experiencing a chemical environment markedly different from what they have always known." Many
technologies in which solvents play a vital role—the rubber, paint, boot
and shoe industries, and many manufacturing concerns in small communities—have relied heavily on a female labor force for the last eighty
years (Hunt 1979).

Two bodies of research suggest a possible relationship between
low-level solvent exposure and women's health. First, two small clinical
studies found some exposure effects similar to the physical and psychological symptoms reported for male workers (Maroni et al. 1977;
Matsushita et al. 1975). The data also showed that the women's physical
and mental health was strongly related to the occupational stress of
monotonous work aand unsanitary conditions. These studies have a
number of methodological limitations, arising from small samples and
non-blind-test situations in which the interviewer's knowledge of
whether or not a woman was solvent-exposed could have influenced
the findings. Nevertheless, the studies are important because they suggest that we must evaluate the impact of exposure on women within
the context of their work environments as a whole. In other words, we
must also consider the effects of other occupational stresses when we
interpret exposure-health relationships.

A second important line of evidence comes from unpublished case
reports of occupational stress and accompanying psychological symptoms among female blue-collar workers (described in Colligan and
Murphy 1979; Colligan, Pennebaker, and Murphy 1982). These reports
are often taken as evidence of the outbreak of "mass psychogenic
illness," or epidemics of hysteria in the workplace. Mass psychogenic
illness is defined as "the collective occurrence of a set of physical
symptoms and related beliefs among two or more individuals in the
absence of an identifiable pathogen" (Colligan and Murphy 1979, 82).
During such "outbreaks," workers report physical symptoms that they
believe are due to the physical environment of the workplace. For
example, they attribute onset of headaches and dizziness to a strange
smell or to the introduction of a new solvent at their plant. However,

in the opinion of the investigators, no environmental cause of the symptoms in these cases is ever established. The workers are therefore judged to suffer contagious psychogenic illness, in which one individual's behavior and symptoms are spread through imitation by other workers and the real causes of these symptoms are anxiety and job stress.

It is striking that the workers described in the majority of reports are women employed in jobs involving not only high levels of occupational stress (e.g., repetitive, rigidly paced jobs, pressures to increase production, etc.), but exposure to organic solvents as well. Furthermore, when the National Institute of Occupational Safety and Health (NIOSH) investigated several presumed outbreaks, it was found that in all cases, the most common symptoms were headache, light-headedness, dizziness, sleepiness, and weakness—symptoms already shown to be associated with solvent exposure in experimental and occupational field studies of *male* workers. Thus, it is debatable whether these case reports provide evidence of true mass psychogenic illness or reflect, instead, the investigators' failure to recognize potential effects of solvent exposure at levels below government-prescribed thresholds. The appropriate identification of links between occupational hazards and worker health is an issue of great importance, and we will consider it in more detail shortly.

Aside from these few studies, research on occupational stress effects in female blue-collar workers is sparse. Moreover, we know very little about the *combined* impact that solvent exposure and occupational stress might have on female workers' health. There is some indication that for male workers these two stressors' effects may be synergistic (Ashford 1976; House et al. 1979). In other words, workers experiencing high levels of both solvent exposure *and* occupational stress may be unusually vulnerable to deleterious health effects—more vulnerable than we would expect given knowledge of the stressors' individual impact. However, potentially synergistic effects on areas other than physical health (such as psychological symptomatology and neuropsychological performance) have not been examined, even for men.

We recently completed the first major epidemiologic study of solvent exposure and occupational stress among blue-collar women. The purpose of our research was to determine whether exposure and occupational stress had negative physical, psychological, and neuropsychological effects on a group of women primarily employed as assembly line workers. Because of the findings outlined above, our research was guided by several central concerns. First, given the lack of data on women, we wanted to examine the nature and extent of female workers' solvent exposure and describe their current physical and mental health. Second, we wanted to test whether solvent exposure was related to measures of physical, psychological, and neuropsychological well-being and, in contrast to previous work, examine these relationships after taking other known risk factors of ill health into account. Third, we wanted to compare the impact of solvent exposure and the impact of occupational stress on health, and determine whether the combination of these two sources of stress had a particularly negative, synergistic effect on health.

Methodology

Our study involved female workers employed in two plants in Pennsylvania. One plant produces small appliances and the other manufactures telephone components. Approximately three-quarters of the women had jobs in which they received varying degrees of organic solvent exposure (as we will describe) and one-quarter had jobs with little or no exposure.

David Parkinson and Leslie Dunn conducted extensive negotiations with the labor unions representing nonmanagerial workers at the plants, and we selected eligible workers from union membership lists. In order to be eligible, a worker had to have been employed at the plant for at least six months, and had to be female, eighteen to sixty-five years of age, a native English speaker, and Caucasian. The latter four requirements reflected the dominant characteristics of the work forces in the two plants. We selected all eligible workers from the relatively small work force at the small appliance plant, and we drew a random sample of eligible workers from the larger telephone components plant.

Data collection was completed at the small appliance plant first, and was recently completed at the second plant; our present analyses focus on 168 workers from the former plant who represented 73 percent of the eligible workers at the plant. We were unable to reach a minority of eligible workers because they had unlisted telephone numbers. Of eligible workers with listed telephone numbers, 85 percent participated in the study.

We first sent a letter to each worker that described our study's focus on the health of working people, noted the support of the union, and assured confidentiality of responses. Trained interviewers then arranged and conducted individual, ninety-minute, face-to-face interviews at facilities provided by the union. The interviews included measures of stress, health, and demographic and social support characteristics.

The stress measures we used focused on environmental (solvent-related) stress, as well as perceptions of occupational stress. For the former, women were asked about their current job-related exposure to solvents, including (*a*) what job they held at the plant (e.g., assembly line work, maintenance work), (*b*) how long they had held their current job, (*c*) the chemicals to which they were exposed, (*d*) whether each exposure was from direct contact (e.g., handling solvents) or was in-direct (e.g., from fumes), (*e*) the percentage of work time that they were exposed to solvents, and (*f*) whether and how much protective clothing they typically wore on the job.

To measure occupational stress, the women were asked a series of questions adapted from scales developed by Caplan et al. (1975). We then created three stress indices to use in our analyses. A work-load index was created by z-scoring and averaging four items pertaining to the women's perceptions of work quantity (higher score = greater work load). An abilities underutilization index represented an average of four z-scored items pertaining to opportunity to use skills on the job (higher score = greater underutilization). A job dissatisfaction index repre-sented an average of six z-scored items pertaining to overall evaluation of the job (higher score = greater dissatisfaction).[1]

Health measures included three areas of functioning that previous studies suggest are sensitive to environmental and/or occupational stress: physical health, psychological symptomatology, and neuropsy-chological performance. With regard to physical health symptomatol-ogy, workers were asked whether they were currently experiencing any of forty-three complaints. These fall into seven clusters: somatic com-plaints (e.g., fatigue), respiratory symptoms (e.g., shortness of breath), cardiovascular symptoms (e.g., palpitations), skin problems (e.g., rashes), symptoms of nervous system damage (e.g., loss of memory), urinary tract symptoms (e.g., infections), and reproductive problems (e.g., irregular bleeding).

Psychological symptomatology was measured by the depression, anxiety, interpersonal sensitivity, and obsessive-compulsive subscales from the Hopkins Symptom Checklist (Derogatis et al. 1974). This checklist inquires about symptoms during the week preceding the in-terview. We created a summary index by averaging the items (higher score = greater distress).

The evaluation of neuropsychological performance was more complex. We selected a subset of tests from the longer Pittsburgh Occupational Exposures Test battery, a series of well-known neuropsychological tests that have been administered to over 500 blue-collar workers (Ryan et al. 1987). These tests have been shown to be sensitive to impairments in brain-damaged patients (Lezak 1983). Three major areas were covered. First, we assessed visuoperceptual functioning using the Visual Reproductions test to measure short- and long-term memory for nonverbal, visual information (adapted from the Wechsler Memory Scale, Ryan et al. 1987), and the Boston Embedded Figures test to measure ability and to analyze and synthesize nonverbal visuospatial information (Kapur and Butters 1977). Second, we assessed attention and psychomotor integration using the Trailmaking test to measure attention and visuomotor tracking (Reitan 1958) and the Digit Vigilance test to measure sustained attention (Rennik 1974). Third, we assessed motor speed and manual dexterity using the Grooved Pegboard test (Rourke 1973).

Finally, we included measures of demographic characteristics and social support that are known to be important risk factors for women's mental and physical health (e.g., Brown and Harris 1978; Kasl and Wells 1985; Turner and Noh 1983). We obtained a complete demographic profile on each worker, and in our analyses we statistically controlled the effects of age, level of education, marital status, and number of children under age six. In addition, whether or not a woman smoked was included as a risk factor in analyses of effects on respiratory and cardiovascular symptoms.

We assessed social support from both work and nonwork environments using items adapted from the Caplan et al. (1975) social support scales. We then created three support indices: five items reflecting support from the worker's supervisor were averaged, five items reflecting support from co-workers were averaged, and five items reflecting support from friends and relatives were averaged. For all three measures, higher scores indicate greater levels of perceived support.

Findings

Our first research goal was to describe the nature of our sample of women's occupational exposure to solvents, as well as their mental and physical health. The 168 women represent a stably employed work force. They had worked at the plant for an average of 8.7 years (ranging from 5 to 16 years), and had held their current jobs for an average of 3.5 years (ranging from 1 month to 14 years). The majority (73 percent) held assembly line positions. Table 1 lists the solvents to which women reported they were currently exposed. Interestingly, many women (37 percent) were unable to name at least one of their chemical exposures.

Current exposure to solvents was extensive in our sample. Most of the sample (85 percent) reported current exposure to at least one solvent, and many (43 percent) received multiple exposures. Over half of the women (57 percent) had direct contact (as opposed to indirect and/or no contact) with at least one type of solvent in their jobs. By direct contact we refer to use, for example, of solvents to clean components of appliances or to clean work areas. Approximately half of the sample (51 percent) reported that they were exposed to solvents from 90 to 100 percent of their time on the job. Finally, the majority of women (81 percent) wore at least one item of protective clothing on the job, and these items most often included gloves, aprons, and safety glasses.

In characterizing each woman's current level of exposure, we wanted to take into account both the type and amount of exposure. Therefore, we created an additional, overall exposure index for each woman. We weighted the percentage of time women reported that they were currently exposed by the number of direct exposures they experienced. This index could vary from one (little or no exposure of any kind) to nine (almost constant direct exposure to several solvents).[2] Fourteen percent of the sample received maximum exposure (scores of nine), 37 percent received moderate degrees of exposure (scores from four to six), and the remainder (49 percent) received minimal exposure (scores from one to three).

Before proceeding to examine the relationship between exposure and health, it was important to determine whether our set of questions about exposure were themselves interrelated (as we would hope). Our six key exposure measures included our overall exposure index, as well as the years women had been employed in their current job, the number of solvents to which they were exposed, the number of direct exposures they experienced, the percentage of work time they were exposed, and

TABLE 1. Solvent Exposures among 168 Blue-Collar Women

Solvent	Number of Cases	Percentage of Sample
Methyl Ethyl Ketone	70	42
1,1,1-Trichloroethane	34	20
RTV Silicone Paste	22	13
Solve-All (perchloroethylene)	9	5
Other	6	4
Unknown solvent	62	37

Note: Women listed all solvents to which they were exposed.

the number of protective clothing items they wore on the job. These measures were indeed intercorrelated, particularly the four measures of numbers and type of exposure, percentage of time exposed, and overall exposure (correlations ranging from .36 to .86). However, the items were far from entirely overlapping. In particular, years on the job and the number of protective items worn, two items that were not strongly related to reports of type or amount of exposure (correlations ranging from −.02 to .16), appear to be both conceptually and empirically weaker measures of current exposure.[3]

We note here that all of our data on exposure are based on women's self-reports, and it is critical to evaluate their accuracy. We found that women's reports of the types of solvents used in their departments corresponded quite closely to company-supplied data. The only exception was that the company stated that Solve-All (perchloroethylene) was used in several departments in which many women in the sample were employed. Only 5 percent of the sample listed Solve-All among their exposures. However, as shown in table 1, 37 percent could not name one or more solvents to which they were exposed. By comparing women's reports of their department and job description with the company data on department-related exposure, it appears likely that in the majority of cases where the type of solvent was not known, the women were in fact exposed to Solve-All.

We also attempted to evaluate the accuracy of women's reports about the extent of their exposure. With the assistance of union officials familiar with operations at the plant, we reviewed the women's job and department descriptions to determine whether they could have experienced the amounts of exposure they reported. The women's reports were corroborated by the union officials.

Finally, to describe the women's health, we used our measures of physical symptoms, psychological symptoms, and neuropsychological performance. Although appropriate normative data were not available on the physical health symptoms, it is noteworthy that the majority of women in our sample reported few current symptoms in any of the seven physical health areas (see also the appendix to this chapter). Regarding psychological symptomatology, the 168 women had a range of symptom scores similar to scores found for a normative sample of female community residents (Derogatis et al. 1974; see the appendix to this chapter). The sample distributions on the neuropsychological measures were similar to normative data from a sample of blue-collar nonexposed male workers who had served as a comparison group in an earlier study of lead exposure effects (Parkinson et al. 1986). These data suggest that although the women knew that our study concerned their health, their health responses were not distorted in any systematic way.

Relationships between Solvent Exposure and Health

Our second major research goal was to determine whether exposure was related to health. Thus, we examined correlations of the six exposure measures described above with the three types of health outcomes. In computing these correlations, we statistically controlled four demographic variables—women's age, level of education, marital status, and number of children under age six—because these variables are risk factors for health problems in women.

We found that the associations between exposure and health outcome were strongest for physical symptoms, somewhat weaker for psychological symptoms, and very weak for neuropsychological performance. Specifically, women who reported exposure to greater numbers of solvents, a greater number of direct exposures, a greater percentage of time exposed, and who scored higher on our weighted index of overall exposure were more likely to report somatic complaints, respiratory symptoms, and cardiovascular symptoms (partial correlations ranging from .16 to .23). Workers who wore more protective clothing items reported greater numbers of skin problems (partial correlation = .20). All four of these physical symptom clusters are areas for which we would expect associations, given clinical evidence of exposure-related health effects. Exposure was also related, though less consistently, to reports of greater psychological distress (partial correlations ranging from .09 to .16). Given other findings in the literature, it was surprising that the exposure measures were virtually unrelated to neuropsychological performance.[4]

Unique and Combined Effects of Solvent Exposure and Occupational Stress on Health

Our third group of research questions concerned (*a*) whether the women's perceptions of occupational stress would also bear an important relationship to their health, (*b*) whether their solvent exposure would continue to be related to their health once we took any effects of occupational stress into account, and (*c*) whether the two sources of stress—solvent exposure and occupational stress—would act together to produce synergistic effects on women's health.

We used linear multiple regression analysis to address these questions because of its flexibility and power for examining relationships between a given outcome variable and multiple predictor variables (Cohen and Cohen 1975). These analyses were performed separately for physical and psychological symptoms, the two health areas for which we found simple associations with solvent exposure. Our weighted index representing type and amount of solvent exposure served as the exposure measure. In addition to controlling for demographic risk factors in these analyses, we also included variables reflecting perceptions of work and nonwork social support in order to examine and control for their effects.

We estimated a hierarchical series of four regression models for each health outcome. Thus, we added four groups of predictor variables to the analysis of a given health outcome in four separate steps. First, we included demographic risk factors and the social support measures in order to determine their effects on health. In the second step, we included effects for the three occupational stress indices, controlling for demographic and social support variables. In the third step, we added the weighted solvent exposure index in order to determine its unique impact on health, controlling for the previous groups of variables. Finally, in the fourth step, we included the interactions of the exposure index with each occupational stress measure (e.g., the interaction between the exposure index and work load) to determine whether the exposure-health relationship was affected by the amount of occupational stress that women experienced.

Table 2 presents results of these analyses for four physical symptom areas (the only physical health areas in which we found solvent exposure and/or occupational stress effects) and for psychological symptoms. The size of each regression coefficient in the table reflects the importance of a given predictor in affecting a particular health outcome. Looking first at the predictors entered in the first group, we note several effects for social support: women who thought they received greater support from their supervisor reported both fewer physical symptoms and less psychological distress (as indicated by the statistically significant negative regression coefficients). However, women's reports of co-worker support were related only to their psychological distress levels, and their reports of support from friends and relatives were associated only with fewer somatic complaints.

Regarding the central hypotheses of our study, we found that occupational stress had a somewhat different relationship to physical than to psychological symptoms. Specifically, women who felt that they carried a relatively heavy work load were significantly more likely to report somatic, respiratory, and nervous system symptoms. In contrast, women who were less satisfied with their jobs primarily showed higher levels

TABLE 2. Estimated Standardized Coefficients from Hierarchical Regressions for Physical and Psychological Symptoms: Main Effects[a]

Group	Predictor	Physical Symptoms[b]				Psychological Symptoms[c]
		Somatic	Respiratory	Cardiovascular	Nervous System	
I	Age	.16	.14	.13	.10	.13
	Education	.01	-.06	-.06	.12	-.06
	Marital status	-.16	.03	.12	-.08	-.08
	No. of children < age 6	.09	-.16*	-.01	.10	-.10
	Smoking habits	—	.14	.08	—	—
	Supervisor support	-.21**	-.16*	-.23**	-.20*	-.25***
	Co-worker support	-.03	.00	-.11	-.14	-.15*
	Friend support	-.18*	-.08	.07	-.03	-.09
	R^2 for Group I	.12*	.11*	.10*	.10*	.17***
II	Work load	.18*	.20*	.11	.21*	.03
	Ability underutilization	-.08	-.15	-.04	.03	-.12
	Job dissatisfaction	.19*	.07	.14	.06	.31***
	Increment in R^2	.09***	.07***	.03*	.05**	.08***
III	Weighted exposure index	.16*	.20*	.17*	.05	.10
	Increment in R^2	.03**	.05**	.04**	<.01	.01

$*p < .05$ $**p < .01$ $***p < .001$

[a]See the appendix to this chapter for direction of scoring of each variable.

[b]$N = 165$

[c]$N = 168$

of psychological distress, although they reported somewhat more somatic complaints as well.

Turning to solvent exposure, it is critical to note that our weighted exposure index was a significant predictor of three types of physical symptoms, even after we took occupational stress, social support, and demographic background characteristics into account. However, this was not the case with psychological symptoms. As when we examined just the simple relationship between exposure and mental health, exposure showed only a weak and nonsignificant association with psychological symptoms when we included demographic, social support, and occupational stress variables in our analysis. We also did not find evidence to support the hypothesis that exposure and occupational stress interact to produce synergistic effects on health; all interactions between these variables were small and nonsignificant.

Finally, we note that the solvent exposure–health relationships that we obtained may have been influenced by subjects' beliefs about what health problems are likely to result from exposure. Women may have overreported certain symptoms because they believed such symptoms were caused by solvent exposure. We evaluated this possibility by examining whether women who believed that exposure caused certain kinds of symptoms (e.g., psychological symptoms or respiratory symptoms) were more likely to have those symptoms than were women who did not share this belief. For the three health areas in which we did find solvent exposure–symptom relationships, we found no sizable or statistically significant differences in women's reports of symptoms depending on their beliefs about the effects of solvent exposure. Thus there appears to be no measurable bias due to expectations.

Discussion

Our research makes at least two contributions to the study of working women's health. First, our investigation represents the first systematic attempt to evaluate effects of both solvent exposure and occupational stress in a female blue-collar work force. Second, few prior occupational stress and exposure studies have considered other known risk factors such as social support when analyzing the relationship between occupational hazards and health. Conversely, research on the effects of psychosocial variables on women's health has typically failed to integrate work-related variables among the factors studied. Women are permanent members of the work force. It thus is critical to understand the impact of *both* "traditional" sources of risk and additional risks emerging from today's technologically sophisticated workplace.

Our findings regarding traditional risks for women's health are consistent with an extensive literature; for example, social support from a work supervisor was related in our sample to women's physical and mental health. Most important however, given our research goals, were the exposure and occupational stress effects that we obtained *after* we took these other risk factors into account. We will briefly summarize these effects, consider potential limitations on what we can conclude about these effects, and then discuss implications of our findings for the identification and reduction of solvent-related occupational hazards faced by female blue-collar workers.

First, concerning physical health, our results were similar to other occupational stress studies (e.g., House et al. 1979): we found that women who experienced more stress on the job tended to show more symptoms. However, in addition, we found that reports of current solvent exposure were related to reports of several types of physical symptoms, most notably somatic, respiratory, and cardiovascular complaints. Somatic complaints such as fatigue and headaches have routinely been observed in individuals with even very low levels of sustained solvent exposure (Baker and Fine 1986). But our findings are noteworthy because the consequences of low levels of exposure for other areas of physical symptomatology have rarely been considered in epidemiologic research. The respiratory and cardiovascular symptoms that our subjects reported are similar to those noted in clinical studies of solvent-exposed workers (see Waldron 1981 for a review), and are consistent with findings reported in the few relevant epidemiologic studies (e.g., Elofsson et al. 1980; Hane et al. 1977). Skin irritations among exposed workers have also been noted clinically (Browning 1965), and although we found that type and amount of exposure were only weakly related to reports of skin problems, our workers who reported irritations did wear more protective clothing, a relationship likely to reflect their attempt to cope with solvent-exacerbated symptoms.

Our second set of findings concerns women's psychological symptomatology. We found that solvent exposure was only weakly related to psychological distress, especially after we took other risk factors into account. In contrast, job dissatisfaction remained strongly associated with psychological distress, a relationship we would expect in light of both prior research on occupational stress–psychological distress associations (e.g., Bromet et al. 1988; Cooper and Marshall 1976; Karasek 1979) and the obvious conceptual overlap between measures of current dissatisfaction and current distress.

Although occupational exposures and perceptions of occupational stress may act together to produce particularly negative effects on workers' health, we could find no evidence of such synergistic effects on either physical or mental health for this particular population. However, the synergy hypothesis is a compelling one, and we believe it deserves additional investigation with both female and male samples.

Finally, we were initially surprised that our third area of concern, neuropsychological performance, was virtually unrelated to solvent exposure. A number of studies have shown that exposure affects the kinds of visuoperceptual and psychomotor processes we assessed, even at levels of exposure below government standards (e.g., Elofsson et al. 1980; see Baker and Fine 1986 for a review). A likely explanation for our lack of findings arises from the increasingly stringent government standards for worker exposure in the United States as well as in other countries (Baker and Fine 1986); permissible levels of exposure for women in our study were lower than the permissible levels for subjects in previous epidemiologic studies. Although high levels of solvent exposure clearly do lead to neuropsychological deficits, whether such effects still appear at the very much lower levels now set by the U.S. government is a matter of controversy (Baker and Fine 1986).

Several potential limitations on interpretation of our findings must be borne in mind. First, the study's cross-sectional design, in which we obtained all data in a single interview, precludes conclusive statements that either exposure or occupational stress *caused* the symptoms women reported. However, our design does allow us to assess the *magnitude*, or strength, of relationships between these variables—an important goal in and of itself, given the lack of epidemiologic data available on solvent-exposed female workers.

A related concern involves potential selection bias with respect to which women worked in exposed areas. Hiring regulations are described in the contractual agreement between the union and the company, and no health restrictions are placed on any of the jobs. However, we are not able to rule out the possibility of health status affecting women's choice of higher exposure jobs. Although a cross-sectional study cannot address such bias directly, we did examine and control personal characteristics (e.g., age and education) in our analyses.

Our focus on workers currently employed at the plant introduces an additional source of selection bias. Those women who may have suffered most from exposure or occupational stress may have left the plant. To the extent that our sample included only relatively "hardy" women, we may have underestimated the strength of the relationships of exposure and stress to health. However, we feel that it is unlikely that workers would have voluntarily left their jobs because the plant is located in an economically depressed area of Pennsylvania where jobs are scarce.

A final concern involves the self-report nature of our data. With respect to exposure, while we would have liked to collect industrial hygiene measurements of plant exposures, we were not able to obtain company permission to do so. (Available routine hygiene survey data showed that solvent exposures were within threshold limit values required by the Occupational Safety and Health Administration.) Furthermore, no reliable biological markers exist that we could have used as objective indices of exposure. However, as we discussed earlier, the women's reports of types of exposure and amount of time exposed appear to be reasonably accurate. Concerning potential biases in self-reported health, we could find no evidence that women who believed exposure caused health problems reported more problems. In addition, we noted the similarity between our sample data and normative data on psychological and neuropsychological measures.

The pattern of our results has several important implications for the interpretation of reports of physical and psychological symptoms among female blue-collar workers. Prior descriptions of "mass psychogenic illness" in this population have asserted that physical health complaints—most notably somatic symptoms—were indicative of high levels of psychological distress, presumably brought on by occupational stressors such as heavy work load or repetitive assembly line work. Even though the women workers in these studies who reported physical symptoms attributed their health problems to specific workplace hazards, including most often organic solvent exposures, such attributions have been discounted as representing workers' attempts to rationalize their symptoms; toxic exposures were below government-prescribed levels (as measured by industrial hygienists' environmental air samplings) and thus were viewed by the investigators as too low to cause any health problems. Our results, however, revealed relatively important relationships between exposure at levels below government standards and several areas of physical health complaints. Furthermore, these relationships held for all of the women in our study, not just for those who believed that exposure caused such health problems. And although psychological distress was indeed related to perceptions of occupational stress, distress bore only a weak relationship to reports of exposure.

We suggest therefore that solvent exposure may have been responsible for the "hysterical" symptoms noted in a number of previous studies of female workers. It is a sad commentary on the state of research on working women that terms such as "mass psychogenic illness" have been invoked to explain female blue-collar workers' physical symptoms, while such symptoms have long been known to be associated with toxic exposures in male workers and are not so labeled. This issue of appropriately identifying links between occupational hazards and worker health is critical because employers are unlikely to acknowledge occupational hazards and alter work environments if they believe workers' symptoms do not arise from environmental conditions such as solvent exposure, but rather reflect personal dispositions. To the extent that health problems associated with toxic exposures are interpreted differently for male and female workers, female blue-collar workers—and the unions representing them—may be less successful than their male counterparts in bringing about any needed changes in their work environments.

NOTES

This research was funded in part by National Institute of Mental Health Grant No. MH-39972 and Training Grant MH-15169-09. We wish to thank members of the United Steel Workers of America for their help in implementing the study.
1. Descriptive statistics for these scales and for measures described below are presented in the appendix to this chapter. Details on individual items and internal consistency reliability for all scales are available from Mary Amanda Dew, at Department of Psychiatry, University of Pittsburgh, 3811 O'Hara Street, Pittsburgh, Pennsylvania 15213.
2. Details on construction of this scale are available from Mary Amanda Dew.
3. A table of intercorrelations among the six exposure measures is available from Mary Amanda Dew.
4. A table of all partial correlations between the exposure measures and neuropsychological performance is available from Mary Amanda Dew.

BIBLIOGRAPHY

Ashford, Nicholas A. 1976. *Crisis in the workplace: Occupational disease and injury.* Cambridge, Mass.: MIT Press.
Axelson, Olav, Monica Hane, and Christer Hogstedt. 1976. A case referent study on neuropsychiatric disorders among workers exposed to solvents. *Scandinavian Journal of Work, Environment and Health* 2:14–20.
————. 1980. Current aspects of solvent-related disorders. In *Developments in Occupational Medicine,* ed. Carl Zenz, 237–58. Chicago: Yearbook Medical Publishers.
Baker, Edward L., and Lawrence J. Fine. 1986. Solvent neurotoxicity: The current evidence. *Journal of Occupational Medicine* 28, no. 2: 126–29.

Brown, George, and Tirrell Harris. 1978. *The social origins of depression.* London: Tavistock.

Browning, Ethel. 1965. *Toxicity and metabolism of industrial solvents.* New York: Elsevier.

Bromet, Evelyn J., Mary Amanda Dew, David K. Parkinson, and Herbert C. Schulberg. 1988. Predictive effects of occupational and marital stress on the mental health of a male workforce. *Journal of Organizational Behavior* 9:1–13.

Caplan, Robert, Sidney Cobb, John French, R. Van Harrison, and S. Pinneau. 1975. Job demands and worker health. DHEW (NIOSH) Publication No. 75-160. Washington, D.C.: Government Printing Office.

Cavanagh, J. B. 1985. Solvent neurotoxicity. *British Journal of Industrial Medicine* 42: 433–34.

Cohen, Jacob, and Patricia Cohen. 1975. *Applied multiple regression/correlation analysis for the behavioral sciences.* Hillsdale, N.J.: Erlbaum.

Colligan, Michael J., and Lawrence R. Murphy. 1979. Mass psychogenic illness in organizations: An overview. *Journal of Occupational Psychology* 52:77–90.

Colligan, Michael J., James W. Pennebaker, and Lawrence R. Murphy. 1982. *Mass psychogenic illness: A social psychological analysis.* Hillsdale, N.J.: Erlbaum.

Cooper, Cary, and Judi Marshall. 1976. Occupational sources of stress: A review of the literature relating to coronary heart disease and mental ill health. *Journal of Occupational Psychology* 49:11–28.

Derogatis, Leonard R., Ronald S. Lipman, Karl Rickels, E. H. Uhlenhuth, and Lino Covi. 1974. The Hopkins Symptom Checklist (HSCL): A self-report symptom inventory. *Behavioral Science* 19:1–15.

Elofsson, Stig-Arne, Francesco Gamberale, Tomas Hindmarsh, Anders Iregren, Anders Isaksson, Inger Johnsson, Bengt Knave, Eva Lydahl, Per Mindus, Hans E. Persson, Bo Philipson, Maria Steby, Goran Struwe, Erik Söderman, Arne Wennberg, and Lennart Widén. 1980. Exposure to organic solvents: A cross-sectional epidemiologic investigation on occupationally exposed car and industrial spray painters with special reference to the nervous system. *Scandinavian Journal of Work, Environment and Health* 6:239–73.

Hane, Monica, Olav Axelson, Jan Blume, Christer Hogstedt, Lennart Sundell, and Berit Ydreborg. 1977. Psychological function changes among house painters. *Scandinavian Journal of Work, Environment and Health* 3:91–99.

House, James S., Anthony J. McMichael, James A. Wells, Berton H. Kaplan, and Lawrence R. Landerman. 1979. Occupational stress and health among factory workers. *Journal of Health and Social Behavior* 20: 139–60.

Hunt, Vilma R. 1979. *Work and the health of women.* Boca Raton, Fla.: CRC Press.

Karasek, Robert. 1979. Job demands, job decision latitude, and mental strain: Implications for job redesign. *Administrative Science Quarterly* 24:285–306.

Kapur, Narinder, and Nelson Butters. 1977. An analysis of visuoperceptive deficits in alcoholic Korsakoffs and long-term alcoholics. *Journal of Studies in Alcohol* 33: 2,025–35.

Kasl, Stan V., and James A. Wells. 1985. Social support and health in the middle years: Work and the family. In *Social Support and Health,* ed. Sheldon Cohen and S. Leonard Syme. New York: Academic Press.

Lezak, Muriel D. 1983. *Neuropsychological assessment,* 2d ed. New York: Oxford University Press.

Lindström, K. 1973. Psychological performances of workers exposed to various solvents. *Work, Environment and Health* 10:151–55.

Maroni, Marco, Carlo Bulgheroni, M. Grazia Cassitto, Franca Merluzzi, Renato Gilioli, and Vito Foa. 1977. A clinical, neurophysiological and behavioral study of female workers exposed to 1,1,1-trichloroethane. *Scandinavian Journal of Work, Environment and Health* 3:16–22.

Matsushita, Toshio, Yoshiki Arimatsu, Atsushi Ueda, Kazuko Satoh, and Shigeru Nomura. 1975. Hematological and neuro-muscular response of workers exposed to low concentration of toluene vapor. *Industrial Health* 13:115–21.

Parkinson, David K., Christopher M. Ryan, Evelyn J. Bromet, and Melanie M. Connell. 1986. A psychiatric epidemiologic study of occupational lead exposure. *American Journal of Epidemiology* 123: 261–69.

Reitan, Ralph M. 1958. Validity of the trailmaking test as an indicator of organic brain damage. *Perceptual and Motor Skills* 8: 271–76.

Rennick, Phillip M. 1974. Procedures for repeatable-cognitive-perceptual-motor testing and general neuropsychologic assessment. Unpublished manual, Lafayette Clinic.

Rourke, Byron P., D. W. Yanni, G. W. MacDonald, and G. C. Young. 1973. Neuropsychological significance of lateralized deficits in the grooved pegboard test for older children with learning disabilities. *Journal of Consulting and Clinical Psychology* 41: 128–34.

Ryan, Christopher M., Lisa Morrow, Evelyn J. Bromet, and David K. Parkinson. 1987. The assessment of neuropsychological dysfunction in the workplace: Normative data from the Pittsburgh Occupational Exposure Test Battery, *Journal of Experimental and Clinical Neuropsychology* 9, no. 6: 665–79.

Turner, R. Jay, and Samuel Noh. 1983. Class and psychological vulnerability among women: The significance of social support and personal control. *Journal of Health and Social Behavior* 24:2–15.

Waldron, H. A. 1981. Effects of organic solvents. *British Journal of Hospital Medicine,* December, 645–49.

Appendix: Descriptive Statistics and Direction of Scoring for Major Study Measures

Variable[a]	Mean	Standard Deviation	Scoring
Occupational Stress			higher score = greater stress (z-scored)
Work load	0.00	0.78	
Ability underutilization	0.00	0.72	
Job dissatisfaction	0.00	0.69	
Physical Health Symptoms			
Somatic	1.08	1.30	0 = none; 3 = 3 to 7 symptoms
Respiratory	0.80	1.14	0 = none; 4 = 4 to 7 symptoms
Cardiovascular	0.68	0.76	0 = none; 2 = 2 to 3 symptoms
Skin	0.63	0.77	0 = none; 2 = 2 to 4 symptoms
Nervous system damage	1.14	1.04	0 = none; 3 = 3 to 5 symptoms
Urinary tract	0.24	0.43	0 = none; 2 = 2 to 4 symptoms
Reproductive	0.81	1.09	0 = none; 3 = 3 to 14 symptoms
Psychological Symptoms	1.62	0.42	1 = not; 4 = extremely distressed
Demographic Characteristics			
Age	36.54	9.73	years
Level of education	2.90	0.67	1 = grammar school; 7 = graduate or professional degree
No. of children < age 6	1.26	0.44	total number
Cigarette smoking	1.94	1.10	1 = do not smoke; 4 = heavy smoker
Marital status[b]	—	—	1 = married; 2 = not
Social Support			1 = less; 4 = more support
Supervisor support	3.01	0.64	
Co-worker support	2.55	0.92	
Friend and relative support	3.36	0.62	

[a]Descriptive statistics for neuropsychological tests are available from the first author.
[b]61 percent were married.

Women's Lives against the Industrial/Chemical Landscape: Environmental Health and the Health of the Environment

Lin Nelson

We live in a difficult time, a time when things may get much worse before they get better. Global ecosystems are being stressed to the limit and the human condition as part of these ecosystems is under attack. Women's health is both a victim and a biological marker of environmental decay. As women's lives are more and more shaped by the ecological degradation around them, the environmental movements are being shaped by the activism and analysis women bring to a growing array of ecocrises. Such threats include heightened risks of cancer and the possibility of a mother releasing her body burden of chemicals to her nursing child. But women are also facing down the forces of pollution: by forming some of the most effective grassroots organizations (witness Lois Gibbs's founding of the Citizens' Clearinghouse for Hazardous Wastes); and by formulating feminist perspectives on the past, present, and future of global ecosystems (a significant development is the newly formed WomanEarth Feminist Peace Institute).

The evolution of industrial technologies and technocracies has a profound influence on women's lives, although this influence is sometimes less obvious and less gender-specific than is that of the medical technologies applied to women as patients. The current flood of pollutants has impacts on all life forms—plants, animals, and humanity. As part of the social ecology, women suffer as human beings, and as female human beings. Women have particular concerns because of the persistent gender inequality that has both striking and subtle ramifications for public and private decision making, research, health care, and efforts at ecological restoration. There are also concerns about being—or being seen as—"potential mothers" or "the potentially pregnant"; whether they have children or not, many women will very likely be affected by emerging policies regarding reproductive health and hazardous environments. The "potentially pregnant" model (familiar in industrial settings) may lead to some insights and protections around reproductive health; but, more likely, in a patriarchal context, it may foster a fetus fetish, minimizing the health of women as women (see

347

Bertin in this volume). Finally, women who do choose to birth a child become "an environment" in an ecologically destabilized world; the force of industrial technology insinuates itself into a woman's body, potentially transforming her into a hazardous place for the developing fetus and nursing infant; being this "hazardous place" carries with it all manner of medical, political, ethical, and emotional meaning.

In developing research on women and health, we need to pay particular attention to the industrial backdrop, the technological infrastructure that frames our lives. We have a strong foundation in the examination of women's health in the workplace, thanks to the work of such organizations as the Women's Occupational Health Resource Center and Double Exposure: Women Against Reproductive Health Hazards. We need to link our workplace concerns with those that are more broadly environmental; we need to look at the impacts on women's health of living in proximity to industrial and agricultural processes, using chemical-rich products in the home, and depending upon a contaminated food supply (see Chavkin 1984 for one of the best works to date on this broad approach). For just as women work a double day, women may endure multiple exposures to the products and by-products of modern technology: on the job (be it sweatshop or swank office), in the home, near the dumpsite. For example, a woman printer—systematically exposed to carcinogenic and teratogenic chemicals like formaldehyde and methylene chloride—may also be exposed to asbestos if she is the one who launders her spouse's construction worker clothing; if her neighbors lavish chemicals on their turf, she may suffer an immune system disorder, escalating further her vulnerability to contaminants.

The industrial/chemical world works its way into women's lives with a quiet stealth, with a capacity for unprecedented destruction and disruption that we are only beginning to understand. This chapter is a preliminary effort to establish the need for critical work in this field, to point to efforts underway, and to link (analytically and strategically) the women's movement—and women's studies—with environmental concerns. First, I will briefly suggest how women may be particularly affected by environmental degradation and the key issues in looking at gender in the environmental health context. Next, I will provide an overview of some of the more significant developments—research on current hazards, relevant policies, and emerging activism. The topic of pollution's impact on nursing mothers and infants will provide a case in point of some of the issues explored here. Finally, I will conclude with some thoughts on an activist agenda for future work.

Analyzing Women and Environmental Health: The Need, the Oversight

In coming to grips with "women and environment" in the late twentieth century, we must carefully assess and respect the everydayness of women's lives. Much of the important raging, grieving, and strategizing emerges from women—alone, around kitchen tables, at community rallies—fighting for their lives and those of their families. It comes from the daily basis of women's experiences as mothers, workers, consumers, patients, neighbors, and citizens (Kraus 1986; Freudenberg and Zaltberg 1984). One woman's story reflects that of many others. June Larson, whose daughter was suffering severe reactions to chemicals as a complication of her muscular dystrophy, took on the lawn care entrepreneurs who cavalierly polluted the small town that Larson had sought as a refuge. Through her vigilance, Wauconda, Illinois, passed a precedent-setting ordinance restricting the industry's activities (Shute 1987). Sam Epstein, noted environmental physician, author, and activist, commented, "This modest ordinance may well become the bellwether for the entire nation" (Gottlieb and Wiley 1986, 52). In the Third World, women's daily labors of gathering food, fuel, and water, and tending to the family's health—often in the absence of male family members who are looking for economic opportunities in the cities— has led them to challenge the development policies that have come to mean deforestation, desertification, and widespread pesticide contamination (WorldWIDE 1987; Dankelman 1987). In the United States and around the globe, the movement has sprung in part out of the perennial struggles of women to cope with technologies, techniques, and technocracies.

In order to comprehend and support women's struggles to eke out their daily lives in technologically complex and often polluted environments, we must nourish a complex view of women's lives. That means not getting locked into the authorities' (medical, industrial, governmental) myopic focus on "woman the reproducer" as being at high-risk environmentally. It also means being sensitive to the differences and the connections between our activities as reproducers and producers, as consumers and citizens. The basis for women's actions and analysis varies; and it changes in the course of one woman's struggles— for example, as she transforms from mother-defending-her-young to activist-rallying-her-community.

We also must not let ourselves be mythologized as environmental victims or ecological saviors. These stock images are both inaccurate and unimaginative. The victimization depiction—woman as techno-phobic, biologically weak, and politically ineffectual—only strengthens the hand of patriarchal and patronizing protectionism and blocks the development of appropriate medical, epidemiological, ethical, and political frameworks for tackling environmental disease. While our health is certainly falling victim to environmental degradation, we must not fall victim to our own worst fears, paralyzed while others set the agenda for analysis and action. The savior depiction is incomplete and misses the elaborate evolution of women's relation to industrial environments and the natural world. "Woman as earth protector" imagery can sometimes work to let men off the hook (women will "naturally" clean up the mess); and it may lower our own guard by blinding us to our complicities and to our being manipulated by those who have their own scripts on "women and environment." It is essential then that we do not lapse into seeing ourselves as hapless victims of industrial poisons or annointed planetary angels. Instead we need to focus on women's distinctive experiences, predicaments, struggles, and visions, to critically examine the medical, moral, and political implications of our place in the social ecology.

Ecological Degradation and Disease: Implications for Women's Diagnosis and Treatment

As women have had to tackle doctors and drug companies head on, we now need to examine and influence the work of others who at first glance have only tangential impact on our health. Industrial hygienists, industrial engineers, epidemiologists, toxicologists, detoxification therapists, and lab chemists do not make women's health their business. But women figure into the calculus of their work. Consider for example: lab chemists and epidemiologists who want to "get women's milk" in order to track pollutants through the food chain. Oregon nurse and environmental health activist Kathy Williams—exposed to herbicide spraying—provides this account of being a nursing mother/research subject:

> The sample collectors told me I would be notified within 6 months of the result. Two years later, pregnant again, I was still trying to get the results. After negotiations through my Congressman, the EPA offered me my results—but only if I would sign an agreement not to make the results public. I declined. Although 6 months later the EPA announced that all samples tested negative, a "deep throat" within the agency told antispray activists that there had been positives. (Williams 1987, 4)

Clearly, we must develop ways to assess carefully emerging research activities as they are alternatively offered, withheld, or pressed upon us.

We need to develop a strong perspective on environmental health because of the nature of the diseases involved, the underdevelopment of relevant research, and the traditional gendered practices of conventional medicine. Carcinogens, teratogens, mutagens, asbestos-induced diseases, chemically induced damage to the central nervous system— these are finding a place in the medical curriculum. But there are more "quiet," yet systemic problems that fall under the rubric of ecological illness (EI). Earon Davis, editor of the *Ecological Illness Law Report*, offers this description:

> These illnesses . . . appear to stem from damage to the immune system, from either acute poisoning by toxic chemicals or from chronic, low-level exposures to many substances that ultimately overwhelm the system. The exact symptoms of ecological illness (also known as environmental hypersensitivity disorder, chemically induced immune system disregulation, total allergy syndrome, maladaption syndrome and the twentieth century disease) may vary from person to person, but they generally involve an increasing intolerance to a wide range of chemicals, including ubiquitous substances like formaldehyde, pesticides, natural gas fumes, perfumes and scents, and solvents. The EI victim may experience a wide range of disabling conditions, from a generalized weakness and joint or muscle pain to mental confusion, depression, and even hypertension, lung disease, heart disease, and neurological disorders. (Davis 1986, 34)

When faced with unfamiliar, amorphous patterns of disease, too often physicians explain these away with "diagnoses" such as hypochondria or psychosomatic. Getting accurate diagnoses for ecological illnesses may be more difficult for women than it is for men. It has been demonstrated that women's health complaints are typically more likely to be trivialized and psychologized (Lennane and Lennane 1973). This pattern of discounting women's complaints as not real may be exaggerated in the environmental health arena, in which knowledge and skills are sparse and in which the assignment of environmental diagnoses is politicized, with antienvironmentalists zealously promoting all explanations except those that implicate how American industry does its business. A report on ecological illness notes that women are more likely to tell health practitioners about vague, amorphous EI-type symptoms; also, gender-skewed terms such as neurasthenia, psychogenic, and hysteria find their way into the definition of some EI patterns (Bell 1982). "Female susceptibility," "female chemophobe," "women's

cyclical vulnerability," and "women reactors" are other labels we may
have to reckon with. And so, much work remains to be done to better
understand the physical, emotional, and social aspects of ecological
illness. Finally, as Lois Gibbs and others have observed, women activists' reporting of personal and family health complaints may be held in
contempt by medical authorities as "housewife hysterics" or "housewife research."

Relatedly, the implications for women go beyond diagnosis to treatment. If a woman—either through medical diagnosis or simply personal concern about occupational or environmental exposures—is
worried about her toxic body burden, she may seek treatment. Detoxification treatment at the Health-Med Center in Los Angeles, for example, involves exercise, heat, and vitamin supplements to mobilize
the fat-stored toxins. While clinic staff warn that the procedure is too
risky for pregnant women, it is being touted as a potential reproductive
health promoter that will substantially reduce toxic body burdens in
women prior to conception. This may be true—but it is a much debated
treatment due to questions about medical side effects (such as liver
damage) and the clinic's connection to the Church of Scientology.
Detoxification could be very significant for reproductive health for
both women and men. But in a world where fears about industrial
contamination and reproductive failure are very real, we need to assess
the possible exploitation of soon-to-be pregnant women as a medical
market. Whereas on the one hand mainstream medicine does not give
enough credibility to ecological illness, on the other hand we want to
beware that our fears—justified though they may be—are not preyed
upon and played upon. It is up to us to investigate various detoxification systems, not leaving it merely to the naysayers of the medical
establishment or to the promoters of these newly emerging
systems.

Forces Antagonistic to Feminist Ecology

Another reason for our cultivation of women's environmental health
perspectives is to make sure that imagery and agendas antagonistic to
women do not hold sway. Earlier I noted my concern that we do not
rely on simplistic depictions of women as environmental victim or savior. Other images may also prevail if we do not assert ourselves in this
arena. While some may see women's reproductivity as a victim of
environmental degradation, others see women's reproductive life as the
villain—as perpetrating a population explosion that suffocates life out
of the planet. In an extreme rendition of this scenario, Wolfgang Led-

erer's epistle *The Fear of Women* (1968) carries with it a warning, detailed in the chapter "Planetary Cancer," about the pathological "uterine hunger" of "normal" women who will inundate the world with their progeny; ecocatastrophes can be blamed upon the blindly orgiastic, irrepressible procreativity of the female half of the species (Daly 1987, 290). This view is on the fringe, but it serves to remind us that there are those analysts and activists (many sounding more reasonable than Lederer) who are blind to human-made pestilence, poverty, and pollution, and who myopically hold population—i.e., women whose birthing is not adequately controlled—to be the culprit.

One cultural message that can be very damaging to us all—women and men—is macho survivalism. In this Darwinian script, it is only the weak (in body, mind, and spirit) who fall victim to hazardous environments. This form of institutionalized bravado has certainly allowed American industry to extract much risk-taking labor from the work force. And in the sagas of Love Canal and the community eco-crises that have followed, denial, bluster, and scapegoating have separated the men from the boys, the men from the women, and the men from their own fears. Of course this script is not always played out; but it is familiar enough to have caused much heartache and confusion and to have undermined a militant and effective response to the predicament.

Finally, in the absence of our persistent engagement with environmental policies and politics, special interests will cast women into their various scripts. One example of this is Nuclear Energy Women (NEW), the front group for and auxiliary to the Atomic Industrial Forum (the major nuclear industry lobby). Troubled by women's greater expressed concern (as compared to men's) with nuclear health hazards, the industry concocted a reeducation campaign to lure women back to the atomic fold. Through conferences, lavish weekend retreats for women leaders, and the targeting of women's organizations (from garden clubs to the American Medical Women's Association), NEW has attempted to quell women's "irrational" fears; audiences are warned that women not only stand to gain through nuclear energy—jobs, comforts, security—but will suffer immeasurably in a nonnuclear world stricken by darkness, crime, poverty, urban strife, and global pandemonium. NEW researches women's environmental dreads and dreams, and then casts nuclear energy as the centerpiece of a healthy environment. (For a more detailed analysis of NEW, see Nelson 1984.) It is essential that we comprehend and challenge the organizations, agencies, and arguments that work to diminish our rights to health and our rights to effective participation in ecological politics.

Signs of Change

How is women's studies, particularly the study of women's health, doing with all of this? Much of feminist health education dwells on individual lifestyle and behavioral issues—food, sport, sex. While important, these issues exclude the ecological health and industrial concerns that may be less obvious to or have less direct effect on the relatively affluent college students taking these courses. There are many women—many, if not most, in poor and working-class communities—whose agonies and accomplishments receive scant attention from mainstream and academic feminists. But there is positive movement in the areas of women and science, women and technology, and women and environment. (See Rosser 1986 for a helpful assessment of these fields.)

Our work in women's studies and the various communities of women will be strengthened through the development of environmental health frameworks. For example, the Reproductive Laws of the 1990s Project (based at Rutgers) effectively encompasses the occupational context. It would be fortified further through the inclusion of a broader analysis of the industrial environment, epidemiology, and toxicology as bearing upon reproductive health and rights. A recent feminism and ecology conference (San Diego, Spring 1987) involved historical, theoretical, philosophical, spiritual, and political analyses of women and nature; these explorations are being enriched through the examination of women's health in changing, contaminated environments.

Two encouraging signs are the formation of an Environmental Task Force within the National Women's Studies Association and the founding of the WomanEarth Feminist Peace Institute. At the first Gathering of the American Greens (Amherst, Massachusetts, July 1987), organizers from both of these groups discussed the importance of grounding the "women and environment" question in the examination and support of women's daily struggles for environmental health and the health of the environment.

On the international front there have been some important developments (see WorldWIDE 1987; Dankelman 1987). The Fifth International Conference on Women and Health held in Costa Rica (May, 1987) made environmental health one of the five main areas of examination. And, the first English-language edition of the Latin American and Caribbean Women's Health Network journal had as its feature article a critical examination of occupational and environmental hazards (ISIS 1987). The centrality this issue has for Third World women contrasts with the limited attention environmental health gets in the typical women and health course in U.S. universities.

The Environment, Women, and Children: Current Research, Policies, and Action

While women's environmental health is not yet a well-crafted area of study, there are important developments that demand our attention. There are a growing number of reports—epidemiological, toxicological, clinical, journalistic, anecdotal—on the environmental stress upon women's health, with reproductive health being a prominent topic of concern (Elkington 1985). As epidemiologists are working to refine the study of, for example, the connection between birth defects and proximity to toxic dump sites (Bloom 1981; DePerna 1985), the preliminary reports are sobering. The June, 1984, edition of the *Conservation Foundation Letter* reported the following: many scientists suspect or indict industrial pollutants as contributors to rising infertility, birth defects clusters, miscarriage hot spots, and the unusually early onset of menopause among some women. One researcher commented on the reproductive health predicament: "the womb is more sump than sanctuary" (Conservation Foundation 1984, 5). Dr. Lora Shields's research on the Navajo concludes that the tripling of birth defects in the 1960s can be attributed to the community's contamination with uranium debris. Ojibway women in Grassy Narrows in Ontario have, due to extensive mercury contamination of their foodsupply, given birth to a disproportionate number of disabled and retarded children (Shkilmyk 1986). Women in Silicon Valley, California have called attention to birth defects clusters associated with groundwater polluted from nearby electronics plants, a pattern now under study by the California Department of Health (Ross 1985).

Connected to the issue of reproductive health is the environmental health of children, more often than not born healthy and then faced with hazardous exposures. This is a daunting and compelling issue for women. As the prime care-givers to children, women must negotiate the medical terrain. Furthermore, women are often held responsible for the child's ill-health, when, by force of ignorance or malign intent, medical and political authorities attribute the child's condition to the woman's poor mothering (Gibbs 1982). Blame, guilt, and recrimination play an exhausting part of the emotional complex for women tending to families in threatened communities.

The research on children's environmental health involves a growing number of warning signals: the epidemic of childhood lead poisoning due to gasoline emissions and leaded water systems; childhood leukemia due to chemical exposures (Peters 1987); contact with hazardous substances at school (asbestos, pesticides, paints), on playgrounds (sometimes built on abandoned landfills), and at home (paints, cleansers, insulation materials) that is generating a variety of diseases (Norwood 1980). Accompanying the physical risks posed by such hazards is the emotional toll plaguing children in at-risk communities. Social workers at Love Canal report that depression and even a few suicides among teenage girls were linked to their fears that they—and their children, if they could have any—were destined to be unwell (Freedman 1981; Levine 1982).

Biased Frameworks

In arguing for a steady and systematic look at women and environmental health, I am not taking the position that biological differences place women and men in noncomparable ecological niches; on the contrary, it is important for us to see how the concept of difference vis-à-vis toxics is often used inappropriately and with draconian implications for both men and women. Consider one prominent example of the "toxic gender gap" perspective. In *Toxic Susceptibility: Male/Female Differences,* Edward Calabrese selectively reviews the impact of various hazardous substances; women, it seems, are the relative toxic weaklings (1985). But Jeanne Stellman, founder and director of the Women's Occupational Health Resource Center in New York City, points to the study's methodological weaknesses. Whereas Calabrese reports that women's liver sensitivity puts them at a disadvantage with the chemical dibromochloropropane (DBCP), he neglects to point out that the Office of Technology Assessment recently reported that women are less sensitive than men to the reproductive effects. Whereas Calabrese points to women's blood enzyme system in describing women's comparative susceptibility in response to lead, he neglects to report on the deleterious impact of lead on sperm production. Stellman concludes:

> The data on sex differences are all over the map: sometimes males are more susceptible, sometimes female. But the author does nothing to synthesize this nor come to a conclusion about its implications. He doesn't address the basic issue of species variability but almost pretends that all males and all females respond alike. There is a distribution of responses within each sex, and usually, the variation within the sex is at least of the same order of magnitude as the variation between the sexes (with some exceptions, of course). This book is a disservice to serious debate about regulation and protection of both men and women from toxic substances. (1987, 11)

As the environment becomes hazardous to healthy reproduction and as reproductive technologies expand, we face the serious prospect of increasing social control over women's reproductive rights and civil liberties. Consider the disturbing scenario predicted by Ruth Hubbard: in the arena of "prenatal torts," pregnant women might be found legally responsible for all insults to fetal development, including environmental hazards. Hubbard quotes from attorney Margery Shaw:

> Once a pregnant woman has abandoned her right to abort and has decided to carry her fetus to term, she incurs a "conditional prospective liability" for negligent acts toward her fetus if it should be born alive. These acts could be considered negligent fetal abuse resulting in an injured child. . . . Withholding of necessary prenatal care, improper nutrition, exposure to mutagens and teratogens, or even exposure to the mother's defective intrauterine environment . . . could all result in an injured infant who might claim that his right to be born physically and mentally sound had been invaded. (as quoted in Hubbard 1984, 345)

Governmental Activities

In response to current environmental realities, there have been signs of some attention from government. Some twenty states now have reproductive health monitoring systems, a few (Arkansas and California) directly addressing the industrial contamination question. On the other hand, little work is being done in the federal Department of Health and Human Services, in particular the Public Health Coordinating Committee on Women and Health and the Division of Maternal and Child Health—two of the agencies we would hope would be more interested. The Environmental Protection Agency (EPA) is the most important agency to consider. During the more expansive pre-Reagan years, the EPA had special programs and publications about women and environment; a now-defunct organization Women for Environmental Health emerged from the D.C. circle of female environmentalists. Today there are important developments in the EPA's Office of Reproductive Effects, as researchers attempt to construct models for assessing the various risks to men and women. Gender-specific risk assessment may be of some service (though there are serious questions about the political uses of government-ordained risk-assessment to mask risks from public view). But a "woman as reproducer" model may mean women's general health and men's reproductive health are given inadequate attention. We need to monitor and measure these developments with an eye to the implications for medical treatment, ethical care, and political fairness.

One area of growing concern to many women is now receiving

attention from researchers and to a lesser extent from medical practitioners and policymakers. It is the question of toxic impacts on nursing mothers and infants, an issue that we will now turn to in some detail.

"Would Mother's Milk Pass USDA Inspection?"

Unlike the wide array of environmental concerns that directly influence both men and women, breast-feeding is, of course, women's province. It is a deeply personal—sometimes fulfilling, sometimes taxing—process of nurturance of the young. It is also a highly contested terrain, one in which a range of social customs shapes the experience for mother and child, and infant formula companies have tried to corner the market. The biological and social meanings of breast-feeding are now being complicated by the reports—trickling in since the 1950s with the first accounts of alarming levels of DDT in mothers' milk—that the toxic by-products of modern life are finding their way into the nursing mother. (See American Academy of Pediatrics 1983; Barr 1983; Caprio 1985; Fein 1984; Harris 1977 and 1981; Hart 1987; Jacobsen 1984; Reale 1986; Savage 1984; Smith 1984)

The examination of toxics and lactation is preliminary, sketchy, and hotly debated in certain public health circles. Some of it has become newsworthy: researcher Arnold Schecter asserts that the average American nursing infant receives more dioxin in the first few months of life than is considered safe by the Centers for Disease Control (CDC) for an entire lifespan exposure (Schecter 1986); news of such crises as the spring 1986 heptachlor contamination of the food chain in Arkansas, Oklahoma, and Missouri when nursing mothers were advised that their milk was likely endangering their babies (Farley 1987; Milner 1986; National Coalition Against the Misuse of Pesticides 1986). The CDC rejected Schecter's conclusions and issued a disclaimer, assuring women that their milk is safe. Women facing the tri-state heptachlor scare were given very mixed signals by regional health authorities. Assertions and disclaimers abound on this topic.

The EPA has commissioned or conducted breast milk sampling. Based on 1976 and 1983 assessments, the agency reported that 30 percent of all U.S. women's milk exceeds .5 parts-per-million for polychlorinated biphenyls (PCBs), exceeding the Food and Drug Administration's accepted daily intake (ADI) standards for other foods (Savage 1984). Currently, the EPA is working with the Arkansas Children's Hospital Heptachlor Project to assess the impact of that incident. The World Health Organization (WHO) has issued reports that document the virtual global presence of contaminants in breast milk (World Health Organization 1985a, 1985b, 1986); yet WHO withholds support from some of the more dire warnings issued by some Swedish researchers on the level of toxins in the milk of mothers living in the shadow of European waste incinerators (Rappe 1985a, 1985b). A decade ago in New York State, an Ad Hoc Committee on the Health Implications of PCBs in Mothers' Milk concluded that women who ate fish twice a week should be advised not to breast-feed beyond three months; they urged further research (New York State Health Planning Council 1977). This report lay idle until some Department of Health researchers recently began sampling breast milk in a few New York communities (Bush 1983, 1985).

Reasons for Ineffective Public Health Responses

The somewhat helter-skelter approach of public health agencies to the issue and the inconsistent recommendations offered to the public can be explained in a number of ways. First, it is a very hot item politically: to declare publicly that in a few short decades of industrial pollution we have managed to arrive at the point of universal contamination of mothers' milk is to lend official approval to the most disturbing warnings of ecologists and environmental activists. Second, it is a difficult and expensive area to research, in terms of lab analysis and in finding appropriate control populations. Also, tracking the actual health impacts for the nursing child is proving to be a challenge. We know that today's children are being subjected to toxins in breast milk that excede that of their mothers' generation. Some researchers estimate that a child may be getting up to fifty times her or his mother's body burden of toxins through combined intrauterine and breast-feeding exposures. The World Health Organization estimates that the levels of chlorinated hydrocarbons are ten to fifty times higher in breast milk than in cow's milk or infant formula (World Health Organization 1985a). The most ambitious epidemiological assessment—that of Walter Rogan's prospective study of 900 nursing children—is as yet inconclusive and is subject to serious budgetary and methodological difficulties (Rogan 1985, 1986, 1987). In the balance, it is hard to compare the uncertain risks of toxic exposure with the certain benefits accompanying breast-feeding. After years of challenging corporate control of infant nutrition, prolactation organizations (such as La Leche League) hardly welcome any evidence that in some cases mother's milk may not be best (Mohrbacher 1986).

Finally, the lack of a coherent picture is partly due to people's inclination to protect themselves from the bad—and often conflicting— news on this issue. One doctor commented to me, "I just don't want to know." Many argue that inconclusive and contradictory information only destabilizes further the delicate balance for the nursing mother and infant. One researcher with the Arkansas Heptachlor Project worries about the anguish caused for nursing mothers by the contradictory advice: "I hope that next time, if unfortunately there is a next time, we have our act together." Because of the painful and frightening nature of the toxins/lactation question, there is no coordinated public right-to-know demand. Most environmental groups have paid only occasional attention to the issue; some have used it in an exploitative way (for example, depictions of breasts with "dioxin" stamped on them), to bring attention to their cause, without offering help to nursing women. As counterpoint, some prolactation leaders seem to view environmentalists—sometimes even more than the polluters—as the enemy, accusing them of trying to undermine breast-feeding.

Routes of pollution

What is the source of the contamination? For some women it is workplace exposures (Wolff 1983), for others it is living in the wake of an accident such as the Japanese incident in which PCB-laden fluids contaminated food and resulted in "Yusho syndrome" (sluggishness, motor problems, low IQ, growth impairment, skin disorders) for newborns and nursing infants (Harris 1977). Hawaii has also had a heptachlor/lactation crisis when the pesticide contaminated the food supply (Milner 1986). Some elevated levels of dioxins are attributed to proximity to waste incineration sites (Commoner 1985; Inform 1986; Rappe 1985a, 1985b). For Third World women it is the suffocation of field and home with pesticides (Campos 1979; World Health Organization 1985a, 1985b). But as most researchers will attest, for most women it is not any one exposure or incident, it is the omnipresence of contaminants, particularly through the food chain. One EPA researcher commented to me: "The sad thing is even when something like DDT is banned it is still there, sitting in women's bodies from years of early exposure."

Chlorinated hydrocarbons such as PCBs and polybrominated biphenyls (PBBs) are lipohilic or fat soluble; they concentrate in the body's fat stores, which then become mobilized during lactation. Newborns are at the top of the food chain. Those of us who nurse today's and tomorrow's infants are possibly delivering the results of years of toxic bioaccumulation. One disturbing example of this is that the pollution of the Great Lakes—one of North America's toxic hotspots—is working its way up the food chain to the fish that many women turn to for protein. Some researchers assert that Great Lakes–area children exposed to high levels of PCBs in utero and through nursing may be suffering developmental difficulties (Cobb 1987; Fein 1984). For years now and with increasing restrictions, New York State issues fish advisories that warn nursing mothers to eat Great Lakes fish only rarely, if at all.

Support and strategies for nursing mothers

Many questions persist, and much work remains to be done. First of all, those of us determined to see women as participants and not pawns in the tensions between environmentalists and prolactation groups (an unfortunate tension that distracts from the real assailants on our health) must do the following: we must challenge environmentalists not to sensationalize an already sensitive matter for nursing women; second, we must urge breast-feeding advocates to see that conscionable support of nursing mothers requires a well-informed perspective, one more critical of government environmental policy and industrial polluters than of these who are the bearers of bad ecological tidings. One organization that is on the frontlines of the effort to protect nursing mothers and infants and enlighten the public is the National Network to Prevent Birth Defects; it has issued a very important position paper and is pressing the EPA to make the social ecology of nursing mothers and children the measure of environmental quality; that is, only when human milk is assuredly safe again can we legitimately claim to be protecting the environment (National Network to Prevent Birth Defects 1985).

As we try to reverse the patterns of pollution (the only real solution), practical and painful questions persist for breast-feeding mothers. How can I know to what extent I'm putting my child at risk? How can I judge the tests and advisories? What level of which contaminants is too much? Should I stop after three months or does the heaviest dose come early anyway? If I have a lifelong body burden of contaminants, will changing my diet during pregnancy make any difference? Will my second child get less of a dose? And what about me: do these fat-stored contaminants heighten my risks of breast cancer, and why isn't research being done on this? These and other questions are very pertinent—and some are under study.

In the breach, as researchers scramble for evidence, it is probably not reasonable for most women to avoid or suddenly stop breast-feeding and turn to formulas. Most researchers and the few activist/researchers dealing with this subject (such as Katsi Cook, see below) argue that the benefits still outweigh the risks in most cases (Cook 1985; Rogan 1985, 1986, 1987). And in some parts of the country babies are dying from "blue baby syndrome" due to agricultural chemical contamination of water supplies, which may be used for formulas (Fruhling 1986). We should not allow infant formula promoters to exploit the situation with claims once again of "ours is better."

Emotionally, this is a very burdensome issue. I can attest to this, having read much of this research as I've nursed my daughter. Guilt, uncertainty, feeling polluted and polluting, rage, sorrow are part of the panoply of feelings. Psychologist Sherry Hatcher explored some of this emotional terrain when she questioned about one hundred Michigan mothers about their responses to a PCB incident during which their milk was tested and they were issued a very hazy advisory by public health authorities (Hatcher 1982). She found that some women experienced haunting images, such as "I looked at my body as a dispenser of poisons." Others, especially those with higher contaminant levels, coped through denial, one cavalierly commenting, "You can't cry over spilled milk." None remained untouched. We must do all that we can so that women do not end up feeling that they are the irresponsible, polluted ones or withdraw with hardened resignation about their predicament.

An example of women tackling this with a vision that goes beyond self-recrimination and resignation is the Akwesasne Environment/ Mother's Milk Project. The Mohawk Nation at Akwesasne (along the St. Lawrence River) is at chemical risk due to the deterioration of the Great Lakes and due to the neighboring industries—General Motors and Reynolds Aluminum in particular—spewing contaminants onto Mohawk land and into the water supply. The women, avid fish eaters and concerned about reports such as those noted here, initiated a community-based study of breast-feeding and children (Cook and Nelson 1985). The project involves negotiated relations with the New York State Department of Health, independent laboratories, foundations, universities, and other outside forces. But dealing with outside forces is nothing new to the Mohawks. Katsi Cook, community midwife and project director, describes their efforts:

> Just as native women are returning to breast-feeding (after years of being told it was wrong), it is discouraging that women now have reason to question whether their breast milk is safe. Women feel doubly colonized— by threats to natural resources and our health, and by technological "solutions" that threaten cultural ways. Through Akwesasne Environment, we are working to develop a fuller understanding of our situation, to make well-informed choices, and to strengthen our community. (Cook 1985, 15)

To try to remain sovereign women, as the Mohawk women are struggling to do in the face of tremendous threats to their health and identity, should be the model for the rest of us.

Building an Activist Agenda for Women and Environmental Health

Against the backdrop of late-twentieth-century pollution and amidst the reports of toxic breast milk, infertility, birth defects clusters, and ecological illness, there is much going on that is encouraging and thought provoking. The Mohawk women are part of a widening circle of indigenous people in this hemisphere who are inspiring and instructing others about the links between social oppression and ecological destruction. There is a strengthening network of resistance to the dumping of hazardous products and hazardous waste in the Third World. In the United States, the National Network to Prevent Birth Defects is challenging researchers, health practitioners, policymakers, and the public to examine how business-as-usual in industry and agriculture is casting a toxic shadow over our children. The Nurses Environmental Health Watch is bringing the environmental message into the daily arena of health care and health education, and is urging nurses to speak out against hazardous landfills and to support such campaigns as the United Farm Workers' antipesticide boycott. The Citizens' Clearinghouse for Hazardous Wastes has initiated a new project—Family Stress, Burn-out, and Women as Emerging Leaders—to respond to the tremendous strain women organizers endure as they become frontline risk takers. To bolster such efforts and to push forward the momentum of analysis and action, the National Women's Health Network is preparing a *Resource Guide on Women and Occupational/Environmental Health*.

To move forward, I think we need to develop analyses and take action in a number of ways.

First, women's health—caring for it, teaching about it, research into it, and policies pertaining to it—should always be approached ecologically. If we are to further our understanding of reproductive health, birthing, aging, gynecological health, cancer, and stress, we must extend our view to the broad industrial, technological, and nature-distorted world around us. Without this extended view our health remains decontextualized and medicalized; we risk losing the opportunity to comprehend causes and to enact preventive action.

Research should develop in several directions. The first involves an examination of the technologies of production that cause or contribute to environmental illness. Second, we should look at the technologies and techniques in the medical, epidemiological, and public health fields that are intended to surveil, screen, diagnose, and treat environmental illness. From fertility screening to lab analysis of breast milk to epidemiological assessments of placentas to detoxification treatments, there is an array of processes that may be offered to, withheld from, or forced upon women—with serious implications for reproductive choice, patient's rights, rights-to-privacy, right-to-know, and research subject's rights. Third, we should critically examine the technologies of remediation, the hardware and procedures presented as capable of restoring polluted places or limiting the damage done. One such remedial technology—waste incineration—is, according to European researchers, posing ever heightened risks to breast-feeding mothers and infants (Commoner 1985; Inform 1986; Rappe 1985a, 1985b).

The pace of environmental health research will undoubtedly quicken. We need to monitor those who would monitor us—our fertility, our breast milk, our chemical sensitivities, and so on. We must provide for accurate and effective uses of the "variables" of race, class, and gender as they bear upon ecological illness. We must ensure that research on pressing questions—like those of concern to the nursing mother or about the effectiveness of detoxification treatment for women wanting to bear children—be made high priorities. But we must not let the research control our lives: being activists instead of someone else's data base is crucial. We need to stand firm on informed consent, access to data, participatory research, and other protections.

We must continually assess how the concept of difference is used as a tool in assessing the physical and social ecologies. We do need to know when there are sexual differences in toxic susceptibility (with either men or women being more susceptible, depending on the specific toxin, the nature and timing of the exposure, etc.); and we do need to protect those at special risk. However, we must continue to keep a skeptic's eye on specious theorizing on "difference" and on sex-specific risk assessments that may promote policies of social control (such as the fetal protection policies, see Bertin in this volume) and that may undermine efforts to protect all people and regenerate the environment. We must take an active role in influencing how the EPA, the Centers for Disease Control, and other regulatory and research organizations do their work.

We need to guard against tighter social control, either in the form of "toxic individualism" or techno-fix solutions. By "toxic individualism," I mean such emerging areas as "prenatal torts," in which an individual woman might be held liable for exposing the fetus to hazards,

hazards outside her control. We also need to resist such quick—and hazardous—fixes as the promotion of reproductive technologies (such as in vitro fertilization) as suitable replacements for reproductive systems damaged by toxic exposures. The "not-to-worry about the environment, we have alternatives" school must be revealed as rabidly antiecological.

We must remain ever-vigilant about the agendas others would have us live—whether it is Nuclear Energy Women, eugenicists with master plans about who is fit to bear children, or environmentalists who may insinuate women are "the cause" or adulate us as "the solution." In turn, we need to support the growing number of women who are making major contributions—whether as degreed scientists or as "kitchen table researchers." The special efforts of the Citizen's Clearinghouse for Hazardous Wastes to honor, protect, and strengthen women activists should be applauded.

As we struggle to educate ourselves and others, to conduct and promote the necessary research, and to take action on both insidious and imminent environmental dangers, we must nourish a sensitivity to each other's emotional experience of all this. The experience of feeling threatened by hazardous environments, of feeling polluted, victimized, violated. We need to explore the consequences of feeling like a toxic threat to others—particularly to our own children. The experience of being studied and surveiled as "biological markers," as "monitored reproducers," as "top of the food chain." The experience of being shunned or scapegoated for taking action. We must be able to see in each other the possibility of developing the strength and vision to bring the world to its senses.

BIBLIOGRAPHY

American Academy of Pediatrics, Committee on Drugs. 1983. The transfer of drugs and other chemicals into human milk. *Pediatrics* 72, no. 3: 375–83.
Barr, Mason. 1981. Environmental contaminants of human breast milk. *American Journal of Public Health* 71, no. 2: 124–26.
Bell, Iris. 1982. *Clinical ecology: A new medical approach to environmental illness.* Bolinas, Cal.: Common Knowledge Press.
Bloom, Arthur. 1981. *Guidelines for studies of human populations exposed to mutagenic and reproductive hazards.* White Plains, N.Y.: March of Dimes Foundation.
Bush, Brian. 1985. Polychlorinated biphenyl congeners (PCBs), p,p'-DDE and hexachlorobenzene in human milk in three areas of upstate New York. *Archives of Environmental Contamination and Toxicology* 14:443–50.

Calabrese, Edward. 1985. *Toxic susceptibility: Male/female differences.* New York: Wiley-Interscience.

Campos, Marit, and A. E. Olszyna-Marzys. 1979. Contamination of human milk with chlorinated pesticides in Guatemala and El Salvador. *Archives of Environmental Contamination and Toxicology* 8:43–58.

Caprio, Emma-Lee. 1985. Breastmilk contamination: Tragic Indicator. *Re:Sources* (publication of the Environmental Task Force) 6, no. 1: 3.

Chavkin, Wendy. 1984. *Double Exposure: Women's Health Hazards on the Job and at Home.* New York: Monthly Review Press.

Cobb, Charles E. 1987. The Great Lakes' Troubled Waters. *National Geographic,* July: 2–32.

Commoner, Barry, Thomas Webster, and Karen Shapiro. 1985. Environmental Levels and Health Effects of PCDDs and PCDFs. Paper presented at the Fifth International Symposium on Dioxins and Related Compounds, Bayreuth, West Germany, September 16–17.

Conservation Foundation. 1984. How Serious Are the Hazards to Reproduction? *Conservation Foundation Letter,* May-June, 1–6.

Cook, Katsi. 1985. A community health project: Breastfeeding and toxic contaminants. *Indian Studies,* Spring: 14–16.

Cook, Katsi, and Lin Nelson. 1985. The seven generations: Community epidemiology and environmental protection in indian country: Lessons from a Mohawk women's health project. Paper presented to the annual meeting of the American Public Health Association, Washington, D.C.

Daly, Mary. 1978. *Gyn/Ecology: The metaEthics of radical feminism.* Boston: Beacon Press.

Dankelman, Irene. 1987. *Women and environment: Alliance for a sustainable future.* London: Cambridge Press.

Davis, Earon. 1986. Ecological illness. *Trial,* October: 34–40.

DiPerna, Paula. 1985. *Cluster mystery: Epidemic and the children of Woburn, Massachusetts.* St. Louis: C. V. Mosby.

Elkington, John. 1985. *The poisoned womb: Human reproduction in a polluted world.* New York: Viking Penguin.

Farley, Dixie. 1987. From tainted feed to mothers' milk: A pesticide's devastating journey thru the food chain. *FDA Consumer* March: 38–40.

Fein, Greta. 1984. Intrauterine exposure of humans to PCBs: Newborn effects. *EPA Report* 600-3-84-060.

Freedman, Tracy. 1981. "Love Canal children: Leftover lives to live." *Nation,* May 23: 624–27.

Freudenberg, N., and E. Zaltzberg. 1984. From grassroots activism to political power: Women organizing against environmental hazards. In *Double exposure: Women's health hazards on the job and at home,* ed. Wendy Chavkin, 246–72. New York: Monthly Review Press.

Fruhling, Larry. 1986. Please don't drink the water. *Progressive,* October: 31–33.

Gibbs, Lois Marie. 1982. *Love Canal: My story.* Albany: State University of New York Press.

Gottlieb, B., and P. Wiley. 1986. Defenders of the home. *Sierra*, January-February: 49–52.

Harris, Stephanie, and Joseph Highland. 1977. Birthright denied: The risks and benefits of breastfeeding. New York: Environmental Defense Fund.

Harris, Stephanie. 1981. Health risks and benefits of nursing or bottle-feeding: The limits of individual choice. In *Strategies for public health: Promoting health and preventing disease*, ed. L. Ng and D. L. Davis, 58–178. New York: Van Nostrand Reinhold Co.

Hart, Kathleen. 1987. Is mother's milk safe? Dioxin climbs to the top of the food chain. *Progressive*, March: 32–34.

Hatcher, Sherry. 1982. The psychological experience of nursing mothers upon learning of a toxic substance in their milk. *Psychiatry* 45:172–81.

Hubbard, Ruth. 1984. Personal courage is not enough: Some hazards of childbearing in the 1980's. In *Test-tube Women: What future for motherhood?*, ed. R. Arditti, R. Klein, and S. Minden, 231–55. Boston: Pandora.

Inform. 1986. Europeans disagree over dioxin from burnt garbage. *Inform Report* 6, no. 1: 1.

ISIS. 1987. Campaign against toxic and dangerous agricultural, industrial and consumer products. In *Women's Health Journal* 1:11–15. From the Latin American and Caribbean Women's Health Network. Santiago, Chile: ISIS International.

Jacobsen, Joseph. 1984. The transfer of PCBs and PBBs across the placenta and into maternal milk. *American Journal of Public Health* 74, no. 4: 378–79.

Kraus, Susan. 1986. Those women of Oregon: They've led the way to pesticide reform. *Environmental Action*, May-June: 28–31.

Lennane, K. J., and R. J. Lennane. 1973. Alleged psychogenic disorders in women: A possible manifestation of sexual prejudice. *New England Journal of Medicine* 288, no. 6 (February 8): 288–92.

Levine, Adeline. 1982. *Love Canal: Science, politics and people.* Lexington, Mass.: D. C. Heath Co.

Milner, Anne. 1986. Banned but not forgotten. *Sierra*, July-August: 30–31.

Mohrbacher, Nancy. 1986. Breastfeeding and contaminants. *La Leche League Journal* 2, no. 5: 128–30.

National Coalition Against the Misuse of Pesticides. 1985. Poisoned milk illustrates weak law. *Pesticides and You* 6, no. 2: 1.

National Network to Prevent Birth Defects. 1985. Petition for a breast milk purity strategy. Petition to EPA, March 1.

Nelson, Lin. 1984. Promise her everything: The nuclear power industry's agenda for women. *Feminist Studies* 10, no. 2 (Summer): 291–314.

———. 1987. Nurses take action on environmental health issues. *Listen Real Loud* (publication of the American Friends Service Committee Nationwide Women's Project) 8, no. 1: 6.

New York State Health Planning Council. 1977. Report of the ad hoc committee on the health implications of PCBs in mother's milk. January 7.

Norwood, Christopher. 1980. *At highest risk: Environmental hazards to young and unborn children.* New York: McGraw-Hill.

Peters, J. M. 1987. Childhood leukemia and parent's occupation and home exposures. *Journal of the National Cancer Institute,* July: 39–46.

Rappe, Christoffer. 1985a. Problems in analysis of PCBBs and PDBFs and the presence of these compounds in human milk. Paper presented at the WHO Consultation on Organohalogen Compounds in Human Milk and Related Hazards. Bilthoven, the Netherlands, January 9–11.

————. 1985b. Identification of 2,3,7,8 PCDDs and PDDFs in the environment and human samples. Paper presented to the American Chemical Society's Meeting on Chlorinated Dioxins and Furans in the Total Environment. Miami, April.

Reale, Barbara. 1986. Breast milk contamination: An issue for nurses. *Health Watch* (publication of the Nurses Environmental Health Watch) 7, no. 2: 1.

Rogan, Walter, and Beth Gladen. 1985. Study of human lactation for the effects of environmental contaminants: The North Carolina breast milk and formula project and some other ideas. *Environmental Health Perspectives* 60:215–21.

Rogan, Walter, Beth Gladen, James McKinney, Nancy Carreras, Pam Hardy, James Thullen, John Tingelstad, and Mary Tully. 1986. PCBs and DDE in human milk: Effects of maternal factors and previous lactation. *American Journal of Public Health* 76, no. 2: 172–77.

————. 1987. PCBs and DDE in human milk: Effects on growth, morbidity and duration of lactation. *American Journal of Public Health* 77, no. 10: 1,294–97.

Ross, Lorraine. 1985. Bittersweet vindication: State study confirms birth defect cluster. *Silicon Valley Toxics News* 2, no. 1: 3.

Rosser, Sue. 1984. *Teaching health and science from a feminist perspective.* New York: Pergamon Press.

Savage, Eldon, Thomas Keefe, H. William Wheeler, John D. Tessari, and Michael J. Aronson. 1984. Second national study to determine levels of chlorinated hydrocarbon insecticides and polychlorinated biphenyls in human milk. Report of the Colorado Pesticide Hazard Assessment Project, Colorado State University, Ft. Collins.

Schecter, Arnold. 1986. Comparisons of human tissue levels of dioxin and furan isomers in potentially exposed and controlled patients 15 years after cessation of 2,3,7,8 TCDD environmental contamination. Paper presented to the American Chemical Society National Meeting, New York, April 13–18.

Shkilmyk, Anastasia. 1986. *A poison stronger than love; The destruction of an Ojibway community.* New Haven: Yale University.

Shute, Nancy. 1987. Toxic green: Mothers in arms take on the lawn chemical industry. *Amicus Journal,* Summer: 10–17.

Smith, B. Jill. 1984. PCB levels in human fluid: Sheboygan case study. University of Wisconsin Sea Grant Institute, Madison.

Stellman, Jeanne. 1987. Book review: Edward Calabrese's toxic susceptibility: Male/female differences. *Women's Occupational Health Resource Center News* 8, no. 2: 11.

Williams, Kathy. 1987. Slashburning and herbicides: The politics of caring. *Health Watch* (publication of the Nurses Environmental Health Watch) 7, no. 4: 1.

Wolff, Mary S. 1983. Occupationally derived chemicals in milk. *American Journal of Industrial Medicine* 4:259–81.

World Health Organization. 1985a. *Organohalogen compounds in human milk and related hazards.* Report on WHO Consultation, Bilthoven, the Netherlands, January 9–11. Geneva.

————. 1985b. *The quantity and quality of human milk: Report on the WHO collaborative study on breastfeeding.* Geneva.

————. 1986. *Principles for evaluating health risks from chemicals during infancy and early childhood: The need for a special approach.* Environmental Health Criteria 59. Geneva: WHO, the United Nations Environmental Program, and the International Labor Organization.

WorldWIDE (World Women in Defense of the Environment). 1987. Newsletter and Directory. WorldWIDE, 1250 24th St. NW, Washington, D.C. 20037.

Sustaining Our Organizations: Feminist Health Activism in an Age of Technology

Gail O. Mellow

Feminist cartoonist Nicole Hollander has drawn a cartoon in which two women are sitting at a kitchen table. One woman says to the other, "I'm certainly glad I'm past childbearing age, so that I can continue to work in this vile polluted atmosphere." The other woman replies "Yes, we are indeed privileged to have the opportunity to develop many debilitating illnesses that a less greedy management would have deprived us of." Angry? Absolutely. Funny? Only in a chilling, black humor sort of way. This cartoon, a less-than-conventional form of health advocacy, is symbolic of the creative ways in which women fight for healthy lives for themselves, their children, their families, and indeed, the planet. Hollander is one of many female voices rising in opposition to the variety of health hazards that women face as they live, work, and play in the twentieth century.

The intent of this chapter is to characterize the current status of activism within the women's health movement, to identify evolving strategies and ideologies, to mention some of the hallmark achievements, to review the lessons gained from these achievements, and to outline future challenges. This chapter is written in homage to the strength and courage of individual women, emboldened by their own experiences, who challenge a monolithic health system by joining forces with other women to create vibrant and effective advocacy organizations, and it is aimed at empowering women to work actively on health.

Two Decades in Retrospect

Beginning in the late 1960s, a feminist health movement emerged in this country that said no to "business-as-usual" medicine. Grass-roots activists—small groups of women meeting, sharing information and horror stories, and developing their own literature—began to identify the medical system's failings. These included the medical system's failure to identify the real medical problems that women faced; its development of inadequate research strategies; its overreliance on medical technology; its disease orientation; its lack of female practitioners; and its underlying profit motive (Fee 1983; Ruzek 1978; Rodriguez-Trias 1984).

Early health activism focused primarily on individual solutions to individual or local problems. There was a decidedly antitechnology cast to the early activism; it was common for grass-roots activists to reject any technological answer to a medical problem, including use of drugs, medical technologies, or surgery. But while the first wave of activism was centered on consciousness-raising to identify women's particular health concerns and on political actions to bring public attention to them, we will see that the next phase has moved to more issue-specific actions played out in larger arenas.

Today, the grass-roots organizing of the 1970s has been transformed to include a more complex and comprehensive vision of technology, a more social view of the components of health care, and a more national and international perspective on health advocacy. As with the other components of the women's movement, current organizing encompasses a greater range of targets as well as a greater diversity of race, class, and ethnicity among its participants. Included in this diversity is a variety of approaches to technology.

Looking at feminist health activism over the past twenty years, three important differences can be identified: (1) the nature of the organizations has differentiated; (2) feminist health organizations' relationship to technology has changed; and (3) activists have moved from outside the health system to greater advocacy from within. I will examine each of these changes in order to ground the subsequent discussion of current activism, and I will cull from these historical changes a perspective on the ingredients needed to establish enduring platforms from which to launch future feminist health advocacy.

The Emerging Differences Among Women's Health Organizations

Across the United States, small, local, informally organized groups of women passionately committed to a specific issue still work diligently to create better health for themselves. In Jacksonville, Arkansas groups of mothers mobilized in 1985 around alarming rates of miscarriages and stillbirths in their community attributed to high rates of dioxin contamination. Such local grass-roots organizations are an important component in the overall picture of women's health activism. Yet, as these local organizations remain and proliferate, there is increasing differentiation among feminist health organizations. The movement is now additionally characterized by women's organizations that focus on national and international issues, that are organizationally structured in a formal rather than informal manner, and that employ both defensive and proactive tactics.

Three organizations, the National Abortion Rights Action League (NARAL), the Boston Women's Health Book Collective (BWHBC), and the National Black Women's Health Project (NBWHP), provide examples of the differing nature of women's health organizations. These organizations trace their individual history to smaller, geographically localized actions, and their present national and formal structure complements rather than replaces the local informal groups.

Examining the National Abortion Rights Action League (NARAL) is instructive because NARAL's ability to capitalize on grass-roots organizing illustrates a typical pattern in the development of mainstream women's health organizations. In addition, the recognition of the limitations of NARAL's philosophy and methods was instrumental in spawning other national reproductive rights organizations with a broader scope. Finally, given the political situation of the past two decades, NARAL provides a good example of the way in which defensive tactics are used by women's health organizations.

Access to reproductive technologies and procedures, and limits on sterilization abuses, were among the clearest and most unanimous of the early feminist demands. Abortion rights activism was an organizing tool: many feminist organizations participated in early actions (sit-ins, pamphleting, guerrilla theater, demonstrations) to demand free and safe abortion services. NARAL developed in the early 1970s as it became clear that a national clearinghouse for information and a national presence to lobby for federal legislation was needed.

The grass-roots activities that preceded NARAL's development created an environment in which the rhetoric and feminist perspective on reproductive freedom was widespread among feminist health activists. Because of this, knowledgeable and committed local activists were ready to be attracted to the emerging national organization and were essential to its development. Thus, NARAL could establish local chapters without conducting the basic groundwork that would have been necessary had the grass-roots activities not taken place. Currently, NARAL maintains statewide chapters, allowing it to keep a connection to the local level and to lobby in state legislatures while inspiring national action and defending against assaults from the right.

NARAL's very public and national stance was vital to the formation of other national women's organizations concerned with reproductive rights. Because of NARAL's high and public profile, it was often covered in the mass media as "the" representative of the feminist

stance on reproductive rights. Yet NARAL's philosophy about reproductive rights, particularly with regard to class, disability, and
race/ethnicity was criticized by other feminist reproductive rights activists. New organizations, notably the Coalition for Abortion Rights
and Against Sterilization Abuse (CARASA) and the Reproductive Rights
National Network (R2N2) emerged in part in response to this critique.

CARASA and R2N2 are vocal on the national level in criticizing
NARAL for being a predominantly middle-class, white women's organization, sometimes insensitive to the concerns of women of color
and of poor women. These groups argue that access to abortion can
not be separated from access to all forms of contraception, or from
freedom from forced sterilization. They caution NARAL not to ghet-
toize the problems of Third World women by presuming that forced
sterilization and population control are issues for women of color, while
abortion is the concern of white women. NARAL has also been criticized by women in the disability rights movement, who charge that
NARAL talks about fetuses in a way that exploits women's fears of
disabled children without adequately addressing issues of sterilization
abuse among disabled women. Despite this apparent acrimony, this
dynamic conflict is essential for feminist organizations to refine their
organizational focus, encouraging an ever more differentiated and more
inclusive perspective on specific health concerns.

The critiques notwithstanding, NARAL has contributed much to
feminist health activism through its development and refinement of
"defensive" advocacy tactics. Since 1973, when the *Roe* v. *Wade* Supreme Court decision allowed for abortions within the first trimester,
NARAL has fought to protect a range of reproductive rights from a
dizzying array of assaults. NARAL's defensive efforts have had to be
flexible and vigilant in order to respond to major challenges at the
federal level (for example, the Hyde amendment, passed in 1977, which
prohibited federal funding of abortion services) as well as small but no
less significant challenges at the local level (such as a city referendum
held in 1984, to condemn abortion in Bristol, Connecticut).

To preserve the range of reproductive rights initially granted by
Roe v. *Wade,* NARAL's approach is generally to pursue high-profile
national campaigns. These national campaigns, funded by sophisticated
national mailings, feature professional lobbyists and expert testimony
before Congress. Other feminist activists organizations use different
approaches, even humor, in mounting the defense against the right.
Ladies Against Women, a San Francisco-based theater troupe, dons
pillbox hats and white gloves to descend upon antiabortion groups with
signs that read "Sperm are People TOO!" Collectively, many organizations are defensively engaged in the constant battle to fight the at-

trition of reproductive rights, especially for low-income women, from the local to the national level.

Other groups use a more proactive strategy to advance their work. The Boston Women's Health Book Collective (BWHBC) is one of those organizations. It began in 1969 when a group of women met at a Boston women's liberation conference where health issues were discussed (Beckwith 1985). Meeting after the conference with the express purpose of developing a directory of good doctors in the Boston area, the group found this goal unobtainable. Instead, they began to share their individual frustrations with the existing health care system. The group met regularly and became committed to developing their own sources of information by talking to lay women and medical practitioners. By 1972 a group of twelve had established a collective. Their efforts at fact-finding, blended with personal interviews, resulted in their first book, *Our Bodies, Ourselves,* initially appearing on local bookstands in newsprint and eventually brought out by a major publisher (Beckwith 1985).

We can see the change from a local, informal approach to a globally focused and formalized one after BWHBC's first success. They used the royalties from the wildly successful book to sponsor other grass-roots women's health projects. BWHBC actively supported the development of the National Women's Health Network, an umbrella of women's health organizations established in 1976. They went on to develop several more books and documents (including films) on women's health which are now published in many languages for worldwide distribution. By staying especially sensitive to poor and minority women's health needs and to the international repercussions of United States policies, BWHBC has aggressively directed their proactive advocacy and education to promoting greater health for the widest possible audience.

As its geographical scope widened, and the number of its activities increased, BWHBC also altered its structure from a loose collection of women to a more formal configuration. It has recently formalized its internal organizational structure by appointing a board of directors. This governing entity will continue the efforts of the collective, staffing a resource center, coordinating efforts to produce future publications, and actively bringing health concerns to the general public.

A third organization, the National Black Women's Health Project (NBWHP) demonstrates how quickly local movements can become national with the growing sophistication of the women's health movement. Almost from the start, NBWHP has maintained a simultaneous local and national focus.

The beginnings of the NBWHP, established in 1981 in Atlanta,

Georgia, are representative of the way in which many feminist health organizations develop. Rooted in specific, personal experiences with problems in the health care system, women create organizations to respond to their fresh vision of needed health care practices. The seeds for the NBWHP were planted when Byllye Avery's young husband died of high blood pressure. Avery came to learn that high blood pressure, a disease of epidemic proportions in the Black community, can be managed with self-care and realistic education. Avery became the founder of the NBWHP, where her experience infuses both a perspective on self-care and an understanding of the socio-political grounding of health care into the activities of the Project. Thus, NBWHP acknowledges the special health problems of Black women as integrally tied to the socio-economic problems of the Black family. It emphasizes that poverty, unemployment, family fragmentation, and inadequate education are all forces that make Black people more prone to stress-induced illnesses and higher rates of chronic disease.

The Project distinguishes itself most clearly, however, in its ability to work at the local, national, and international levels. As the Project provides direct services in its local Atlanta neighborhood, it also works to place the concerns of Black women on the national agenda. The National Institutes of Health (NIH) did not consider cervical cancer a communicable disease until the NBWHP consulted with NIH about their experiences with women in the Atlanta community. The national presence of the NBWHP is also maintained through conferences and distribution of materials; it has established over fifty-two local self-help chapters across the country. NBWHP's latest educational film, *On Becoming a Woman,* which shows mothers and daughters in workshops held by NBWHP talking about menstruation, sex, and relationship issues, has received rave reviews. Its strongly interactive stance—direct experience providing health care, and then advocacy work to bring this experience to national attention—is one of the creative and important dynamics that still fuels the national women's health movement with the vitality of the grass roots. Finally, the NBWHP is holding a 1989 international conference on Black women's health to be held in the Caribbean, illustrating its international focus and activities.

Many other examples exist of the varieties of organizational structure of women's health organization. Sometimes formal and national, sometimes small and informal, and often with feet planted at both ends of this continuum, organizations continue to develop structures and strategies to create real options for women's health. The National Women's Health Network, the Federation of Feminist Women's Health Centers, and other formally organized and nationally focused health organizations function to bring women's health concerns to public attention, to develop service delivery systems that promote health, and to educate broadly on the feminist issues in health care. At the same time, women still meet in living rooms to discuss the latest problem with their community health clinic.

From "Luddite" to Appropriate Technology

In the weaving districts of England in the mid-nineteenth century, a workers' movement emerged that has given its name to individuals unilaterally opposed to technological transformations. As weaving machines were installed in shops, a group of weavers attacked and destroyed these machines, frequently scrawling antagonistic notes from a fictitious Ned Ludd—thus the term *Luddites*. Although Luddite has come to mean opposition to any new technology, a closer look at history reveals that the Luddites were selective in their destruction of weaving machines, attacking only those machines in shops where their introduction lowered wages or displaced workers. Thus the Luddites' focus was not antitechnology, but against the negative impact of the use of such technology. Over time, the women's health movement has seen a change in ethics from a near absolute rejection of technology, in line with the common meaning of Luddite, to an ethic of knowledgeable choices about appropriate technology much more akin to the real legacy of the Luddite movement.

Early pamphlets from the women's health movement show a decidedly Luddite approach to technology, using the common meaning of the term. Yet given the reality of women's experience with the health care system's widespread and excessive reliance on medical technology, this critique was appropriate. Cast in this light, these activists were closer to the more historically accurate meaning of Luddite. Moreover, these early, lacerating critiques of medical technology provided an important impetus to resist traditional medical care. Books such as *Lunaception* (Lacey 1975) purporting to regulate ovulation with the moon and therefore make the "rhythm" method of birth control reliable or *Spiritual Midwifery* (Gaskin 1977), which promotes lay attendance during normal childbirth, were grounded in a strongly antitechnology ethos. Antitechnology stances are still present in the movement: for example, the international organization Finnrage is totally opposed to the use of high-technology reproductive procedures such as in vitro fertilization in all circumstances.

Early activists also promoted self-care as a response to the health care system, but this required highly committed women with enough time and patience to learn to examine themselves. For example, the Los Angeles Feminist Women's Health Center developed systems for gynecological self-examination in the 1970s (Ruzek 1978). More recently, however, the way in which self-help is defined has changed. Today, self-help is more likely to mean that women actively participate in choices and develop and share information about the technology that supports their health care.

The National Women's Health Network defines self-help as an activist approach to health, with self-help differentiated from self-care, and seen as a way to initiate and control health and "validate ourselves" (National Women's Health Network 1980, 2). There are many instances of working with, instead of unilaterally against, medical technology. The Women's Cancer Resource Center in San Francisco provides information to cancer patients so that they can more fully participate in decisions about chemotherapy and surgical techniques (Selleck 1988). The Moroccan Association of Women and Health provides a service through which women get needed information about the side effects and efficacy of prescription drugs they have received (Tudiver 1986). Thus the evolving feminist health perspective is that technology may be used, but only to the extent that it is determined appropriate by the consumer as well as the attending health professional, who fully discloses the technology's benefits and liabilities.

The testing of the cervical cap, primarily by feminist health clinics, in order to secure Food and Drug Administration (FDA) approval in the United States is an example of the emergence of an empowering dynamic that allows control of technology. Because feminists actively established the criteria by which the medical establishment evaluated this technology, they implicitly outlined the parameters for appropriate medical technology. The cervical cap is deemed appropriate by feminist health activists because it is less disruptive to the body than other birth control technologies; it can be inserted for several days at a time, requiring less planning; it requires less spermicide and only one application at each insertion, so it is less expensive than other technologies; and it can be fitted by nurse practitioners. These benefits suggest a definition of appropriate medical technology: the technology is available to all women (not just women from a particular race or class), it can be administered by nonphysician practitioners outside of traditional medical settings, it is minimally disruptive to the body, and it works with instead of against the body's natural functioning.

A network of feminist health clinics in conjunction with the National Women's Health Network also used the testing of the cervical cap to frame the kinds of questions that should determine whether or not a new medical technology is deemed good for women's health. They required an evaluation that included women as fully informed participants in the efficacy trials, that considered all changes resulting from the technology as effects rather than labeling some as effects and others as side effects, and that incorporated clients' stated concerns about sexuality, pregnancy, and work into its assessments. By framing the questions about efficacy and safety, and by creating and implementing the evaluation research methodology, feminists put their concerns at the center of the process. This is a good model process, for it promotes "appropriate" medical technology while making women more equal partners in the decision-making structure of medical science. This process might be contrasted with the development and implementation of in vitro fertilization (IVF) techniques. Women are denied the most basic information about IVF and even statistics about how success rates are measured are generally obscured. (See Beck-Gernsheim in this volume; Corea 1985)

Increasing Activism from the Inside

The final historical change to be considered in this retrospective is the emergence of activism from within the formalized medical system. There is growing resistance from women inside traditional medical fields to standard health care delivery. Female activists from nursing and the allied health professions, from physicians' groups, from free-standing feminist clinics, and from traditional health advocacy agencies are increasingly the driving forces behind changes in health care.

Nurse practitioners have been especially active in the last decades. Part of the activity stems from claiming (or reclaiming) a central role in the delivery of services. Nurse practitioners' demands to provide direct service to women in clinics across the country have made a dramatic difference in many women's lives. This is seen especially in nurse-midwives' role in promoting home birth as an option for women to reassert female control over the increasingly medicalized birth process (DeVries 1985, Oakley 1984). Their success can be measured by the strength of resistance to their efforts. To use but one of many possible examples, the powerful Massachusetts Medical Society, joined by well-heeled insurance companies in the early 1980s, battled a bill allowing nurse-midwives to practice in free-standing birth centers. But the Massachusetts Nurse Practitioners Association linked with other vocal groups and convinced the state legislature to override the governor's veto. These battles continue as physicians' groups and insurance companies try to limit nurse practitioners' ability to provide direct care, and to deny them insurance coverage.

Nurses have also been active on a variety of fronts. One emerging focus is on environmental issues. The Nurses Environmental Health Watch (NEHW) directs much of its attention to hazards in the workplace, both for the nurses themselves and for the patients they treat. This group is involved with public policy questions, and with building coalitions with community activists. ". . . NEHW members find they are often the only health practitioners at public hearings and demonstrations" (Nelson 1987, A–6). Cassandra, a radical feminist nurse's network started in 1984, provides support for feminists within the nursing profession. Through their newsletters, network, and meetings, this group pushes for a feminist analysis of the role of nursing within the medical community. Both the nurse practitioners and the nurses' organizations show the breadth and the depth of commitment to creating change from within the health care system. Much remains to be done, however, as many other allied health professions (recreational therapists, respiratory therapists, pharmacists, epidemiologists, toxicologists) lack even a single feminist health advocacy organization.

Women physicians are also creating change within the traditional medical profession as their numbers increase substantially. In 1969, 9 percent of the first-year medical students were female, but by 1987 the figure had risen to 37 percent (Klass 1987). Only 8 percent of all physicians were women in 1970, but projections indicate that women will be 20 percent of all physicians by the year 2000 (Rix 1987). These numerical increases notwithstanding, female physicians work under a number of constraints in their attempt to effectively alter traditional health care systems.

One difficulty female physicians face is the ideology of "professionalism" within medicine. Doctors are taught to be experts, working within carefully drawn parameters to limit the interpersonal nature of the patient/doctor relationship, and paying more attention to those unique problems that draw most heavily upon their technological expertise (Fowlkes 1983). Thus professionalism is at odds with a feminist approach to health care, which requires the relationship of doctor to patient to be one of mutuality. Female physicians will continue to be pulled by these opposing forces until traditional medicine becomes more responsive to a feminist critique.

Another problem for women physicians is their exclusion from high status and leadership positions. Despite the fact that women comprise almost three-quarters of all health care practitioners, only 6 percent of all women health care workers hold top-level administrative positions (Harris 1984). Women continue to be slotted into certain specialities (pediatrics, not surgery; general practice, not cardiology), and to lack the sponsorship of older physicians that is critical to their movement into effective policy and leadership positions (Lorber 1984). Working from the inside creates some latitude to affect the system, but women physicians still need to be activists in their efforts to link to each other and to the women who are their patients.

Yet there is some evidence that women physicians are transforming the standards of care. In part, this change is based on women's traditional valuing of relationships. As one female dean of a medical school notes, "For the women [physicians], relationships with patients are very important, a very positive thing." (Klass 1987, 48). Additionally, the change comes from an unwillingness to function within medicine's traditional power hierarchies. One female physician reports, ". . . you prepare to walk into that room to talk to a couple about their dying baby. [How do you acknowledge] their grief and the failure of medicine to help, while retaining the authority you need as a doctor? And how much authority do you need anyway?" (Klass 1987, 48). The presence and actions of these women has shaken up traditional habits. Perhaps unintentionally, often without an organizational basis, these physicians are beginning to create a practice of medicine that incorporates some of the feminist principles that health activists have demanded for years.

Feminists have also begun to claim the "inside" of the medical profession by creating alternative free-standing health care clinics. With over 1,000 free-standing feminist health care centers existing in the United States at any one time (Simmons et al. 1984), these alternative sites influence the way a community offers health care out of proportion to their numbers. The centers frequently offer not only a full range of reproductive and gynecological services, but also educational sessions on taking control of one's health, thus setting an example that becomes difficult for area clinics and hospitals to ignore. By welcoming nurse-practitioners and supportive health care personnel (nutritionists, exercise physiologists, pharmacists) feminist health clinics promote preventive health care maintenance. Their wholistic perspective on well-being puts into action the movement emphasis on self-help and informed use of technology. By moving their ideas directly into the full-blown practice of medicine and health care delivery, feminists can control completely their ability to provide feminist health care. This new way of "becoming" the inside, however, can lead to parallel systems whereby alternative systems function for some fortunate women, while many women are left with the inadequacies of ordinary health care.

New ways of mobilizing around health care issues are also emerging from women within traditional professional health organizations. The American Medical Women's Association, the women's caucus of the American Psychological Association, and the women's caucus of the American Public Health Association, to mention a few, all battle the subtle sexism that bars women from policy-making and authority positions within their own fields. Groups such as Committees on Occupational Health and Safety (COSH) at the state level have responded to internal pushes to pay attention to gender as it relates to health advocacy. For example, the New York COSH develops educational materials about VDT terminals, pregnancy, and workers' rights (Pinsky 1987). By working from within these systems, feminist health activists avoid the exhaustion associated with establishing an independent organization, but they also face the internal resistance of organizations that rarely take women's health issues seriously.

An encouraging new development is the linking of women inside and outside professional organizations through alliances of grass-roots activists and professional women. This can be seen particularly in environmental activism. Lois Gibbs, a community activist from Love Canal (an upstate New York neighborhood contaminated by toxic wastes) worked with epidemiologist Beverly Paigan to document the extent of the harm done to people living in her neighborhood (Levine 1982). Jesse Deer-in-Water, organizer of Native Americans for a Clean Environment, worked with Canadian epidemiologist Rosalie Bertell to prohibit Kerr-McGee's spraying of nuclear waste on company farmland as fertilizer (Bleifuss 1987). These liaisons provide a powerful catalyst for change, although there are inherent strains within the linkage. Professional women are unaccustomed to the harassment and job threats that accompany work with direct political implications. Grass-roots women can be estranged from their community as their alliances with the professional cadre become more pronounced (Fowlkes, private conversation, 1988).

Yet another way to characterize the increasing influence of feminist health advocates within traditional systems is to examine women in administrative and legislative branches of government. Legislation for abortion rights, policies against sterilization abuse, legal recourse for diethylstilbesterol (DES) exposed women, federal mandates for pharmaceutical information disclosure, and other administrative actions to protect women's health are often drafted by sympathetic women within federal agencies or legislative offices. Activists within these agencies take seriously their need to be informed and up-to-date on women's issues, as demonstrated by the Congressional Caucus for Women's Issues series of briefings in 1987 on "Women, AIDS and

Lupus," "Teenage Pregnancy and Family Planning," and "Domestic Violence During Pregnancy."

The increasing presence of activists within the health care system is seen both at the level of changes in direct service (by nurse practitioners, nurses, physicians, and alternative site practitioners), and in policy development (by women in traditional health organizations, and women in government). By definition, working from within a system limits the potential for radical changes, and yet the efforts of these activists have had profound effects on the way in which health care policy and health care delivery have responded to the feminist critique of medicine and medical technology.

Sustaining Our Organizations: The Politics of Empowerment

The traditional health care system, both in the United States and throughout the world, is an embedded power structure. Like all power structures, it will not easily or readily give up its vested interest in maintaining the status quo. To sustain ourselves and our organizations, feminist health activists must be fully versed in the politics of empowerment, learning with each struggle what works and what doesn't as we face the increasingly complex issues surrounding women, health, and technology. To do so, it is critical that the hard-won knowledge of individual feminist health organizations is not lost. Yet much of the wisdom has disappeared as organizations fold, and the knowledge is buried in the files of defunct organizations or the minds of burned-out activists. In the final section of this chapter, the lessons learned from the achievements of activist health organizations will be reviewed, and then some ideas about the issues looming in our future will be discussed. Throughout this discussion, the focus will be on ways to create and nurture enduring feminist health organizations.

Lessons from the Achievements of Feminist
Health Organizations

It is evident from the foregoing review that effective strategies to fight for women's health have been developed and achieved by a myriad of differing organizations. What lessons can be derived from the good fights these organizations have mounted? Although hundreds of organizations could provide rich accounts of individual struggles, pointing out strategies to avoid or pursue, three major themes emerge. The first is that activist organizations have learned to be inclusive, both about the women for whose health they advocate, and about the definitions of "health." Second, activists have become effective in pushing for administrative policy or legislative solutions for specific health care problems. Finally, as the increasing complexity of health advocacy is recognized, the need to maintain organizations that survive over the long run surfaces as one of the pivotal issues for the 1990s and beyond.

Any review of the feminist health movement demonstrates how activists increasingly include all women (by age, by race/ethnicity, by class, by ability, by sexual preference) as the beneficiaries of their advocacy. For instance, lesbians have worked actively in the past decades to produce a medical community that is aware of and responsive to the unique needs of lesbians and gay men. Although the AIDS crisis has mobilized many within the homosexual community to focus on health care and related education, the movement has also increasingly placed demands on medical establishments, particularly on the training of doctors, so that heterosexuality is not presumed by health care services. U.S. organizations and organizations throughout the world no longer restrict their focus tó women within their own countries. For instance, under the leadership of Fran Fishbane, DES Action, Inc., whose initial activities centered on lobbying, legislative monitoring, and supporting individual lawsuits on behalf of DES-exposed mothers and children in the United States, now has an international reach, translating its information into Spanish for Latin American countries, and establishing shared projects with Canada and the Netherlands (Tudiver 1986).

The movement has also taught us to broaden our ideas about what constitutes health and health care, and how to more fully mesh what is discovered from other areas into health care activism. For example, activists demand that the care given to children, especially within emergency room protocol, be sensitive to the prevalence of incest and the sexual abuse of children.

Activists have increasingly considered mental health as a component of overall physical health, and significant achievements in the field of mental health have occurred, although these changes are painted against a background of intransigence from the psychological community. Feminist psychotherapy, unheard-of twenty years ago, is now a viable alternative for women requesting therapy. Additionally, routine understanding of such issues as harassment, assault, and the sexual abuse of children has dramatically improved the mental health field's ability to be truly therapeutic for women. The challenges in this field are still large: e.g., training of therapists still neglects women's mental health needs, overuse of psychotropic drugs for female clients continues (Swift 1986), and electroshock technology is making a resurgence as a treatment for depression, that quintessentially female complaint.

Activists have also created opportunities for the inclusion of alternative health care providers, such as herbalists, acupuncturists, or massage therapists. The Venezuelan Alliance of Women Doctors, formed in 1977 to promote women's access to health education and supportive services, has recently researched the use of indigenous plants (usually free for the picking) to respond to specific female health needs (Tudiver 1986). Some alternative insurance carriers now provide coverage for these nontraditional health care providers. The Worker's Trust Health Plan of the Association for Democratic Workplaces covers chiropractic, acupuncture, homeopathic, and naturopathic medicine in addition to standard coverage in a plan that does not have sex-biased rate structures. This awareness of the need to include the widest range of participants and the most complex and comprehensive definitions of health care must be solidified as we move toward a feminist health agenda for the next millenium.

The second powerful lesson is derived from organizations that successfully forged real change by using administrative policy or legislative initiatives. In doing so, they have combatted health care technologies, thus effectively thwarting the technological imperative of emerging technologies within traditional medicine. The activist response to toxic shock syndrome is indicative of the sophistication of the feminist health movement in this regard. In the early 1970s, feminist health activists questioned the contents of tampons, which trade secrecy laws allowed to remain unknown. In the late 1970s, incidents of toxic shock syndrome, particularly deaths associated with the syndrome, aroused the feminist health care community to greater activity. In 1980–81, the Coalition for Medical Rights of Women, based in New York City, began to question the relationship of absorbency in tampons and toxic shock, and distributed information about the connection to their members. By 1984, the Boston Women's Health Book Collective began an intensive effort to put pressure on the FDA to label absorbency on tampons, and by mid 1985, companies were labeling absorbency levels of tampons so that consumers could make more informed choices about this product (Olesen 1986).

Other examples of the effectiveness of organizations that pressure federal agencies is seen in the success of the National Women's Health Network, which in the 1970s thwarted the Upjohn Corporation's efforts to get Depo-Provera approved by the FDA as a contraceptive, or the actions taken to redress the harm created by the Dalkon Shield (See Yanoshik and Norsigian, in this volume). These lessons show us that not only must feminist health organizations remain alert monitors of federal, state, and local agencies, but that activists must move even more strongly into the administrative structures that support and shape mainstream medicine. The Food and Drug Administration, the American Medical Association, and the Centers for Disease Control are but a few of the regulatory agencies that are critical in determining the nature of health care for women. The pattern of identifying an issue, creating public interest, pressuring federal agencies, and receiving legislative or industry response is an example of how the feminist health movement has begun to successfully challenge the medical establishment by working with systems of government in the United States.

More compelling than these lessons, however, is the need to create feminist health advocacy organizations that will endure, that can withstand the forces of co-optation, and that nurture their activists. Because feminist health advocacy is over its first blush, when women discovered the excitement of defining what is healthy for themselves, we are now faced with the need to attack head-on the intractable issues that stand in the way of real health for women. This means tackling the systems of health care financing, including insurance companies and the capitalist model of health care delivery. It means understanding the forces of poverty, of entrenched sexism and racism, that undergird all mainstream health care systems and agencies. It requires that we begin to integrate advocacy that to date has followed separate yet parallel paths, and that we address environmental and occupational health issues. And finally, it means using the existing technology to our advantage. Thus, the problem of creating enduring structures that can go the distance in challenging powerful opponents becomes the starting point for the next decades of struggle. This problem, one feminist health organizations have in common with the feminist movement as a whole (Bunch 1987), requires that organizations move with as much flexibility, creativity, and force as can be mustered. I will begin with a discussion of the need for and the problems in establishing long-term organizations, and end with a discussion of some of the challenges for these hearty organizations to surmount in the coming years.

Think of what past experiences tell us about what happens when our organizations are short-term. A group of North Carolina feminists who used their own bodies to teach medical students how to perform pelvic examinations so as to protect unsuspecting women in hospitals from being used for practice (a high burn-out project if there ever was one!) is no longer in existence (Scully 1983). A group of women in Hartford, Connecticut, ran a phone-in campaign to document sexual abuse of women by physicians. Three years after the project ended, the medical examining board disbarred *one* of the many physicians whose abuse of clients they had documented. Without longer-lasting organizations, we cannot sustain the vigilance necessary to fight entrenched groups within traditional medicine.

As organizations succeed in their attempts to make permanent their demands for change, the forces of co-optation swell to undermine what activists have achieved, as Whatley and Worcester (in this volume) and others (e.g., Morgen 1986) have shown. Sometimes, feminist health achievements have become marketing tools. A new volume entitled *Marketing Women's Health Care* (Dearing et al. 1987) blatantly divides women's health care into three parts: "Marketing Redefined"; "Innovative Women's Services in the Reproductive Years"; and "Innovative Women's Services Before and After Childrearing." It cautions hospitals that the awakened female consumer knows to ask questions and expects certain things from a hospital—so hospitals better make sure that they have the *right products!* This is *not* the kind of success feminists envision. Another example of co-optation is noted by Sandra Morgen (Bookman and Morgen 1988). A group of multiethnic, predominantly low-income women linked with a local women's center in the 1980s to fight the closing of a neighborhood health clinic by using a variety of tactics, including demonstrations and lawsuits. However, when the doctors finally reopened the clinic, they successfully used the local power structures (including the media) to indicate that they were not responding to the pressure tactics of the organizers, but rather were acting out of their own wisdom and generosity. This hollow victory demoralized the activists, and their group fizzled.

Our need for enduring structures is especially apparent as we examine the complexity of the interrelationship between health care, women, and technology. The feminist health care movement must pursue technologies that provide preventive and wellness support, while simultaneously developing a democratic and participatory feminist ethic for the screening of choice-limiting technologies. Technologies that drain financial resources in the service of the few over the needs of the many must be avoided. Only an intelligent, long-lasting collection of feminist organizations can mount the kind of careful monitoring and struggle needed. We cannot make changes unless feminists are able to fully participate in establishing policy and making laws that govern technology's use. When we consider that 47 percent of all sitting federal judges have been appointed by Ronald Reagan, we can begin to understand the magnitude of our mission.

What is needed for an organization to endure? It needs a solid funding base, administrative acumen, political savvy, skill in using media, and effective outreach and educational campaigns. Perhaps as important, it needs to build effective leadership and to nurture those activists who face the stress and potential burn-out of facing powerful opponents while remaining open to the crises of individual women victimized by the system.

There are certainly examples of organizations that have achieved this stability. Exciting efforts are emerging to nurture those who put their bodies and their lives on the line to fight for real health care for women. The Citizen's Clearinghouse for Hazardous Wastes recognized the toll that women pay as health activists. Their project, "Family Stress, Burn-Out and Women as Emerging Leaders," was developed in response to the family disruption that occurs as women, many of whom have never been organizers before, try to combat what may be the major employer in an area. The project's outreach has documented that domestic violence appears to increase for women who are activists. Further, activist organizations must create strong and powerful leaders to move organizations forward. Although feminists internally struggle with their desires not to recreate the entrenched hierarchical power structures of other organizations, activist organizations without effective leadership mechanisms do not sustain themselves (Gardner 1983).

Developing the organizations themselves is a sometimes overwhelming task. But if achieved, what lies in wait for these tough, resilient organizations? The debate about the appropriate agenda for the future women's health movement will undoubtedly evolve as it has in the past, producing a synthesis of different organizational perspectives and philosophies, responses to emergent technologies and a multifaceted vision of women's health within the framework of the current political situation. But there are central concerns that must be addressed if the feminist health movement is to move beyond the all-too-familiar scenario of fighting spontaneous brushfires, perhaps most evident in the area of reproductive rights, where feminists have fought for decades without ever gaining the upper hand in framing the terms of the debate. The final section of this chapter attempts to outline some of the core questions that must be answered.

Remaining Challenges

Despite its fluctuations, and the attempts to co-opt its force and focus, the feminist health movement has forever altered the face of health care in the United States. Activists have had a dramatic impact on the general awareness of and knowledge about women's health issues, on the structure of health care delivery, and on local, state, and federal health policies (Baumgard 1986). Many of the struggles articulated in the preceding sections of this chapter are not finished. Meanwhile, additional challenges have emerged, including insurance health care financing, integrating health activism with other feminist actions, expansion of the international linkages among organizations, environmental and occupational health, and using technology to our benefit.

The system of health care financing, well outlined in Kathryn Ratcliff's chapter in this volume, requires a comprehensive overhaul of the health care system. This activism must go head-to-head against the profitable proliferation of health care delivery. A key component of the economic activism has to do with insurance and its effect on (1) who has access to service; (2) sex discrimination in levels of access to health care (i.e., if women tend to be in those jobs with nonexistent or limited health care insurance, sex discrimination in access is a given); (3) who provides medical care; and (4) what types of technologies are used.

Because women are disproportionately the poor in this country and others, because they often lack the kinds of employment that provide real insurance health benefits, and because they lack the social support of services like childcare, a feminist health movement must address the high cost of health care for all people. Women's poverty, lack of education, and marginalization from mainstream health care delivery services make them especially vulnerable. Poor women are all too often seen as easy guinea pigs for experimental drugs or new medical technologies, such as the widespread testing of birth control devices that routinely occurs in countries like Puerto Rico. Only by eradicating women's poverty and illiteracy can we ensure that these issues never again determine women's access to good health care and appropriate medical technology.

Insurance coverage will be one of the pivotal health care concerns of the next decade. Over 35 million Americans lack medical insurance, with women much more likely than men to lack coverage (Worcester 1988). This is particularly true when we examine women's medical coverage for maternity care: more than 25 percent have no maternity coverage, and over half a million of the women who lack coverage give birth each year (National Women's Law Center 1987). Even if covered, women usually pay higher premiums for medical coverage, despite the fact that this coverage often does not include many routine care needs, from physician care attendants to routine examinations to contraceptive use. Of course, low-income women, and women who work part-time, rarely have any coverage at all. The Boston Women's Health Book Collective has been particularly vehement of late in efforts to establish a National Health Insurance Plan to ensure provision of health care for all Americans, and it must be made clear that a national health system is a women's issue. Poverty, malnutrition, and illiteracy dictate that the movement give voice to the people with the least access to any health care system. A transformed health care system that responds to the vision and needs of those rarely served must be our future goal. Thus, activist efforts must be grounded in a complex sociopolitical understanding that recognizes diverse cultures, nations, and economic issues as we articulate new structures of health care.

The movement's efforts must continue in struggles to break physicians' exclusive license to provide certain services, to revamp medical training systems, and to challenge the medical establishment's monopoly of provision of health care services. For example, if physicians and insurance companies succeed in their efforts to limit nurse-practitioners' attendance at births through limits on licensure and denial of liability insurance, we have lost an important struggle in the de-medicalization of birth. How liability is construed by insurance companies, who seem able to insure nuclear power plants but not real health care for women, is embedded in this fight. A particularly horrifying case unfolded in Washington, D.C., in 1988, when a twenty-seven-year-old terminally ill cancer patient was forced to undergo a caesarean section. She knew the operation would in all likelihood kill her, and it was against the expressed wishes of herself, her husband, her parents, and her physician. The court ruled that the hospital needed to protect itself from *potential* liability, and ordered the caesarean. Neither the mother nor the twenty-six-week-old fetus survived the surgery (Ratterman 1988). Where a woman's right to bodily integrity ends, and the profit-driven imperative to avoid liability and therefore advocacy for a technology such as fetal surgery begins, is but one of the unsettled, and unsettling, questions to be answered. Feminists must be the ones to articulate the real concerns; we must not allow insurance companies' wishes to be the motor that drives policy development in this area.

Other important questions are derived from the need to more fully mesh the complex range of feminist health concerns. Feminists have been particularly successful in creating agencies to cope with and combat male violence against women, including battered women's shelters and rape crisis centers that offer medical and mental health care for women previously at the mercy of unenlightened emergency room staff. Yet the movement to end violence against women has thrived, for the most part, independently from the health movement. Despite the fact that these services are examples of how the medical establishment can respond to the demands of grass-roots activists outside of the system, and even though they routinely employ significant numbers of feminist health care practitioners within the system, better ways of integrating each movement's perspectives into the other's ongoing actions should be developed.

Activists must also continue to knit together the ways in which poverty, illiteracy, and racism detrimentally affect women's health care. Achieving adequate levels of care for poor women, particularly preventive or "wellness" care, requires activists to understand the social and political dynamics of the health care delivery system. We must remind ourselves that the feminist model of health care, including ethics of autonomy, self-care, and participatory decision making, remains viable as services are sought for underserved populations. There are some excellent examples of how this can be achieved. With seed money from the Ms. Foundation, a group of Chicana women from the Santa Cruz Women's Health Center equipped a van with a laboratory, examination rooms, educational materials, and health care providers and literally delivered health care door-to-door in southern California. Such innovations empower women to manage their own health, and to view their health problems as solidly rooted in their culture and their environment. As the Jefferson and Hall chapter (in this volume) makes apparent, we must include issues of race and class in all examinations of health technology. In particular, while guarding against abuses in the use of the emergent reproductive technologies—in vitro fertilization, artificial insemination, fetal surgery, surrogacy, electronic fetal monitors, prenatal testing—activists must not neglect issues of access and affordability for all women. These are but a few examples of the kinds of integration necessary to keep up the momentum on inclusion started by feminist health activists. Each demands that organizations link with each other, continue to educate themselves and their membership, and remain open to the need to continually evolve and redefine our understanding of our issues.

How to best move forward with international efforts is another core question for the future. Women in industrialized countries must remain vigorous in using their privilege to provide information and technical assistance to women in nonindustrialized countries who are exploited by the technology and wholesale use of western medical practices (Yanoshik and Norsigian, in this volume). Conferences such as the International Consultation on Micro-Chip Technology: Its Impact on the Lives of Women Workers held in Manila (October 1986) is an example of how organizations can link across countries. This conference was a collaborative effort of the Participatory Research Group of

Canada, the Women's Program of the International Council for Adult Education, and the Center for Women's Resources, the Women's Center, and the Kilusan ng Manggagawang Kababaihan (KMK) (Women Workers Movement) of the Philippines. Tudiver (1986) reports that women's health networks have been created in over twenty countries, and that these networks are starting to make international links. The newly formed Latin American and Caribbean Women's Health Network links over 250 women's health groups to other national networks in Europe and North America. These efforts form a good beginning, but the need in this area is great.

Connected to the need to develop potent links between nations is the question of how to bring environmental and occupational health issues more centrally into constructions of what constitutes a health care system. This is especially important for United States groups, because of the ways in which our toxic chemicals are indiscriminately dumped abroad, and the ways in which occupational hazards are exported along with other forces of exploitation of labor. Environmental health issues pose a particularly difficult challenge because cause-effect relationship and temporal lag of cancer onset make high-profile activism difficult. As Lin Nelson's chapter makes clear, women are at the forefront of these environmental fights, but they must clarify women's role in the struggle for a hazard-free environment.

As more women enter the paid labor force, particularly in nontraditional jobs, and as protections offered by federal health agencies and unionization decline, issues in occupational health remain an area of visible activism. As chapters in this volume (see Bertin) demonstrate, occupational health issues are the focus of several organizations. Initiatives to date tend to be "single-issue" in their focus on occupational health. Double Exposure: Women Against Reproductive Health Hazards works to change reproductive hazards stemming from the workplace as well as the community. Women of All Red Nations (WARN) combines a critique of occupational hazards of uranium mining with its deleterious impact on the community's health. Occupational health of health care workers takes on new dimensions with the rising incidence of AIDS victims. Groups of primarily female health care technicians have been actively developing systems of humane care at the same time as groups of primarily male physicians debate the ethics of refusing professional care to AIDS patients (Spencer 1988). The charge, however, is not to let these issues remain separate from the health movement as a whole.

Finally, we must learn to use technology to our advantage. Organizations must think about how high technology can be used to make *real* education about health available, instead of the empty advice that fuels the "fitness craze." Weston and Ruggiero (1985–86) found many instances of health and diet information in popular women's magazines, but little attention to the serious health problems women actually experience. Organizations must work intensively with researchers to translate scholarship to the general public in such a way as to inspire action.

Organizations must learn to more effectively use such technologies as computer-generated data bases and computer mailing lists to build a national and international constituency. Especially important is the need to create innovative ways to control the media. One example of our continual struggle in this effort involves Accutane, a drug used to control acne, and one that causes severe birth defects. Since 1982, when the Food and Drug Administration approved use of Accutane without requiring a pregnancy test or informed consent from women of childbearing age, health activists have demanded that the FDA require dermatologists to sign an affidavit promising to use Accutane safely (Endor 1988). Yet when the FDA responded to this pressure, the news releases read that the *FDA* acted upon the findings of its advisory committee, and a spokesperson commented "*We* believe *we* can do the job with these innovative approaches. . . ." (Hartford Courant 1988, emphasis added). This type of news coverage leaves the average female reader believing that the FDA is doing a good job in protecting her health, rather than understanding that the FDA blocked any action on this drug for six years until activists made that position untenable.

Thus, the emerging challenge is to move beyond headline-grabbing issues of reproductive technologies, and to talk about systemic change for women's health. This means confronting the structure of profit making within hospitals and health clinics, the access of all people to health care insurance, the impact of catastrophic illness on the well-being of families, the use of women as unpaid health care workers for the elderly and the disabled. It means continuing to heighten awareness of hidden problems—alcoholism, aging, disability. And it means working toward a world where gender does not predict one's ability to be healthy, active, and well. Because many women still echo the words of Fannie Lou Hamer, "I'm sick and tired of being sick and tired," feminists must continue to be in the forefront of health activism. We owe it to ourselves and to our movement.

394   Healing Technology

BIBLIOGRAPHY

Baumgard, Alice. 1985. Women's health: Directions for the 80s. *Health Care for Women International.* 6:267–76.

Beckwith, Barbara. 1985. Boston women's health book collective: Women empowering women. *Health Care for Women* 10, no 1: 1–9.

Bleifuss, Joel. 1987. Kerr-McGee lays waste to eastern Oklahoma. *In These Times,* August 19–September 1, 12–13.

Bookman, Ann, and Sandra Morgen, eds. 1988. *Women and the politics of empowerment.* Philadelphia: Temple University Press.

Bunch, Charlotte. 1987. *Passionate politics.* New York: St. Martin's Press.

Campbell, Margaret. 1973. *Why would a girl go into medicine?* Old Westbury, N.Y.: Feminist Press.

Coombe, Jeanne, and Margaret Drolette. 1977. Discrimination: The case of the female dental student. *Women and Health,* July-August, 12–21.

Corea, Gena. 1985. *The mother machine.* New York: Harper and Row.

Dearing, Ruthie, Helen Gordon, Dorolyn Sohner, and Lynne Weidel. 1987. *Marketing women's health care.* Aspen, Col.: Aspen Publishers.

DeVries, Raymond G. 1985. *Regulating birth: Midwives, medicine and the law.* Philadelphia: Temple University Press.

Fee, Elizabeth. 1983. *Women and health: The politics of sex and medicine.* New York: Baywood Publishing Co.

Fowlkes, Martha. 1983. Katie's place: Women's work, professional work, and social reform. *Research in the Interweave of Social Roles: Jobs and Families.* 3:143–59.

————. 1988. Private conversation with the author.

Gardner, Barbara. 1983. Longevity, women's leadership, and women's centers. Paper presented at the National Women's Studies Conference, Ohio State University, Columbus, June.

Gaskin, Ina May. 1977. *Spiritual midwifery.* Summertown, Tenn.: Book Publishing Company.

Harris, J. 1984. Women in medicine: Making a difference in health policy. *Journal of the American Medical Association* 39, no. 3: 77–79.

Hartford Courant. 1988. New warnings ordered for acne drug. January 14.

Lacey, Louise. 1975. *Lunaception: A new revolutionary, natural way to control your body and fertility.* New York: Warner Books.

Levine, Adeline. 1982. *Love Canal: science, politics, people.* Lexington, Mass.: Lexington Books, D.C. Heath Co.

Lorber, Judith. 1984. *Women physicians: Careers, status and power.* New York: Tavistock Publications.

Morgen, Sandra. 1986. The dynamics of co-optation in a feminist health clinic. *Social Science and Medicine* 23, no. 2: 201–10.

National Women's Health Network. 1980. *Self-Help,* Resource guide 7/8. Washington, D.C.

National Women's Law Center. 1987. *Women without health insurance.* Washington, D.C.

Nelson, Lin. 1987. Nurses take action on environmental health issues. *Listen Real Loud* 8, no. 1: A–6.

Oakley, Ann. 1984. *The captured womb: A history of the medical care of pregnant women.* Oxford: Basil Blackwell.

Olesen, Virginia. 1986. Analyzing emergent issues in women's health: The case of toxic shock syndrome. *Health Care for Women International* 7, no. 1–2: 51–62.

Pinsky, Mark. 1987. *The VDT book: A computer user's guide to health and safety.* New York: NYCOSH.

Scully, Diana. 1983. *Men who control women's health.* Boston: Houghton Mifflin Co.

Selleck, Denise. 1988. A women's building: And much more. *Guardian* 40, no. 26: 3.

Simmons, Ruth, Bonnie J. Kay, and Carol Regan. Women's health groups: Alternatives to the health care system. *International Journal of Health Services* 13, no. 4: 619–34.

Spencer, Frank. 1988. The AIDS obligation. *Hartford Courant.* Jan. 14.

Swift, Carolyn. 1986. Pain killers and tranquilizers: The use of prescription drugs to mediate normative transitions and situational crises. Paper presented at the Women, Health, and Technology Conference, Storrs, Conn. October 19.

Tudiver, Sari. 1986. The strength of links: International women's health networks in the eighties. In *Adverse effects: Women and the Pharmaceutical industry,* ed. Kathleen McDonnell, 187–214. Toronto: Women's Press.

Rix, Sara. 1987. *The American woman: A report in depth.* New York: W. W. Norton and Co.

Ruzek, Sheryl. 1975. Emergent modes of utilization: Gynecological self help. In *Women and health care: Research implications for a new era,* ed. V. Olesen, 80–85. Washington, D.C.: Government Printing Office.

Ratterman, Donna. 1988. Forced cesarean kills mother. *Off Our Backs* 17, no. 1: 1.

Weston, Louise, and Josephine Ruggiero. 1985–86. The popular approach to women's health issues: a content analysis of women's magazines in the 1970s. *Women and Health* 10, no. 4: 47–62.

Worcester, Nancy. 1988. Insurance: It's time for a real change. *Network News,* May/June, 3.

Resources

Reproductive Rights

Abortion Rights Mobilization, 175 Fifth Ave., Suite 712, New York, NY 10010

American Civil Liberties Union, Reproductive Rights Project, 132 West 43rd St., New York, NY 10036

Catholics for a Free Choice, 2008 17th St. NW, Washington, D.C. 20009

Coalition for Abortion Rights and Against Sterilization Abuse, 17 Murray St., 5th floor, New York, NY 10007

The Committee to Defend Reproductive Rights, 2845 24th St., San Francisco, CA 94110

Double Exposure: Women Against Reproductive Health Hazards, P.O. Box 1342, Brookline, MA 02146

Indian Women United for Social Justice, P.O. Box 38743, Los Angeles, CA 90038

Mexican American Women's National Association (MANA), L'Enfant Plaza Station NW, P.O. Box 2356, Washington, D.C. 20024

National Abortion Federation, 900 Pennsylvania Ave. SE, Washington, D.C. 20003

National Abortion Rights Action League, 1424 K St. NW, Washington, D.C. 20005

National Organization for Women (NOW) Reproductive Rights Task Force, 425 13th St. NW, Suite 723, Washington, D.C. 20004

Religious Coalition for Abortion Rights, 100 Maryland Ave. NE, Suite 307, Washington, D.C. 20002

Reproductive Rights National Network, 17 Murray St., 5th Floor, New York, NY 10007

Environmental Health

Citizens' Clearing House for Hazardous Wastes, P.O. Box 926, Arlington, VA 22216, (703-276-7070)

Nurse's Environmental Health Watch, RCU Box 1277, New York, NY 10185

WARN (Women of All Red Nations), P.O. Box 3386, Rapid City, SD 57709

Women and Environments, Centre for Urban and Community Studies, 455 Spadina Ave., Toronto, Ontario, M5s 2G8, Canada

Women-Environment-Sustainable Development, Netherlands IUCN Committee, Damrak 28-30, 1012 LJ Amsterdam, The Netherlands

WorldWIDE—World Women in Defense of the Environment, 1718 P St. NW, Suite 813, Washington, D.C. 20036.

Pregnancy and Birth

Caesarean Prevention Movement, P.O. Box 152, Syracuse, NY 13210

Coalition to Fight Infant Mortality, Box 10436, Oakland CA 94610

Environmental Risks and Pregnancy Teleconference, March of Dimes Birth Defects Foundation, 1275 Mamaroneck Ave., White Plains, NY 10605

International Association of Parents and Professionals for Safe Alternatives in Childbirth, P.O. Box 267, Marble Hill, MO 63764

Midwives Alliance of North America, c/o Concord Midwifery Service, 30 South Main St., Concord, NH 03301

National Association of Childbearing Centers, Box 1, Route 1, Perkiomenville, PA 18074

National Network to Prevent Birth Defects, Box 15309, Southeast Station, Washington, D.C. 20003, (202-543-5450)

National Women's Health Organizations

Black Women's Health Project, Martin Luther King Community Center, Suite 157, 450 Auburn Ave. NE, Atlanta, GA 30312

Cassandra: Radical Feminist Nurses Network, P.O. Box 341, Williamsville, NY 14221

Coalition for the Medical Rights of Women, 2845 24th St., San Francisco, CA 94110

DES Action National Office, Long Island Jewish Hillside Medical Center, New Hyde Park, NY 11040

Endometriosis Association, c/o Bread and Roses Women's Health Center, 238 West Wisconsin Ave., Milwaukee, WI 53202

Gay Nurses' Alliance, 44 St. Mark's Place, New York, NY 10003

National Black Women's Health Project, 1237 Gordon St. SW, Atlanta, GA 30310

National Latina Health Project, P.O. Box 7567, Oakland, CA 94601, (415-534-1362)

National Women's Health Network, 224 7th St. SE, Washington, D.C. 20003, (202-543-9222)

Native American Women's Health Education Resource Center, P.O. Box 572, Lake Andes, SD 57365, (605-487-7072)

Women's Cancer Resource Center, The Women's Building, 3543 18th St., San Francisco, CA 94110

Women, Health, and Technology

Project on Women and Technology, University of Connecticut, 417 Whitney Rd., U-181, Storrs, CT 06268, (203-486-4738)

Women and Technology Project, 315 S. 4th St., Missoula, Montana 59409

International Women's Health Networks

International Baby Food Action Network, c/o Doug Clement, 1701 University Ave. SE, Minneapolis, MN 55414

International Childbirth Education Association, Box 20048, Minneapolis, MN 55420

International Contraception, Abortion, and Sterilization Campaign, 374 Grays Inn Rd., London WCI, England

Latin American and Carribean Women's Health Network, c/o ISIS International, P.O. Box 25711, Philadelphia, PA 19144

Rural Women's Social Education Center, 15/1 Periya Melamaiyur, Vallam Post, Chingleput 603 002, South India

Occupational Health

COSH groups: Coalitions of Committees for Occupational Safety and Health typically link unions, activists, and health professionals in a community. To find local or national COSH groups, contact:

MassCOSH, 718 Huntington Ave., Boston, MA 02115

NYCOSH, The New York Committee for Occupational Safety and Health, 275 Seventh Ave. 25th Floor, New York, NY 10001, especially for VDT information

Women's Occupational Health Resource Center, School of Public Health, Columbia University, 600 W. 168th St., New York, NY 10032

Violence Against Women

National Coalition Against Domestic Violence, P.O. Box 15127, Washington, D.C. 20003-0127, (202-293-8860)

Women Against Violence Against Women, 543 N. Fairfax Ave., Los Angeles, CA 90036

Disabilities and Illness Groups

Disabled Lesbian Alliance, Room 229, 5 University Place, New York, NY 10003

Lesbian Illness Support Group, c/o Nancy Johnson, P.O. Box 1258, New York, NY 10001

Contributors

Glenn Affleck is a professor of psychiatry at the University of Connecticut Health Center. He is currently director of the social and behavioral teaching program in the medical school. His major research interests include coping with serious illness and victimization.

Elisabeth Beck-Gernsheim is professor of sociology at the University of Giessen in West Germany. She is the author of *The Baby Question*, a book on the difficult dilemmas confronting women who have to decide for or against having children. She is also author of *The New Motherhood*, a book on the changes in norms and realities of motherhood as a social institution and *A Divided Life*, which is about conflict between work and family.

Susan E. Bell is an associate professor of sociology at Bowdoin College and research fellow in sociology at the Laboratory in Social Psychiatry, Harvard Medical School. She has written a number of articles about DES, medicalization, and the development, diffusion, and social impact of medical technology.

Joan E. Bertin, an attorney, is associate director of the Women's Rights Project of the American Civil Liberties Union. She specializes in pregnancy and sex discrimination law and has done extensive work on reproductive hazards in the workplace. She represented the women workers at the American Cyanamid Company who challenged that company's sex-based exclusionary policy after some women submitted to sterilization surgery to protect their right to jobs.

Evelyn J. Bromet received her Ph.D in epidemiology from Yale University and is currently professor of psychiatry and behavioral science at the State University of New York at Stony Brook. Her research has focused on longitudinal studies of schizophrenic and alcoholic patients, mental health effects of acute and chronic stress, occupational mental health, and measurement issues.

Mary Amanda Dew received a Ph.D. in social psychology from Harvard University and completed postdoctoral training in psychiatric epidemiology at the University of Pittsburgh. She is currently an assistant professor of psychiatry, psychology and epidemiology at the University of Pittsburgh School of Medicine. Her research interests center on the mental and physical health effects of chronic stress and on issues in research design and analysis.

Leslie O. Dunn received a M.P.H. in health services administration from the University of Pittsburgh. She is currently senior research program coordinator in the Department of Psychiatry at the University of Pittsburgh School of Medicine. Her research interests center on assessment techniques in psychiatric diagnoses and the prevalence of depression in populations with chronic stress.

Myra Marx Ferree is professor of sociology at the University of Connecticut. With Beth Hess, she authored *Controversy and Coalition: A New Feminist Movement* (1985) and edited *Analyzing Gender* (1987). Her current interests include women's reactions to the division of household labor, the feminist movement in West Germany, and class and gender consciousness among working-class women. She was a member of the editorial board of *Women, Work and Technology: Transformations* (1987).

Judith Fifield is a research associate in the Department of Behavioral Sciences at UCONN Health Center, an R.N., and a doctoral candidate in the Sociology Department at the University of Connecticut. Her dissertation research, funded by a traineeship from the Arthritis Foundation, examines the effects of gender and class on illness outcomes in rheumatoid arthritis. Her other interests include gender and stratification research and cross-national issues in health.

John C. Fletcher is professor of biomedical ethics and professor of religious studies at the University of Virginia, Charlottesville. He was formerly Chief of the Bioethics Program at the National Institutes of Health.

Lynne C. Garner received her Ph.D. in sociology from the University of Massachusetts. She is a director of quality assurance for the Connecticut Department of Mental Health, and her work focuses on developing outcome measures to assess programs.

Elaine J. Hall is a doctoral candidate in the Sociology Department at the University of Connecticut. Her research interests include the determinants and shape of abortion attitudes (the topic of her Master's thesis) and the portrayal of women in introductory sociology textbooks. She is currently engaged in dissertation research on the way gender affects the institutional, organizational, and interactional processes of waiters and waitresses.

Judith R. Kunisch is an R.N. and holds a Master's of Business Administration. She develops and teaches courses on the subject of health care business. Currently, she is project manager of a citywide prevention of low birthweight project in Hartford, Connecticut.

Alice Lind is an R.N. and is the nursing care coordinator for a new residential program for persons with AIDS in Seattle, Washington. Active in the Washington Chapter of the American Nursing Association she frequently gives talks on nursing ethics.

Gail O. Mellow has a Ph.D. in Social Psychology. She is director of the Women's Center at the University of Connecticut, and cochair of the Project on Women and Technology. She served as a member of the editorial board on *Women, Work, and Technology: Transformations* (1987).

Julien S. Murphy is an assistant professor of philosophy at the University of Southern Maine. Her publications in continental philosophy and philosophy of medicine include articles on abortion, IVF–Embryo Transplant technology, and AIDS.

Lin Nelson is an activist, teacher, and researcher concerned with women and occupational and environmental health. Presently she is codirector of the Central New York Council on Occupational Safety and Health and cochair of the National Women's Health Network Committee on Occupational and Environmental Health.

Judy Norsigian is a member of the Boston Women's Health Book Collective, and coauthor of the new edition of *The New Our Bodies, Ourselves*. She has been on the Board of the National Women's Health Network for more than eight years and active in the women's health movement since 1971. Her special interest is in women's reproductive health concerns.

Laurie Nsiah-Jefferson is currently a doctoral candidate at the Johns Hopkins University School of Public Health. She is a health consultant who writes and speaks across the country on minority women's health issues. She is currently involved in the Black Women's Health Project, and the Healthy Mothers Healthy Babies Coalition both nationally and locally, and has served on the board of directors of the Elizabeth Blackwell Health Center for Women in Philadelphia. She has also been a member of the Massachusetts Department of Public Health Task Forces on Cervical Cancer and on Breastfeeding and has recently completed working on the Reproductive Laws in the 1990s Project with Rutgers University Law School.

David K. Parkinson, M.D., M.S., received his training at Oxford University in England as well as Harvard University. He is currently professor of preventative medicine and director of the Division of Occupational Medicine at the State University of New York at Stony Brook. His research has focused most recently on the epidemiology and prevention of occupational disease.

Carol A. Pfeiffer, Ph.D., is a medical sociologist in the school of medicine at the University of Connecticut. She is currently director of the Clinical Skills Assessment program. Her other interests include coping with chronic illness, gender role issues, and professional socialization.

Glenda D. Price is the dean of Allied Health Professions at the University of Connecticut. She is a clinical laboratory scientist with a special interest in the modification of health professional education toward a greater focus on the humanities.

Kathryn Strother Ratcliff is assistant professor of sociology at the University of Connecticut and holds a joint appointment in the Department of Community Medicine, UCONN Health Center. Her research interests are applied sociology and health sociology. Within health sociology her speciality areas include psychiatric epidemiology, the mental health impact of unemployment, and perinatal health care systems.

Susan Reisine is associate professor of behavioral sciences and community health at the UCONN School of Dental Medicine. She is currently director of the education/community/health services research component of the UCONN Multipurpose Arthritis Center. Her major research interests include the social impacts of chronic health conditions.

Christopher M. Ryan received a Ph.D. in psychology from the University of California, Berkeley. At the present time he is an assistant professor of psychiatry at the University of Pittsburgh School of Medicine. His current research focuses on the neurobehavioral consequences of toxic chemical exposures and various medical diseases in both children and adults.

Richard C. Tessler is a medical sociologist on the faculty at the University of Massachusetts in Amherst. He is also a staff associate in the Social and Demographic Research Institute where for the past five years he has directed a NIMH-sponsored research training program in the area of mental health services. He has a long-standing interest in the interface between health and society. Currently he is studying the recognition of depression by Anglo and Hispanic adults.

Dorothy C. Wertz is research professor of health services at Boston University School of Public Health. She is conducting a thirty-nation survey of ethics in medical genetics and reproductive technologies, together with John C. Fletcher. She is author of *Lying In: A History of Childbirth in America,* an enlarged edition (1989), and of *Ethics and Human Genetics: A Cross-Cultural Perspective* (1989).

Mariamne H. Whatley has a Ph.D. in biological sciences. She is an assistant professor with a joint appointment in the Women's Studies Program and the Department of Curriculum and Instruction at the University of Wisconsin, Madison. She teaches women's health and biology and is coordinator of the health education program. Her main area of research involves a feminist critique of health and sexuality education and curricula. She is a founding member of the Wisconsin affiliate of the National Women's Health Network.

Nancy Worcester has a Ph.D. in nutrition from the University of London. She teaches women's health in the Women's Studies Program at the University of Wisconsin, Madison, is the state education coordinator for the Wisconsin Coalition Against Domestic Violence, and is chair of the board of the National Women's Health Network. She was active in the women's health movement in England, participated in the 1984 USA-Nicaragua Health Colloquium, and she organized and/or led health study tours to China (1978, 1983), Cuba (1981), and Grenada (1983).

Barbara Drygulski Wright is associate professor of German in the Department of Modern and Classical Languages at the University of Connecticut. She was lead editor of *Women, Work, and Technology: Transformations* (1987). She is currently working on ways to use video technology in foreign language instruction.

Kim Yanoshik is a doctoral candidate in the Sociology Department at the University of Connecticut and is a Health Science Fellow in the Department of Community Medicine at UCONN Health Center. Her dissertation research is concerned with the social construction of premenstrual syndrome (PMS) and women's menstrual experiences. Her other interests include mental health, women's health activism, and women's status cross-nationally.

Index